ISODOSE ATLAS

Series in Radiology

VOLUME 5

Series ISBN 90 247 2427 9

ISODOSE ATLAS

for use in radiotherapy

Edited by

Gy. Németh M.D., C.Sc. (med.)
Department of Oncoradiology, Weil Emil Hospital, Budapest

H. Kuttig Dr. med. habil.
Professor of Radiology
University Department of Radiology
(Czerny Hospital), Heidelberg

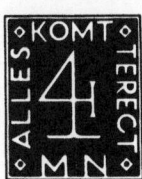

1981

MARTINUS NIJHOFF PUBLISHERS

THE HAGUE / BOSTON / LONDON

Distributors:

for the United States
and Canada

Kluwer Boston, Inc.
190 Old Derby Street
Hingham, MA 02043
USA

for all other countries

Kluwer Academic Publishers Group
Distribution Center
P.O. Box 322
3300 AH Dordrecht
The Netherlands

for Hungary, Albania,
Bulgaria, China,
Cuba, Czechoslovakia,
German Democratic Republic,
Democratic People's Republic
of Korea, Mongolia, Poland,
Roumania, Soviet Union,
Democratic Republic of Vietnam,
and Yugoslavia

Akadémiai Kiadó
P.O.B. 24
H-1363
Budapest
Hungary

This volume is listed in the Library of Congress Cataloging in Publication Data

ISBN-13: 978-94-009-8278-9   e-ISBN-13: 978-94-009-8276-5
DOI: 10.1007/978-94-009-8276-5

English translation by K. Takácsi-Nagy

Joint edition published by

MARTINUS NIJHOFF PUBLISHERS
P.O.B. 566, 2501 CN The Hague, The Netherlands
and
AKADÉMIAI KIADÓ
P.O.B. 24, H-1363, Budapest, Hungary

Copyright © Akadémiai Kiadó, Budapest 1981
Softcover reprint of the hardcover 1st edition 1981

Contents

Preface

When compiling the present atlas our aim has been to provide the practising radiotherapist with a handbook which would help him to plan the radiation therapy of tumours of individual organs. Apart from a few exceptions, all isodose charts in this atlas show dose distributions resulting from external irradiation. Combination of external irradiation with intracavitary radium therapy is presented in the treatment of carcinoma of the uterine cervix, in which case the two techniques are complementary.

The immense material of the pertinent literature could, naturally, not have been included in the atlas. As a result of scrupulous selection, the isodose charts shown may not invariably be the optimum ones, and some of them may not be the most modern. However, the usefulness of the information they provide has made us to keep them all the same.

We did not intend to change the original charts in any way and standardization of the isodoses was not undertaken. Radiation parameters are given in the figure captions and, if available, information has also been provided on the phantoms used by the authors.

Naturally, the isodoses presented will not automatically apply to all situations and all apparatuses without due attention to the individual patient and technical details such as penumbra and source diameter. They merely serve as a starting point and will help to save time and work during treatment planning also with the computer.

It has been another important consideration of ours to provide help for those radiotherapists who have no access to all the modern equipment on the market. An exact reproduction of the techniques is in most cases possible on the basis of the information provided in the captions, but if this were insufficient, the exhaustive reference list makes it possible to check in the original publication.

It is a further aim of the present atlas to stimulate radiotherapists to improve the existing techniques and devise new, more effective ones.

The Editors

Abbreviations

A	anterior
CR	centre of rotation
FAD	focus to axis distance
FID	focus to isocentre distance
FSD	focus to skin distance
HVT	half-value thickness
L	left
P	posterior
R	right
SAD	source to axis distance
SSD	source to skin distance

Skin

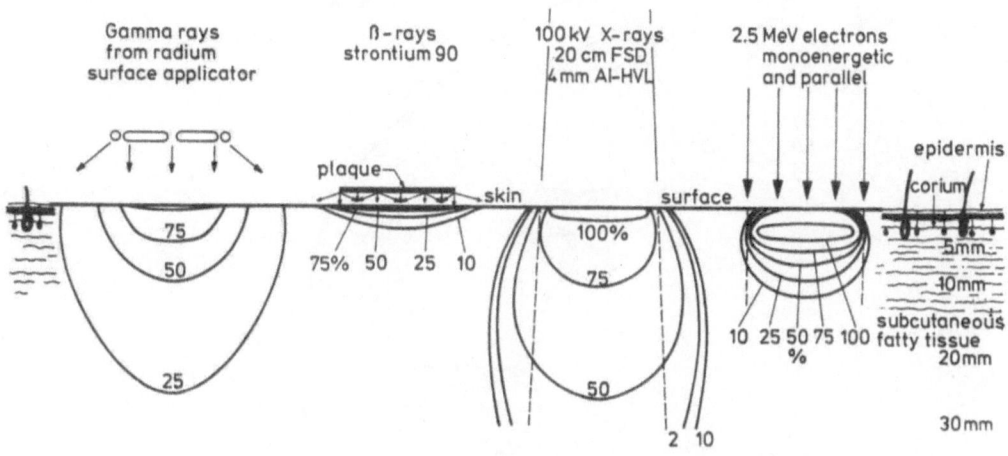

Fig. 1. Isodose distribution in the skin using different forms of irradiation
226-Ra
90-Sr
X-ray (100 kV, HVT 4 mm Al, FSD 20 cm)
(Wright et al. 1956)

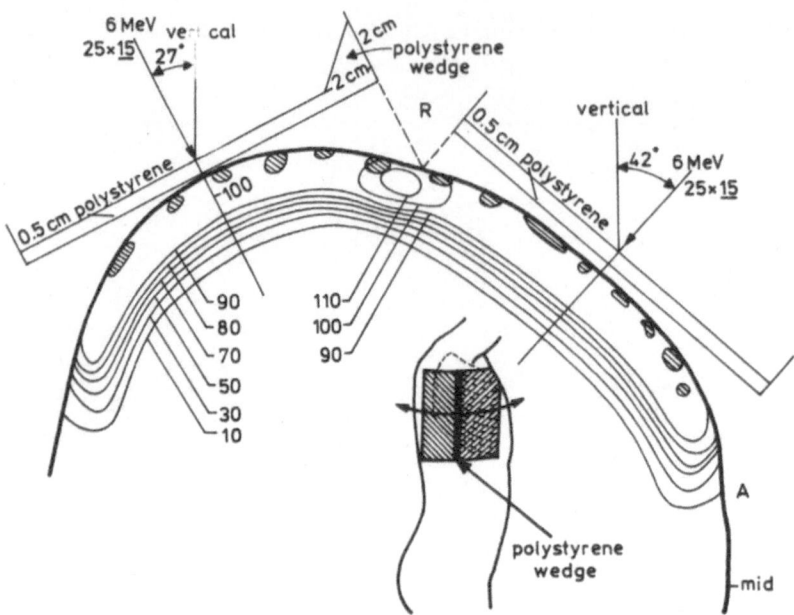

Fig. 2. Electron beam therapy (6 MeV) of multiple metastases in the skin of the thoracic wall through two stationary fields using a 45° wedge filter and two polystyrene absorbers
FSD 90 cm
field size 15 × 25 cm each
Inhomogenous phantom with skeleton
(Laughlin 1967)

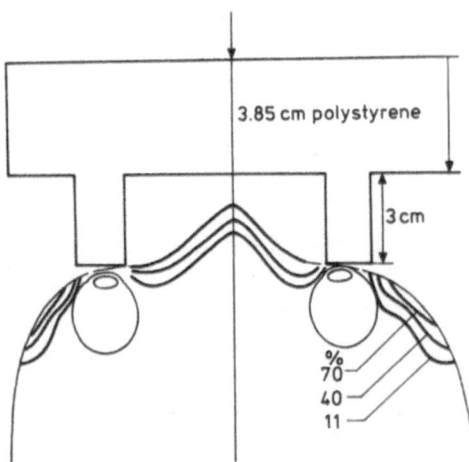

Fig. 3. Electron beam therapy (10 MeV) of the facial skin through a stationary ventral field with polystyrene absorber in a case of mycosis fungoides (protection of the crystalline lenses with additional absorbers 6 cm long and 1 cm thick)
FSD 90 cm
field size 15 × 15 cm
Inhomogeneous phantom
(Kitagawa 1962)

Head and neck

Orbit

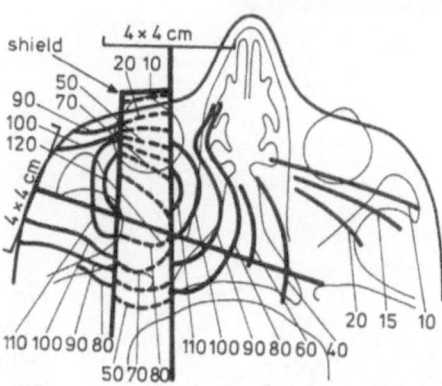

Fig. 4. X-ray therapy (220 kV) of the orbit with two stationary fields (protection of the lens with a lead rubber shield 2 mm thick, diam.15 mm)
    HVT 1.5 mm Cu
    FSD 50 cm
    field size 4 × 4 cm each

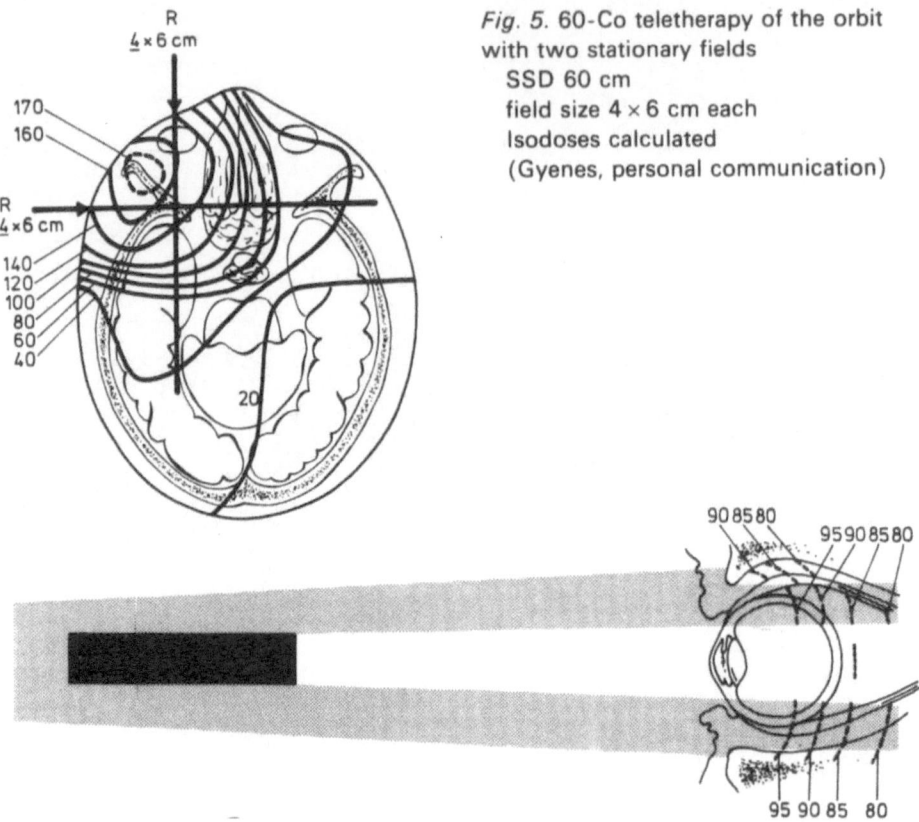

Fig. 5. 60-Co teletherapy of the orbit
with two stationary fields
SSD 60 cm
field size 4 × 6 cm each
Isodoses calculated
(Gyenes, personal communication)

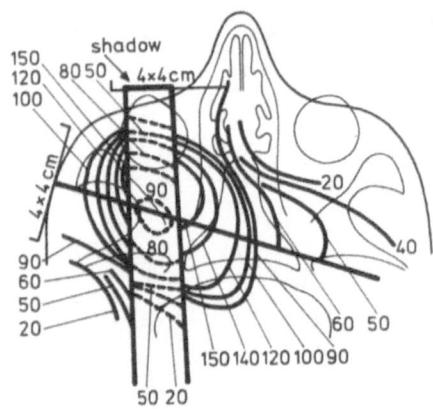

Fig. 6. High-energy X-ray therapy
(2 MV) of the orbit through two
stationary fields (protection of the
lens with a 7 cm long lead insert
interposed in the central
beam—indirect protection,
"shadow method")
FSD 67 cm
field size 4 × 4 cm each
(Lederman 1957)

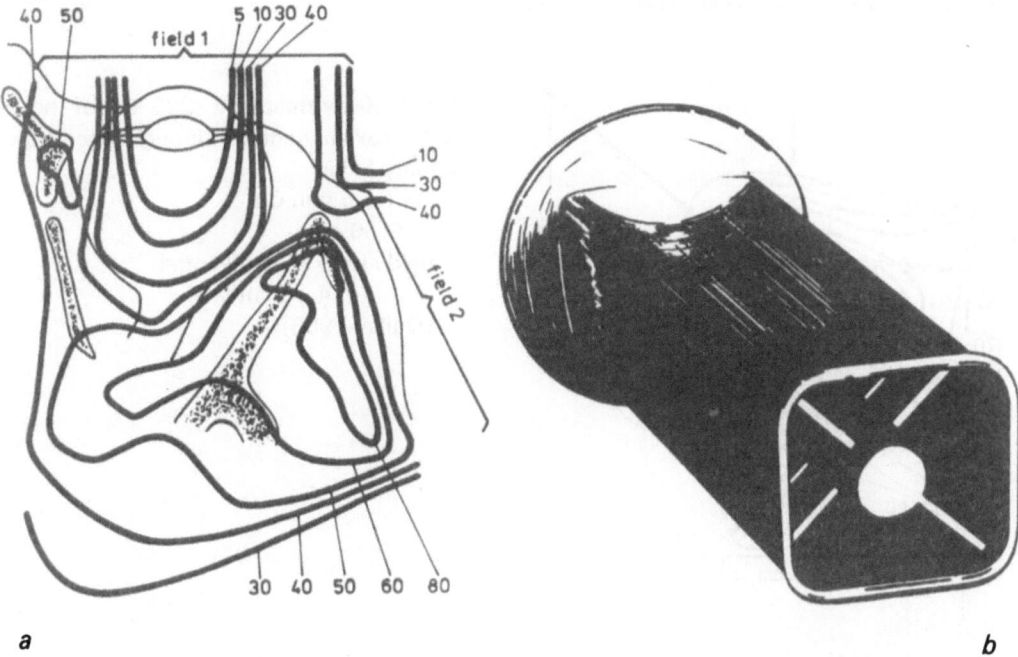

a

b

Fig. 7. a Electron beam therapy (15 MeV) of the orbit through two stationary fields
b Protection of the lens with a 4 × 4 cm tube having a 4.5 cm long 1.5 cm diam. absorber
nucleus fixed to the tube in its axis by means of plastic pegs
    FSD 100 cm
    field size 4 × 4 cm frontal with protective tube
          3 × 6 cm tilted temporal field
    Phantom: cranium filled with Plastika ®
    (Becker and Baum 1960)

Fig. 8. Electron beam therapy
(10 MeV) of the eye and peri-
bulbar connective tissue using
the protective tube shown in Fig. 7b
    FSD 100 cm
    field size 4 × 4 cm
    Phantom: bone plus plastic
    (Kärcher et al. 1971)

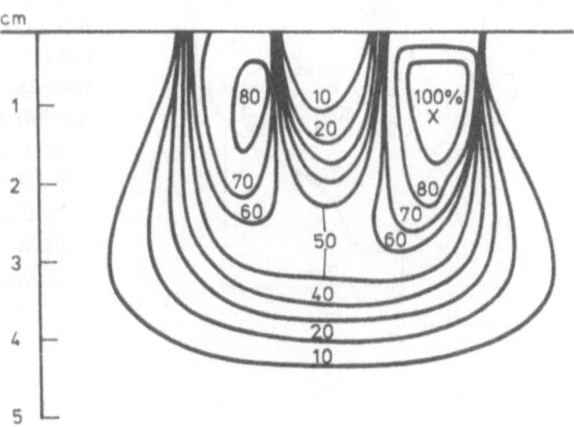

Nasal and paranasal sinus

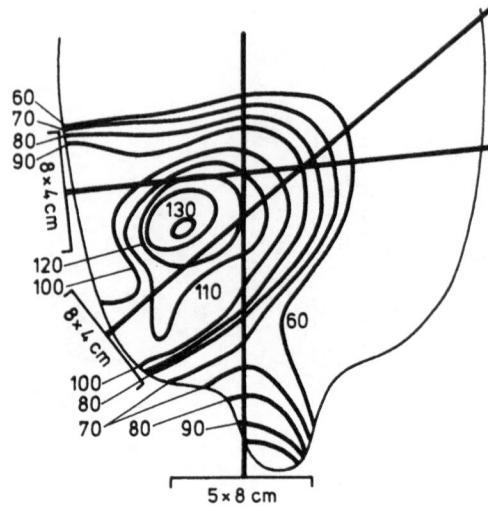

Fig. 9. X-ray treatment (220 kV) of the right maxillary antrum through three stationary fields
   HVT 1.5 mm Cu
   FSD 50 cm
   field size 5 × 8 cm ventral
                  4 × 8 cm lateral
   (Dalley 1959)

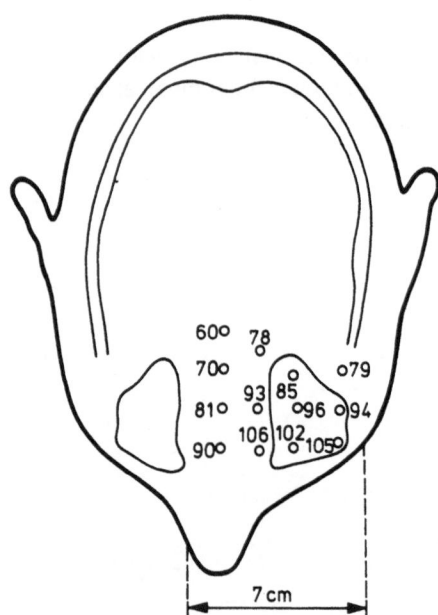

Fig. 10. 60-Co teletherapy of the left maxillary antrum, entire nasal cavity, ethmoid cells, frontal sinus, and sphenoid sinus through a central stationary field (part of the left eye is shielded with a 3 cm × 1.5 cm × 5.4 cm lead block)
   SSD 50 cm
   field size 7 × 8 cm
   Alderson–Rando phantom
   (Zwicker and Felix 1972)

Fig. 11. 60-Co teletherapy of the left maxillary antrum, entire nasal cavity, ethmoid cells, frontal sinus, and sphenoid sinus through two stationary fields (protection of lenses the same as in Fig. 10)
   SSD 50 cm
   field size 7 × 8 cm ventral
          5 × 8 cm lateral
   Alderson–Rando phantom
   (Zwicker and Felix 1972)

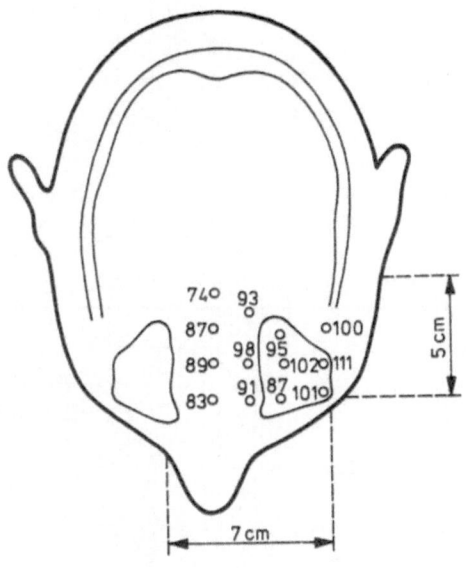

Fig. 12. 60-Co teletherapy of the left maxillary antrum with two stationary 10° wedge filter fields
   SSD 50 cm
   field size 5 × 6 cm
   (Burkell and Watson 1956)

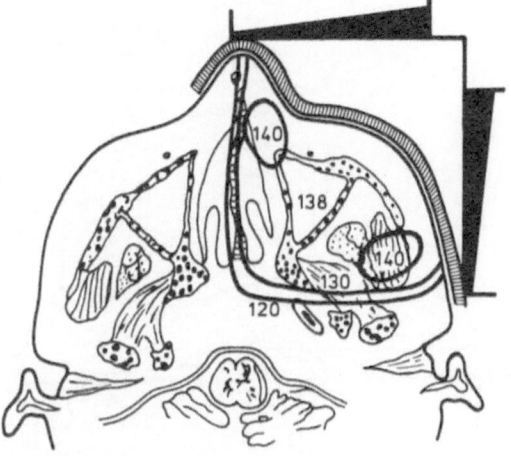

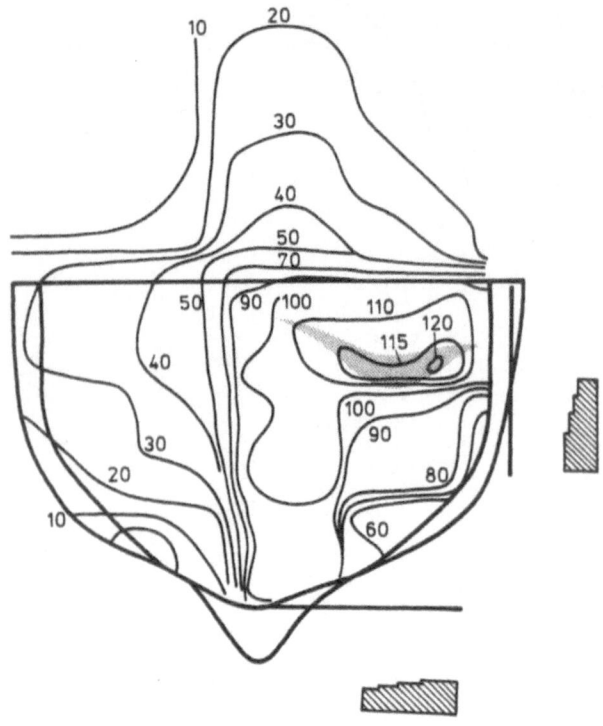

Fig. 13. Postoperative 60-Co teletherapy of the left maxillary antrum, ethmoid and sphenoid sinuses through two 45° half-wedge filtered fields
SSD 50 cm
field size 6 × 8 cm each
Water phantom
(Fletcher 1956*a*)

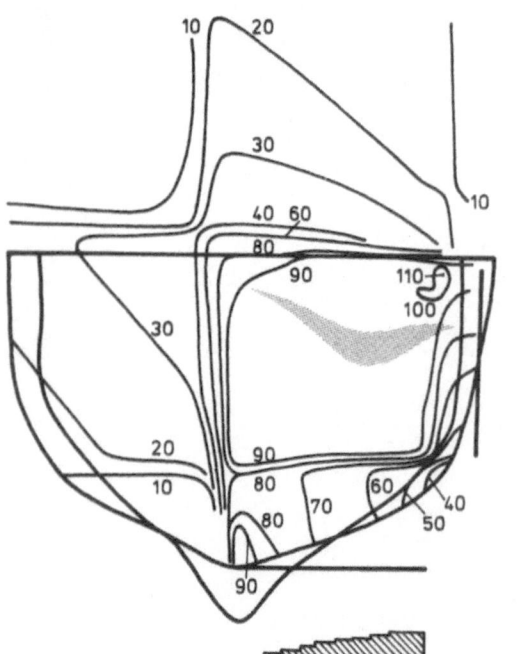

Fig. 14. 60-Co teletherapy of the left maxillary antrum, ethmoid and sphenoid sinuses through two 45° full-wedge filtered fields
SSD 50 cm
field size 6 × 8 cm each
Water phantom
(Fletcher 1956*a*)

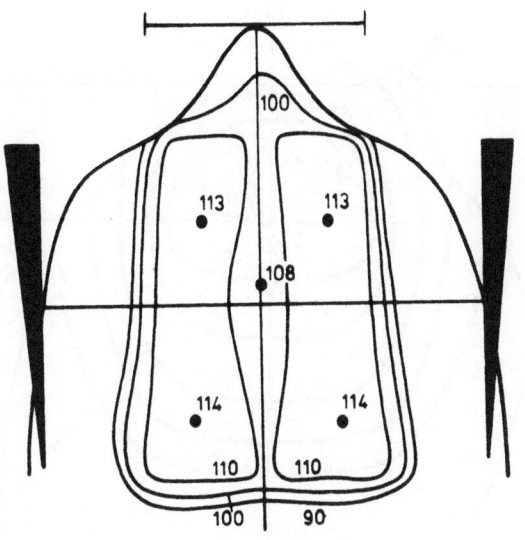

Fig. 15. 60-Co teletherapy of the entire nasal sinus, ethmoid cells, frontal and sphenoid sinuses through a stationary ventral open field and two opposing lateral fields with 60° wedge filters (50% of the total dose to the ventral field and 25% to each lateral field)
 SSD 70 cm
 field size 6 × 8 cm ventral
  8 × 8 cm lateral
 (Boone et al. 1968)

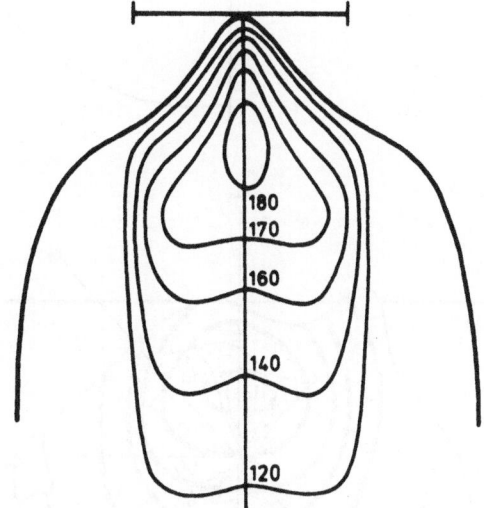

Fig. 16. 60-Co and electron beam treatment of the nasal, ethmoid and sphenoid sinuses through a single stationary ventral field
 60-Co:
  SSD 70 cm
  field size 6 × 8 cm
 22 MeV electron beam:
  FSD 80 cm
  field size 6 × 8 cm
 (Boone et al. 1968)

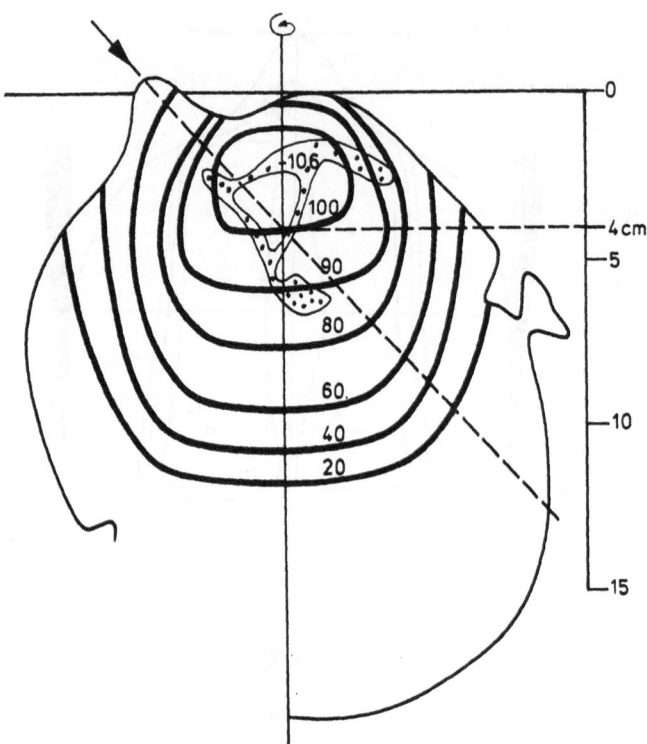

Fig. 17. 60-Co conical
rotation treatment of the
right antrum using a 16.8°
copper wedge filter
  SSD 70 cm
  axis depth 4 cm
  angle of incidence 45°
  field size 6.7 × 6.7 cm
    on the surface
  Pressdwood phantom
  (Castro and Whitcomb
    1963)

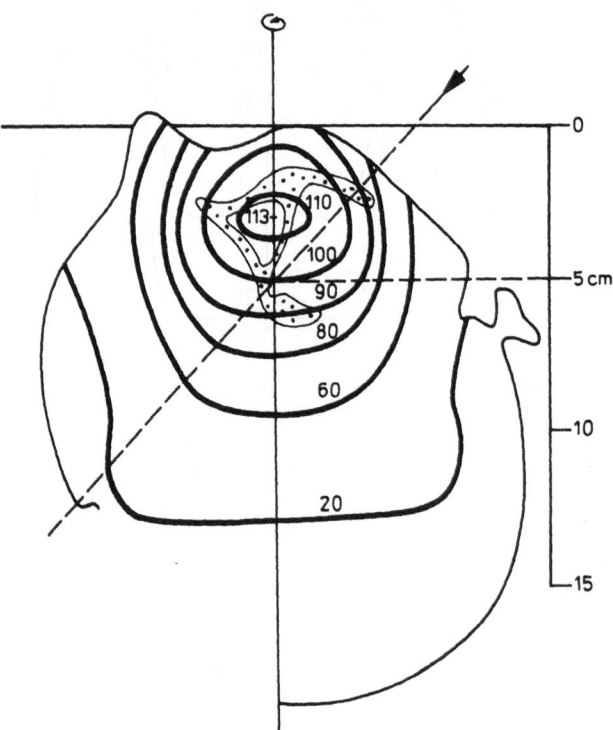

Fig. 18. 60-Co conical
rotation treatment of the
right maxillary sinus
  SSD 70 cm
  axis depth 5 cm
  angle of incidence 45°
  field size 6 × 6 cm
    on the surface
  Pressdwood phantom
  (Castro and Whitcomb
    1963)

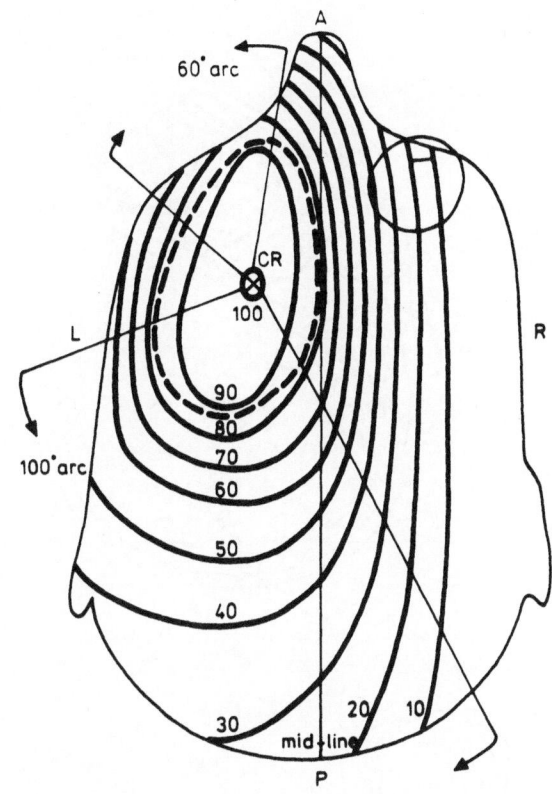

Fig. 19. One-centre two-arc
60-Co rotation treatment of
the left antrum
   SAD 75 cm
   axis depth 4 cm at 270°
   arcs: 60° ventral
         100° dorsal
   field size 6 × 10 cm each
   (Gough 1962)

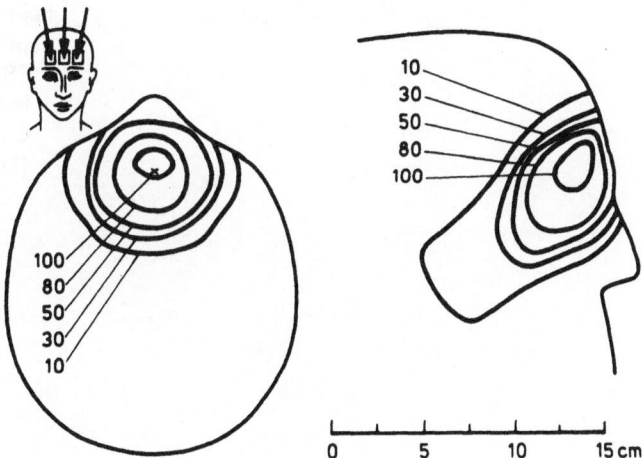

Fig. 20. 60-Co tele-
therapy of the ethmoid
sinuses through three
frontal fields (40° down-
ward tilt of the central
beam of all three fields
and 70° backward tilt of
the lateral fields.
Reference point at 2.5 cm
depth in the ethmoid
sinuses)
   SSD 50 cm
   field size 4 × 4 cm each
   Calculated isodoses
   (Fornusek et al. 1972)

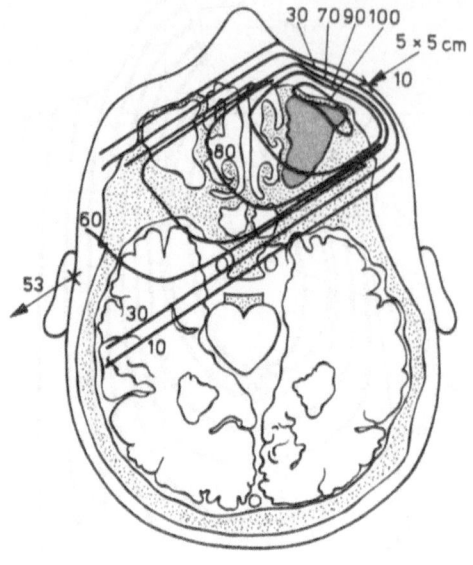

Fig. 21. High-energy X-ray
(8 MV) irradiation of the left
antrum through a stationary
ventrolateral field
    FSD 100 cm
    field size 5 × 5 cm
    Calculated isodoses
    (Morrison et al. 1956)

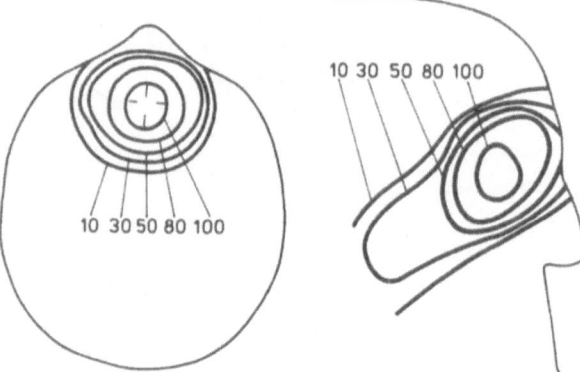

Fig. 22. High-energy X-ray
(42 MV) treatment of the
ethmoid sinuses through three
temporal fields (40° downward
tilt of the central beams of the
intraorbital field and both
supraorbital fields and 70°
downward tilt of the supraorbital
fields. Reference point at 2.5 cm
depth in the ethmoid sinus)
    FSD 100 cm
    field size 4 × 4 cm each
    Calculated isodoses
    (Fornusek et al. 1972)

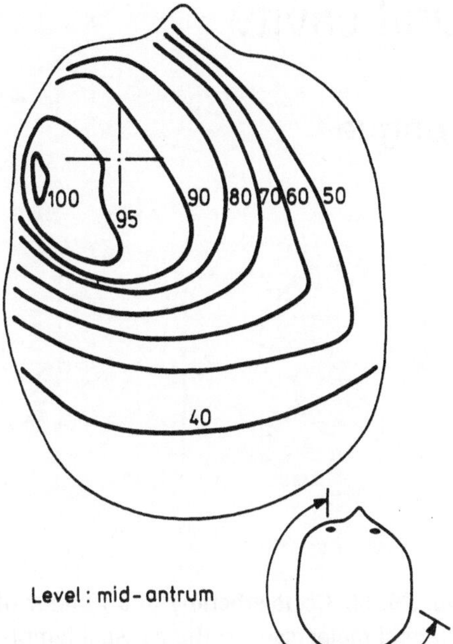

Fig. 23. High-energy X-ray (2 MV) arc (260°)
therapy of the left antrum
    SAD 100 cm
    axis depth 4 cm (at 270°)
    field size 8 × 6 cm
    Pressdwood phantom
    (Friedman et al. 1959)

Level: mid-antrum

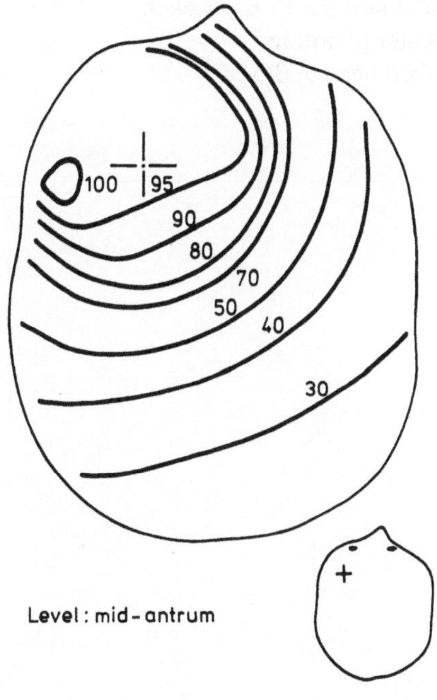

Fig. 24. Rotation therapy (360°) of the antrum
with 2 MV high energy X-rays
    SAD 100 cm
    axis depth 4 cm at 270°
    field size 8 × 6 cm
    Pressdwood phantom
    (Friedman et al. 1959)

Level: mid-antrum

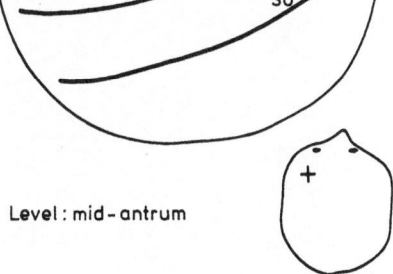

Oral cavity

Tongue

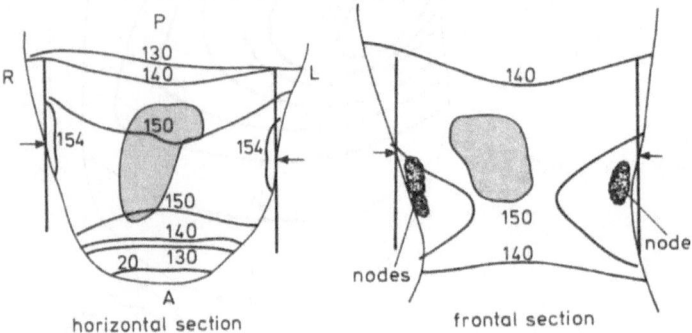

horizontal section   frontal section

Fig. 25. 60-Co teletherapy of a tumour of the tongue with
bilateral metastases to the cervical lymph nodes, through
two opposing stationary fields
   SSD 60 cm
   field size 9 × 11.5 cm each
   Water phantom
   (Fletcher 1956*a*)

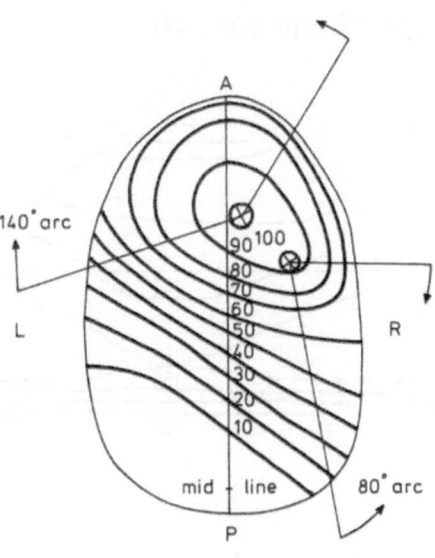

Fig. 26. Two-centre two-arc 60-Co teletherapy of the tongue
  SAD 75 cm
  distance of axes 2.5 cm
  arcs: 140° ventral
          80° right
  field size 6 × 10 cm each
  (Gough 1962)

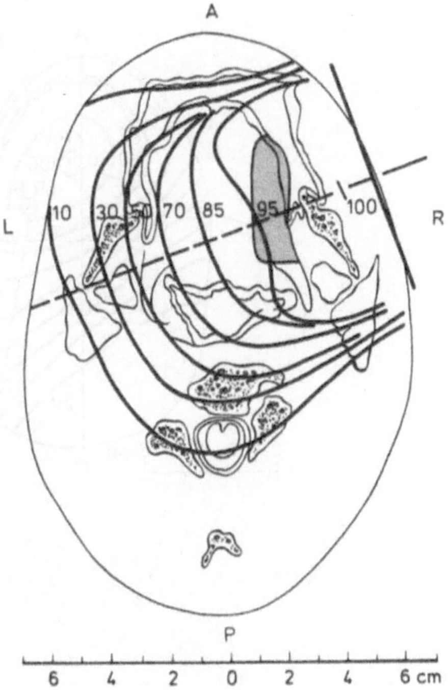

Fig. 27. Electron beam (22.5 MeV) therapy
of a tumour on the right lateral border of
the tongue through a stationary field
  FSD 90 cm
  field size 8 × 16 cm
  Water phantom
  (Perry et al. 1962)

Floor of the mouth

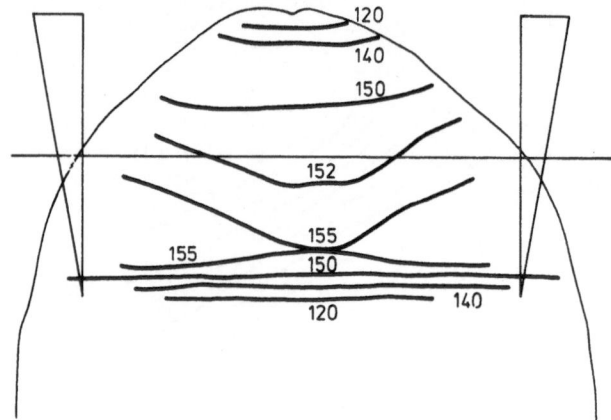

Fig. 28. 60-Co teletherapy of the floor of the mouth through two opposing stationary 30° wedge fields
    SSD 73.3 cm
    field size 6 × 6 cm each
    (Campos et al. 1971)

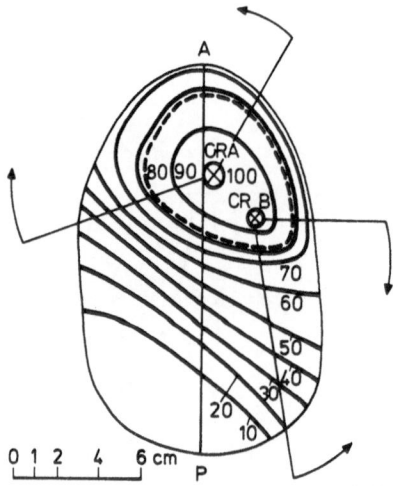

Fig. 29. 60-Co teletherapy of the left side of the floor of the mouth using the two-centre two-arc technique
    SAD 60 cm
    distance of axes 2.5 cm
    axis depth:
        ventral axis, 5 cm
            from ventral
        dorsal axis, 3 cm
            at 90°
    arcs: 140° ventral
            80° dorsal
    field size 6 × 10 cm each
    Calculated isodoses
    (Howarth and Wilson 1961)

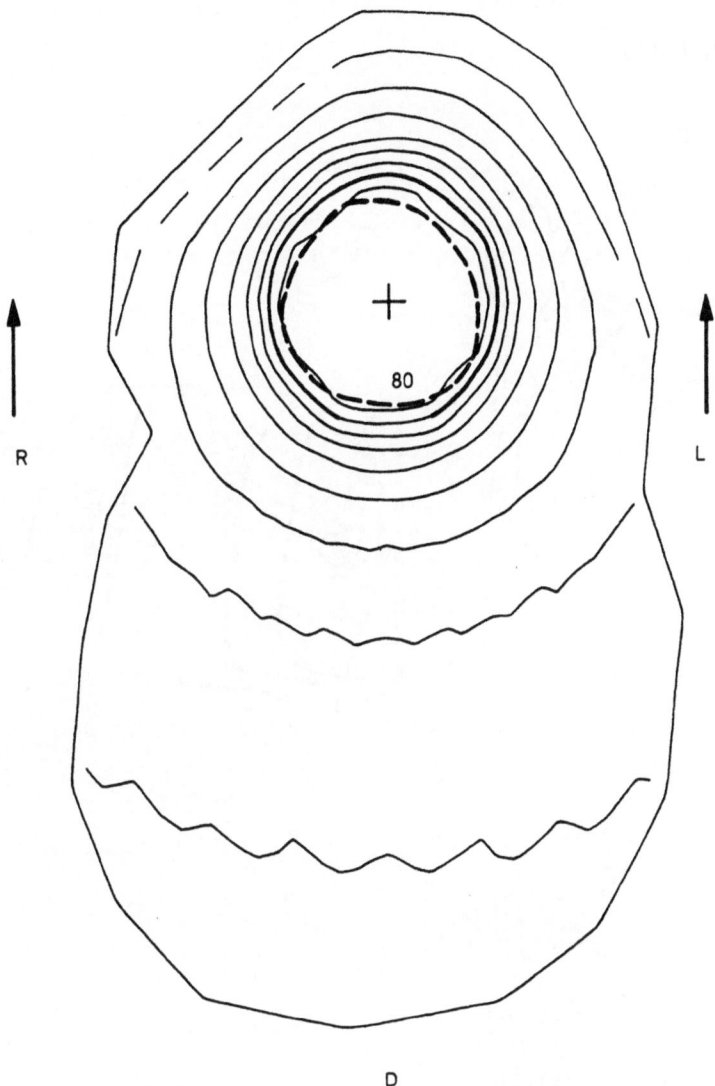

Fig. 30. High-energy X-ray (42 MV) arc (180° — ±90°) therapy
of the floor of the mouth
  FAD 120 cm
  axis depth 5 cm
  field size 4 × 4 cm
  Computer calculated isodoses

Gingiva

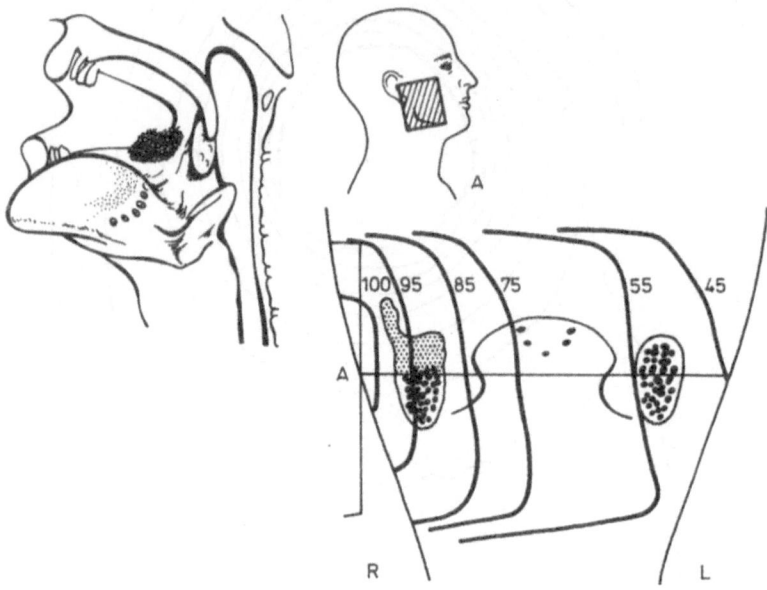

Fig. 31. 60-Co
teletherapy of the
right retromolar
trigone
  SSD 60 cm
  field size
    8 × 9 cm
  (Fletcher et al.
    1959)

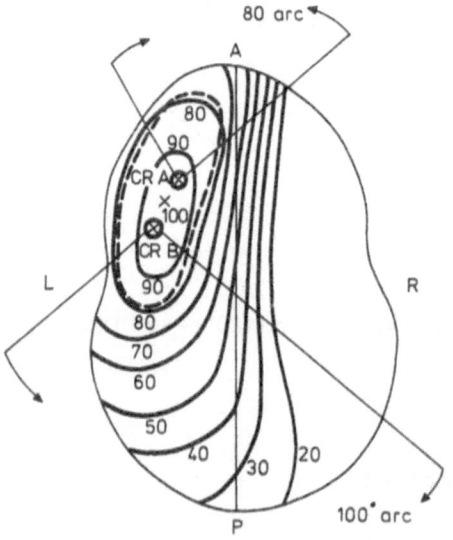

Fig. 32. Two-centre two-arc 60-Co
rotation cycling for carcinoma of the
alveolar margin
  SAD 75 cm
  distance of axes 2.5 cm
  arcs: 80° ventral
        100° dorsal
  field size 4 × 8 cm each
  (Gough 1962)

Fig. 33. Electron beam (30 MeV) therapy of a tumour of the left retromolar trigone (metastases in the ipsilateral submandibular and cervical lymph nodes) through a stationary field with a 3 cm thick bolus over the submandibular and cervical lymph nodes
  FSD 200 cm
  field size 10.5 × 10.5 cm
  Pressdwood phantom
  (Zatz et al. 1961)

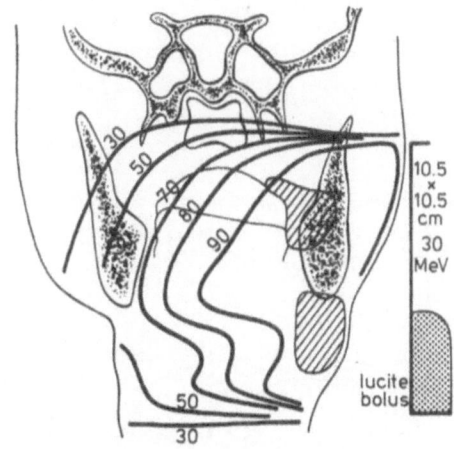

Buccal mucosa

Fig. 34. X-ray (8 MV)· irradiation of a buccal tumour through a stationary field
  FSD 100 cm
  field size
    7 × 6 cm
  (Morrison et al. 1961)

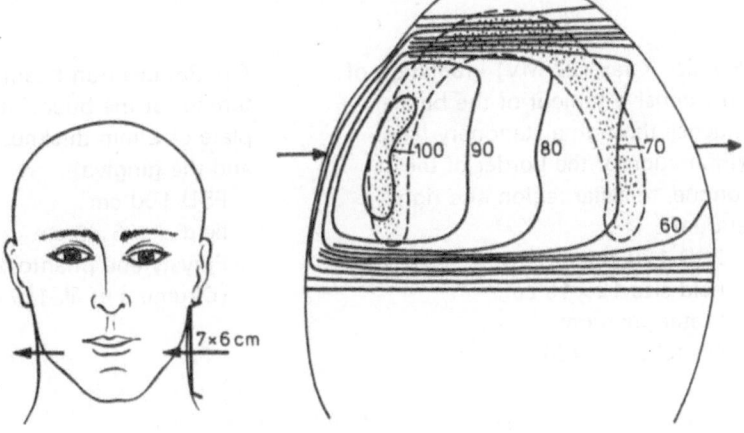

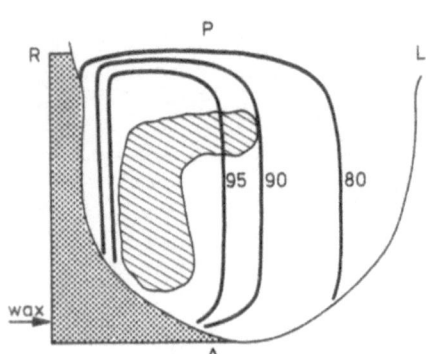

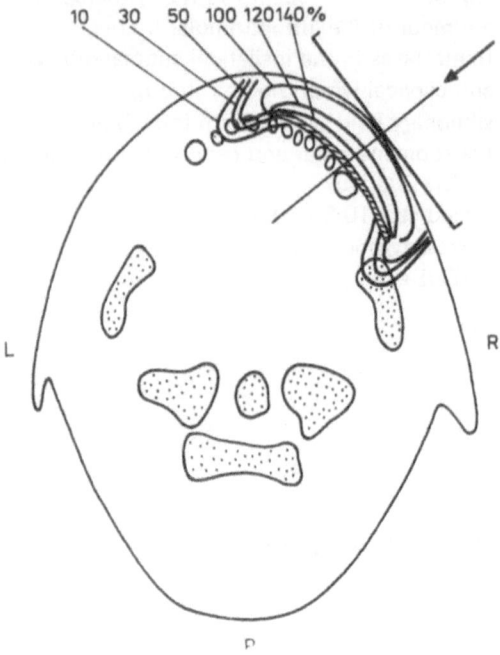

Fig. 35. X-ray (22 MV) irradiation of an extensive tumour of the buccal mucosa through a stationary field. (Infiltration of the border of the tongue, tonsillar region and right antrum)
    FSD 120 cm
    field size 12 × 15 cm
    Water phantom
    (Fletcher 1956b)

Fig. 36. Electron beam (10 MeV) therapy of a tumour of the buccal mucosa (with a lead plate of 2 mm thickness between the tumour and the gingiva)
    FSD 100 cm
    field size 6 × 8 cm
    Polystyrene phantom
    (Okumura et al. 1971)

Pharynx

Nasopharynx

Fig. 37. X-ray (200 kV) irradiation of the
nasopharynx through four stationary fields
(protection of the eyes with lead plates of
3 mm thickness)
    HVT 1 mm Cu
    FSD 60 cm
    field size 5 × 6 cm each
    Mix-D phantom
    (Nordberg and Olivecrona 1966)

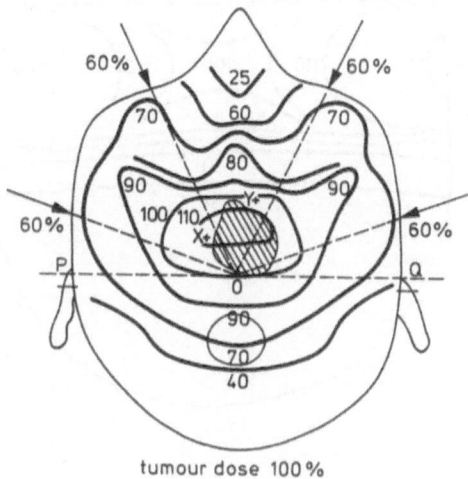

tumour dose 100%

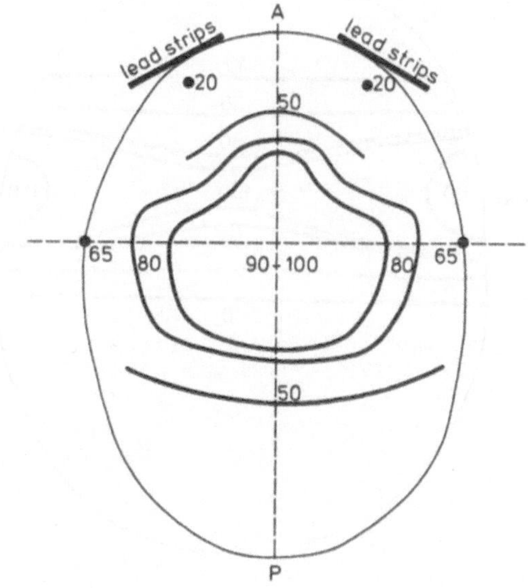

Fig. 38. Rotation (360°) therapy with
250 kV X-rays of the nasopharynx (eye
protection with lead strips)
    HVT 1.7 mm Cu
    FAD 85 cm
    axis depth 8 cm (in the midline)
    field size 6.5 × 8.5 cm at axis
    Calculated isodoses
    (Robbins and Tsien 1958)

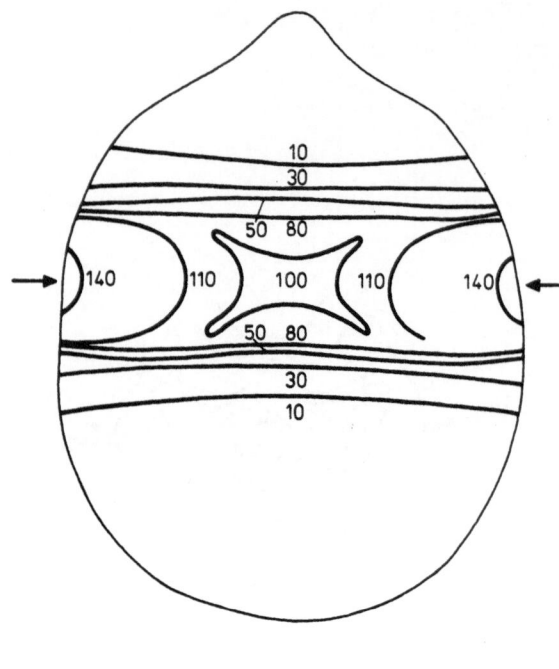

Fig. 39. 137-Cs teletherapy of
the nasopharynx with two
opposing stationary fields
  SSD 25 cm
  field size 6 × 4 cm on the
    surface
  Calculated isodoses
  (Fornusek et al. 1972)

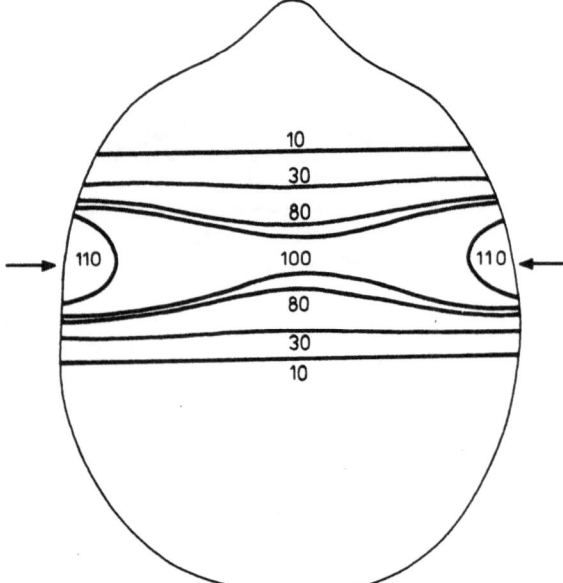

Fig. 40. 60-Co teletherapy of
the nasopharynx with two
opposing stationary fields
  SSD 50 cm
  field size 6 × 4 cm on the
    surface
  Calculated isodoses
  (Fornusek et al. 1972)

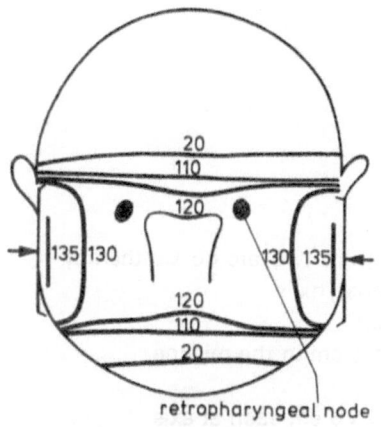

Fig. 41. 60-Co teletherapy of the nasopharynx and retropharyngeal lymph nodes through two opposing stationary fields
SSD 60 cm
field size 6 × 9 cm each
Water phantom
(Fletcher 1956a)

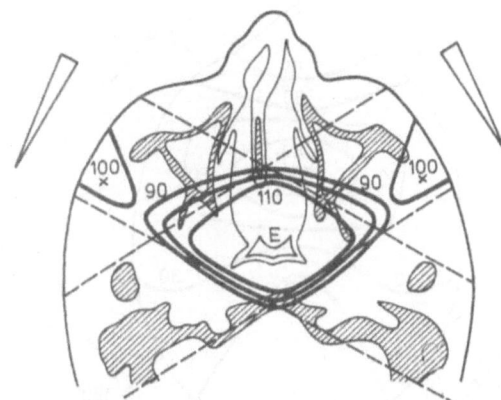

Fig. 42. 60-Co teletherapy of the nasopharynx through two wedge filtered (15°) fields
SSD 50 cm
field size 4 × 6 cm each
(Kuttig and Herbig 1965)

Fig. 43. 60-Co teletherapy of the nasopharynx and retropharyngeal lymph nodes through four stationary fields
SSD 50 cm
field size 5 × 7 cm ventral
6 × 9 cm lateral
Water phantom
(Fletcher 1956a)

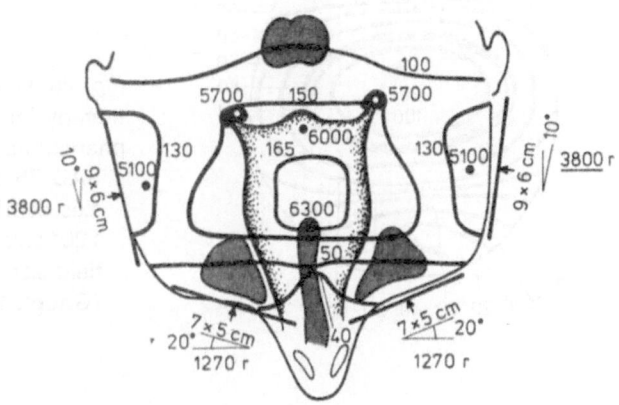

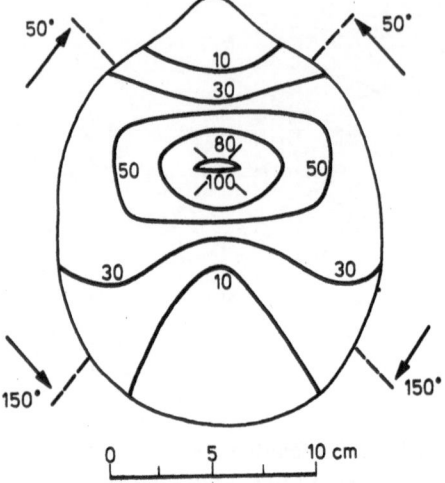

Fig. 44. One-axis two-arc 60-Co therapy
of the nasopharynx
  SAD 60 cm
  axis depth 8 cm in the midline
  100° arcs
  field size 4 × 6 cm each at axis
  Calculated isodoses
  (Fornusek et al. 1972)

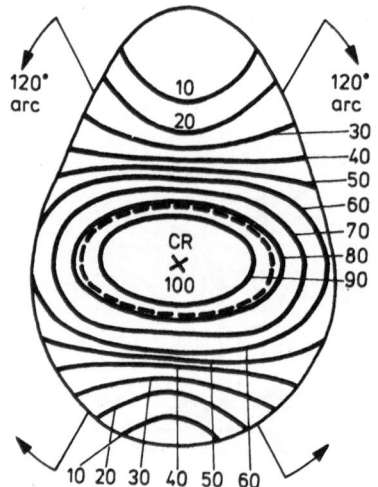

Fig. 45. One-centre equi-arc rotation
therapy for carcinoma of the nasopharynx using a rotating 60-Co unit
  SAD 75 cm
  axis depth 8 cm in the midline
  120° arcs
  field size 6 × 8 cm each
  (Gough 1962)

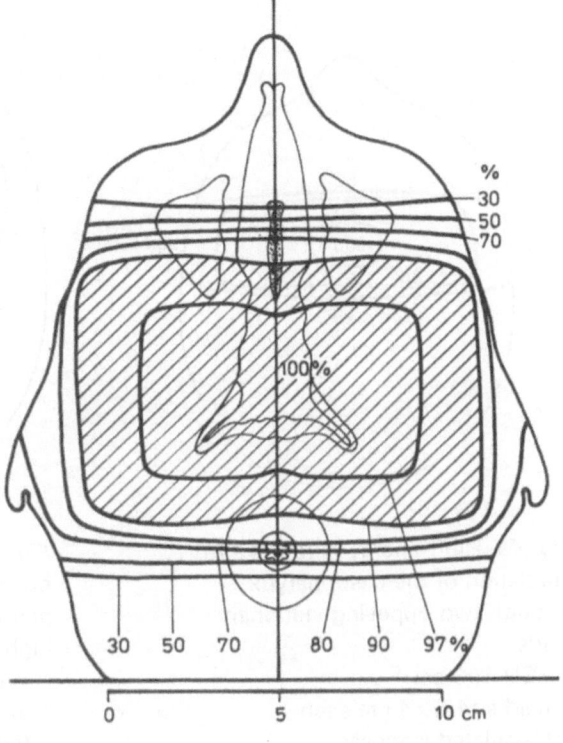

Fig. 46. High-energy X-ray (16 MV) irradiation of the nasopharynx through two opposing stationary fields
  FSD 60 cm
  field size 9 × 7 cm in target volume
  Calculated isodoses (Gauwerky and Frommhold 1973)

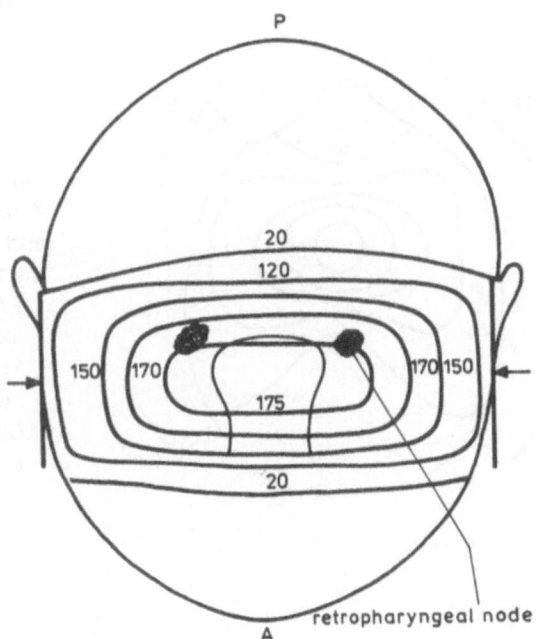

Fig. 47. High-energy X-ray (22 MV) irradiation of the nasopharynx through two opposing stationary fields
  FSD 80 cm
  field size 6 × 8 cm each
  Water phantom
  (Fletcher 1956*b*)

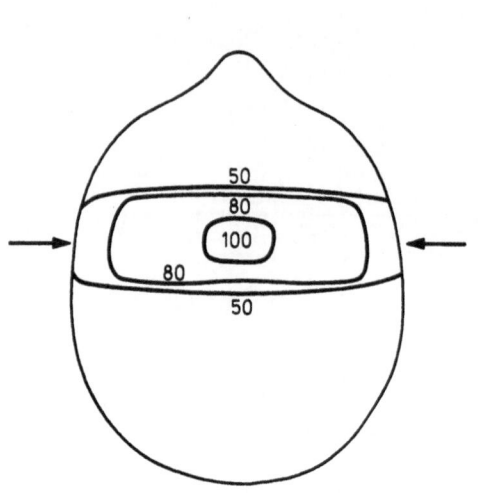

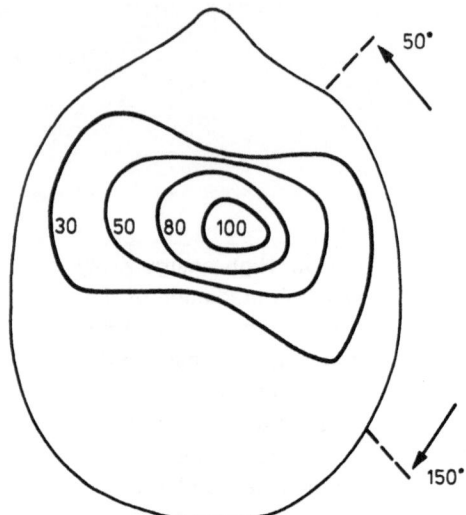

Fig. 48. High-energy X-ray (42 MV) irradiation of the nasopharynx through two opposing stationary fields

    FSD 100 cm
    field size 6 × 4 cm each
    Calculated isodoses
    (Fornusek et al. 1972)

Fig. 49. Arc therapy (100°) of the naso- pharynx and the apical area of the petrous part of the left temporal bone with 42 MV high-energy X-rays

    FAD 120 cm
    axis depth 8 cm in the midline
    field size 4 × 6 cm at axis
    Calculated isodoses
    (Fornusek et al. 1972)

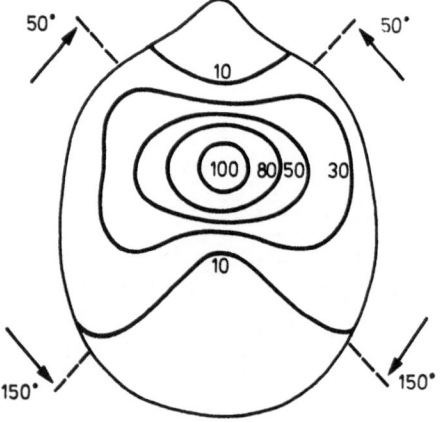

Fig. 50. One-axis two-arc high-energy X-ray (42 MV) therapy of the nasopharynx and the apical area of the petrous part of the temporal bone

    FAD 120 cm
    axis depth 8 cm in the midline
    100° arcs
    field size at axis 4 × 6 cm each
    Calculated isodoses
    (Fornusek et al. 1972)

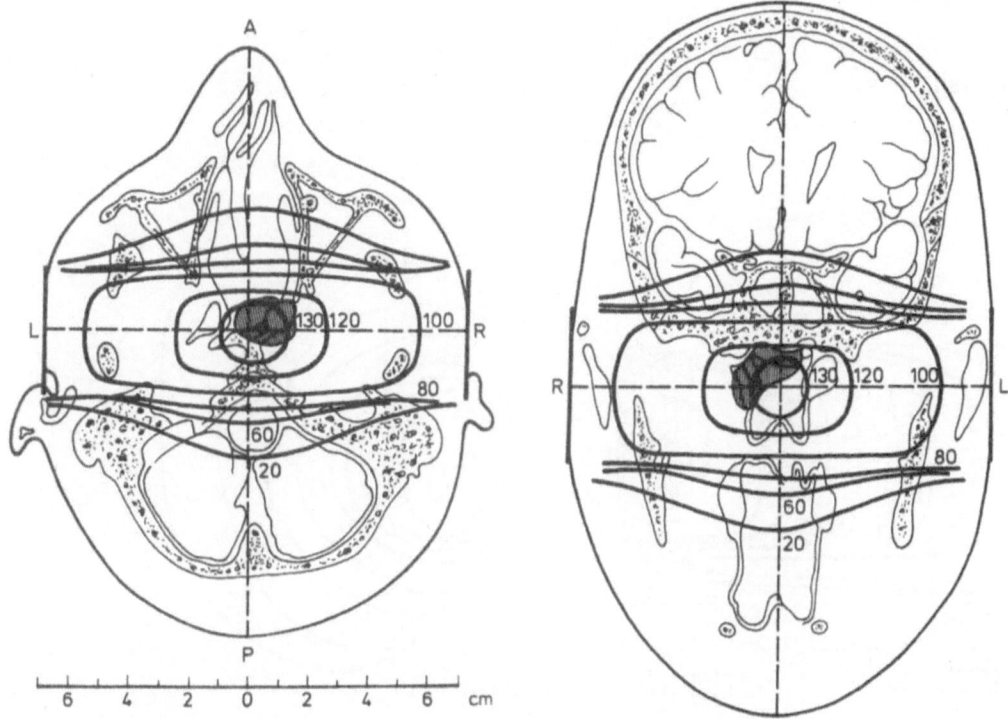

Fig. 51. Electron beam (24 MeV) therapy of the nasopharynx through two opposing stationary fields (horizontal and frontal sections)

 FSD 90 cm
 field size 4 × 5 cm each
 Water phantom
 (Perry et al. 1962)

Oropharynx

Tonsil

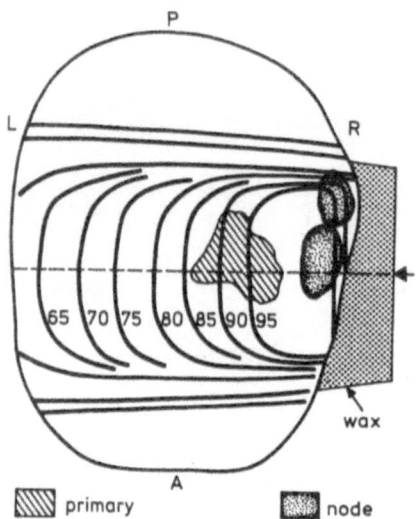

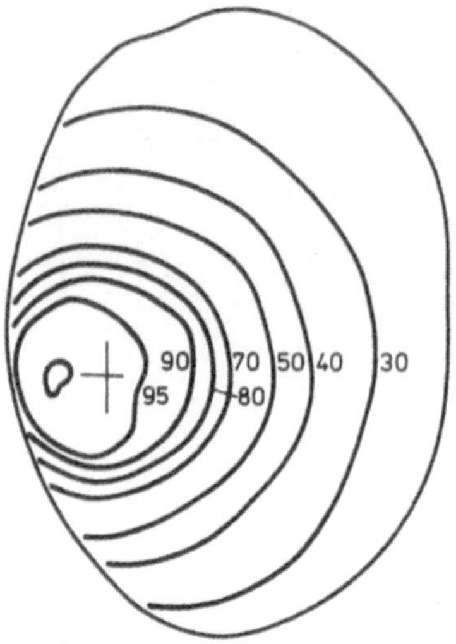

Fig. 52. High-energy X-ray
(22 MV) irradiation of a right
tonsillar tumour (with metastases in the cervical lymph nodes)
through a stationary field
  FSD 80 cm
  field size 8 × 10 cm
  Water phantom
  (Fletcher et al. 1959)

Fig. 53. Rotation treatment
(360°) of the tonsil with 2 MV
high-energy X-rays
  FAD 100 cm
  axis depth 3 cm at 270°
  field size 6 × 8 cm
  Pressdwood phantom
  (Friedman et al. 1959)

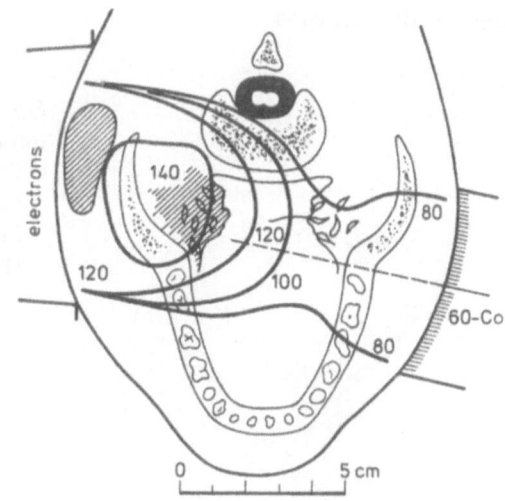

Fig. 54. Combined electron beam (17.5 MeV) and 60-Co teletherapy of the right tonsil
  Electron beam:
    FSD 100 cm
    field size 8 × 8 cm
  60-Co:
    SSD 50 cm
    field size 6 × 8 cm
  (Van Vaerenbergh et al. 1969)

Uvula

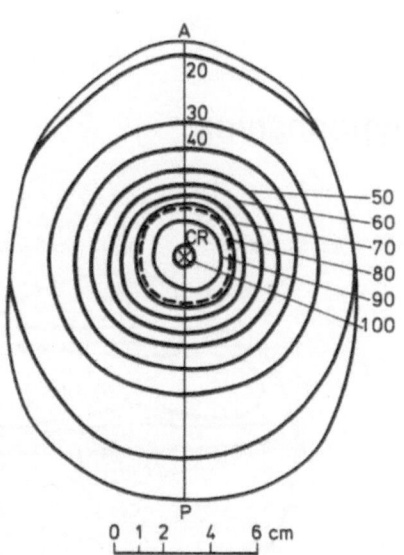

Fig. 55. 60-Co rotation treatment (360°) of the uvula
  SAD 60 cm
  axis depth 8.5 cm in the midline
  field size 4 × 8 cm
  Calculated isodoses
  (Howarth and Wilson 1961)

Base of the tongue

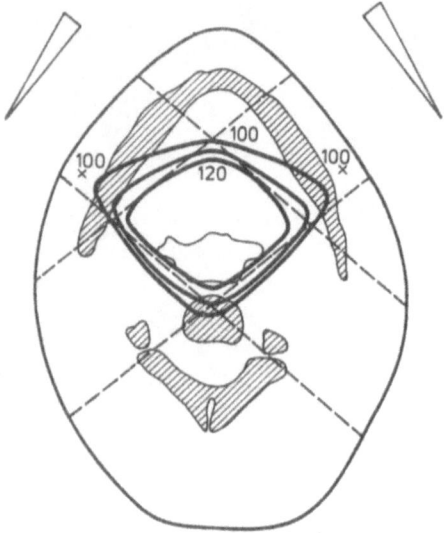

Fig. 56. 60-Co teletherapy of the base of the tongue through two 15° wedge filtered fields
  SSD 50 cm
  field size 4 × 6 cm each
  Plexiglas phantom
  (Kuttig and Herbig 1965)

Hypopharynx

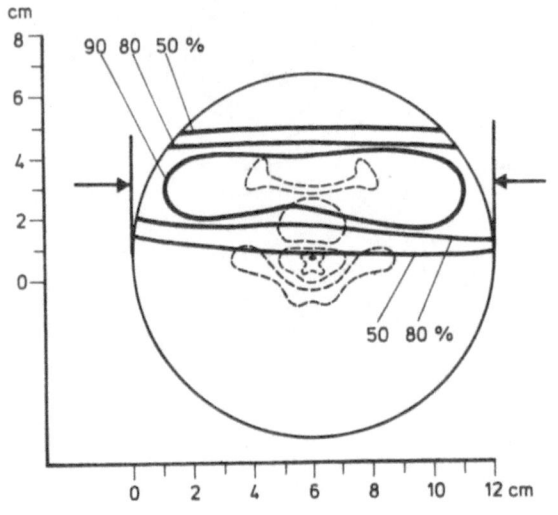

Fig. 57. 60-Co teletherapy of the hypopharynx through two opposing stationary fields
  SSD 65 cm
  field size 4 × 10 cm each
  Mix-D phantom
  (Németh and Wulff 1970)

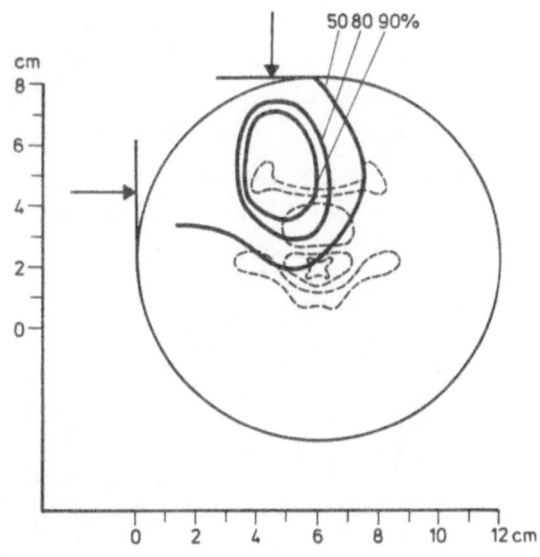

Fig. 58. 60-Co teletherapy of the hypopharynx through two opposing stationary fields
  SSD 65 cm
  field size 3 × 6 cm ventral
           4 × 6 cm lateral
  Mix-D phantom
  (Németh and Wulff 1970)

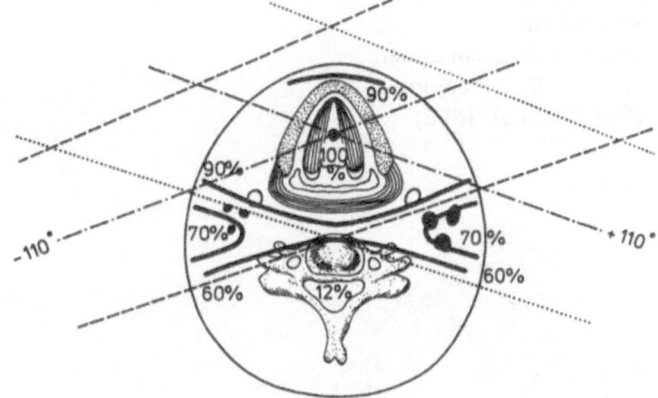

Fig. 59. 60-Co teletherapy of the hypopharynx through two stationary fields (a tilt of 10° of the fields caudally)
  SSD 65 cm
  field size 6 × 17 cm each
  angle of incidence 110°
    on both sides
  Calculated isodoses
  (Schuhknecht and Tietze 1970)

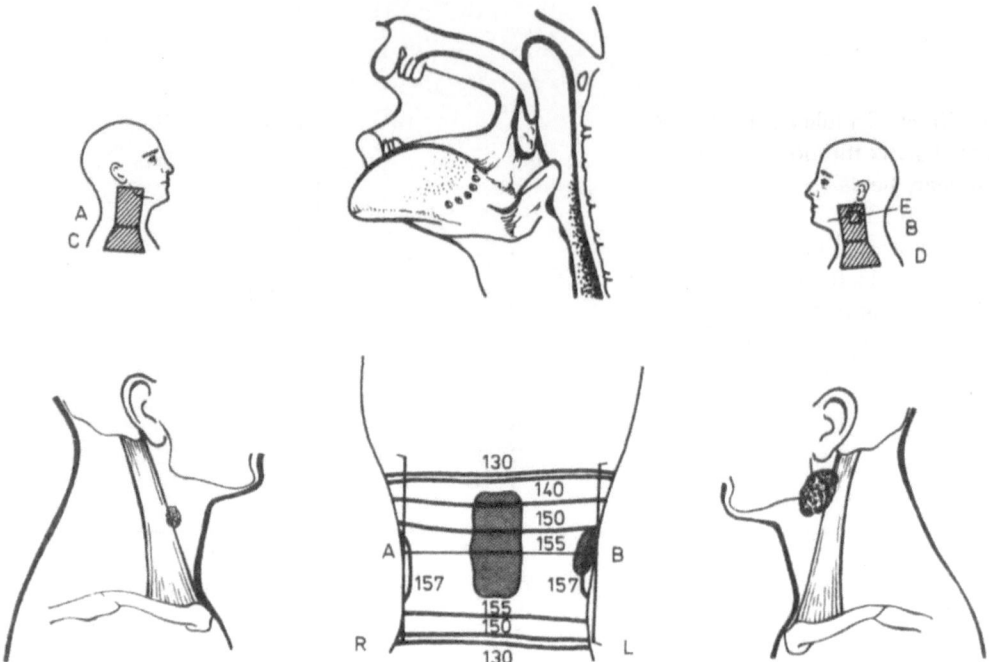

Fig. 60. 60-Co teletherapy of a tumour of the posterior hypopharyngeal wall (with cervical lymph node metastases on the left side) through two opposing stationary fields
   SSD 60 cm
   field size 9 × 8 cm upper
             8 × 13 cm lower
   (Fletcher et al. 1959)

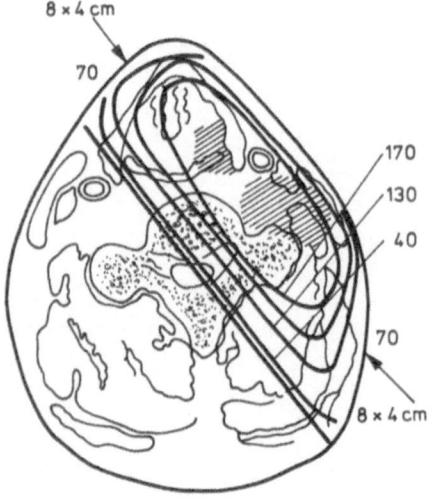

Fig. 61. High-energy X-ray (8 MV) irradiation of a tumour of the right hypopharynx (with ipsilateral cervical lymph node metastases) through two opposing stationary fields
   FSD 100 cm
   field size 4 × 8 cm each
   Calculated isodoses
   (Morrison et al. 1956)

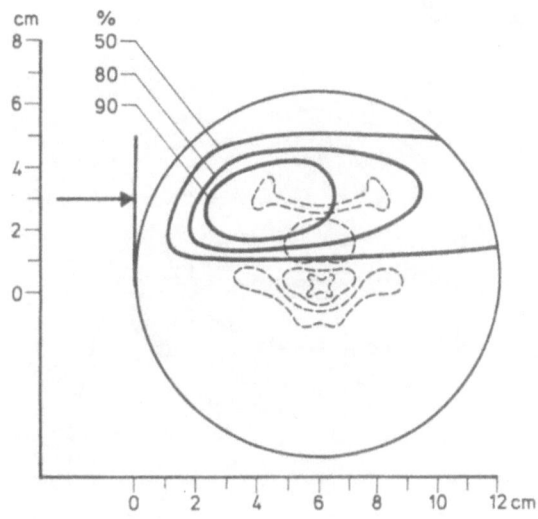

Fig.62. High-energy X-ray (15.5 MV) irradiation of the hypopharynx with one stationary field
    FSD 65 cm
        tissue compensating filter No. 3
        field size 4 × 10 cm
    Mix-D phantom
    (Németh and Wulff 1970)

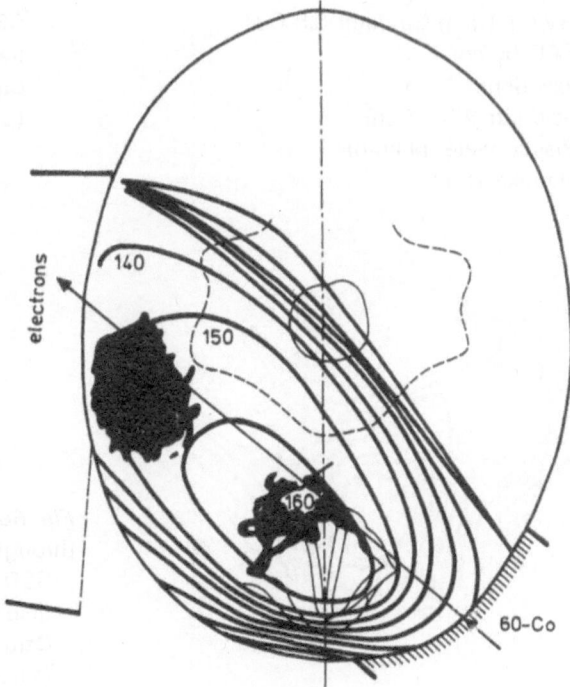

Fig. 63. Combined electron beam (17.5 MeV) and 60-Co tele-therapy of the right pyriform sinus and cervical lymph node metastases
    Electron beam:
        FSD 100 cm
        field size 8 × 12 cm
    60-Co:
        SSD 50 cm
        field size 4 × 12 cm
    (Van Vaerenbergh et al. 1969)

Larynx

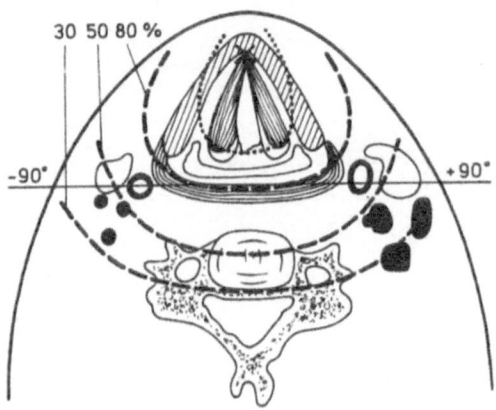

Fig. 64. X-ray (200 kV, 20 mA) arc (180°) therapy of the larynx
HVT 1.1 mm Cu, filter 0.5 Cu
FAD 50 cm
axis depth 4 cm
field size 4.5 × 5 cm
Plastic-water phantom
(Franke 1957)

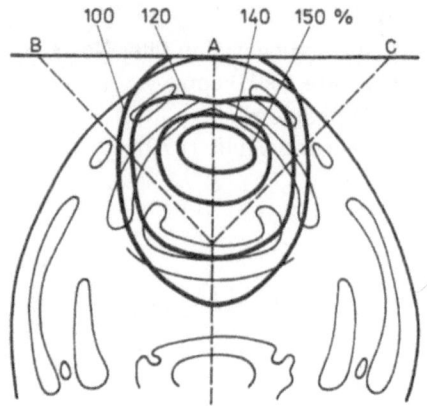

Fig. 65. 137-Cs teletherapy of the larynx through three stationary fields
SSD 20 cm
field size 3 × 6 cm each
Calculated isodoses
(Lintner et al. 1964)

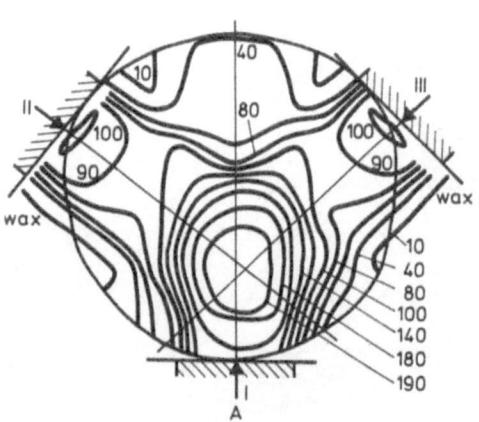

Fig. 66. 60-Co teletherapy of the larynx through three stationary fields
SSD 80 cm
field size 5 × 5 cm each
Calculated isodoses
(Smith and Lott 1958)

Fig. 67. 60-Co tele-
therapy of the larynx
through three stationary
fields (dose to the ven-
tral field is 50% of those
to the lateral fields)
SSD 80 cm
field size
6 × 7 cm each lateral
4.5 × 6 cm ventral
Calculated isodoses
(Malinowski
and Wasilewski
1968)

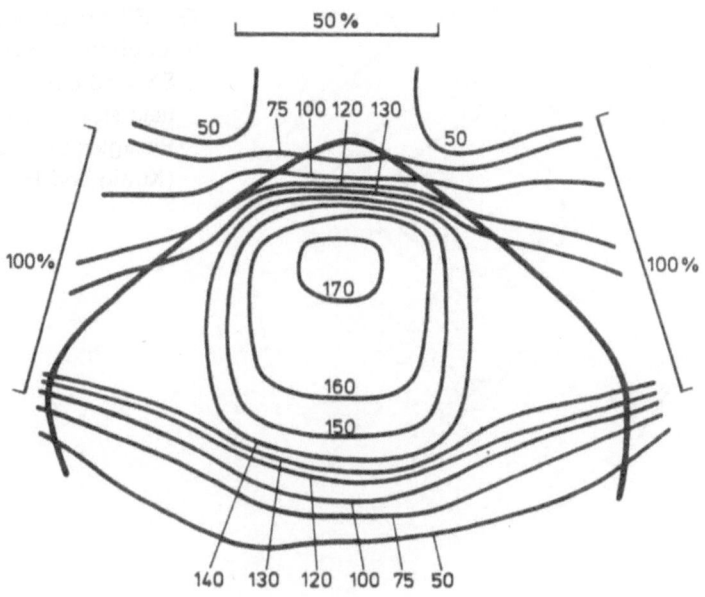

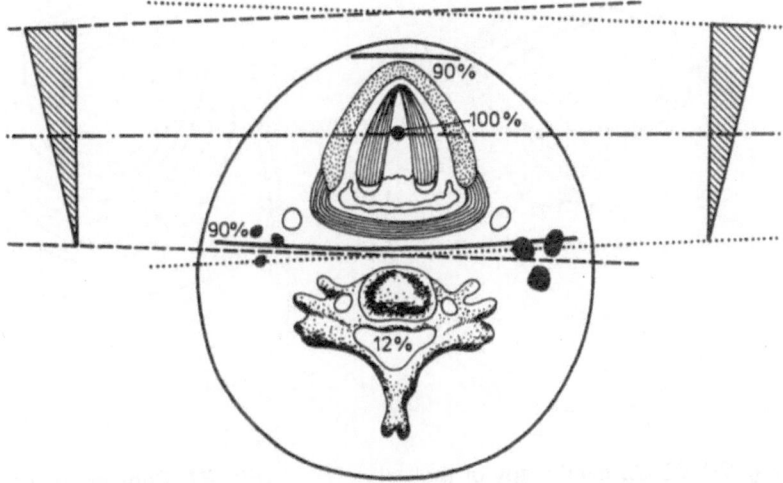

Fig. 68. 60-Co teletherapy of the larynx through two 14° wedge fields
SSD 65 cm
field size
5 × 7 cm each
Calculated isodoses
(Schuhknecht and Tietze 1970)

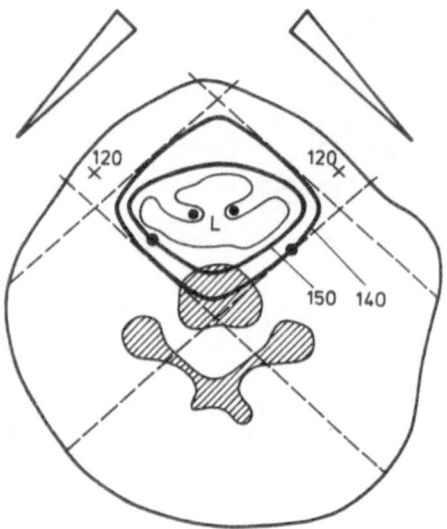

Fig. 69. 60-Co teletherapy of the larynx
through two 15° wedge fields
  SSD 50 cm
  field size 4 × 6 cm each
  Plexiglas phantom
  (Kuttig and Herbig 1965)

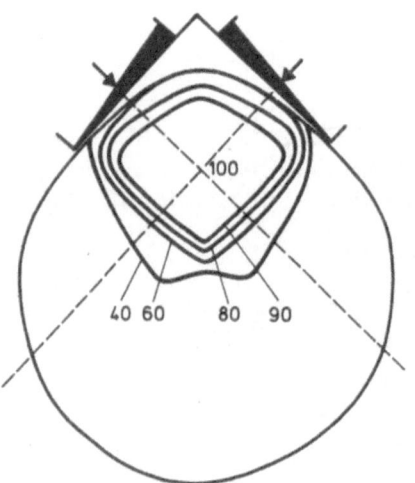

Fig. 70. 60-Co teletherapy of the
larynx through two 10° wedge fields
  SSD 50 cm
  field size 5 × 5 cm each
  (Burkell and Watson 1956)

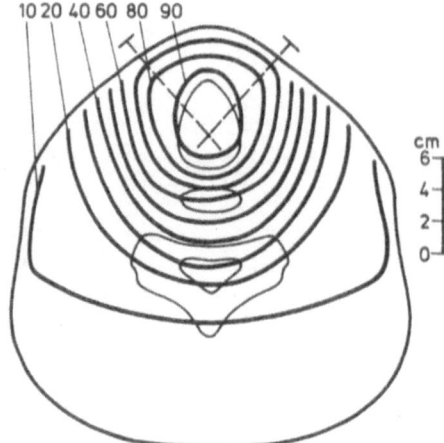

Fig. 71. Convergent-beam 60-Co
irradiation of the larynx
  SAD 75 cm each
  axis depth 2 cm each
  angle of convergence 30° each
  angle of axes 84°
  field size 4 × 4 cm each at the axis
  (Ratner et al. 1967)

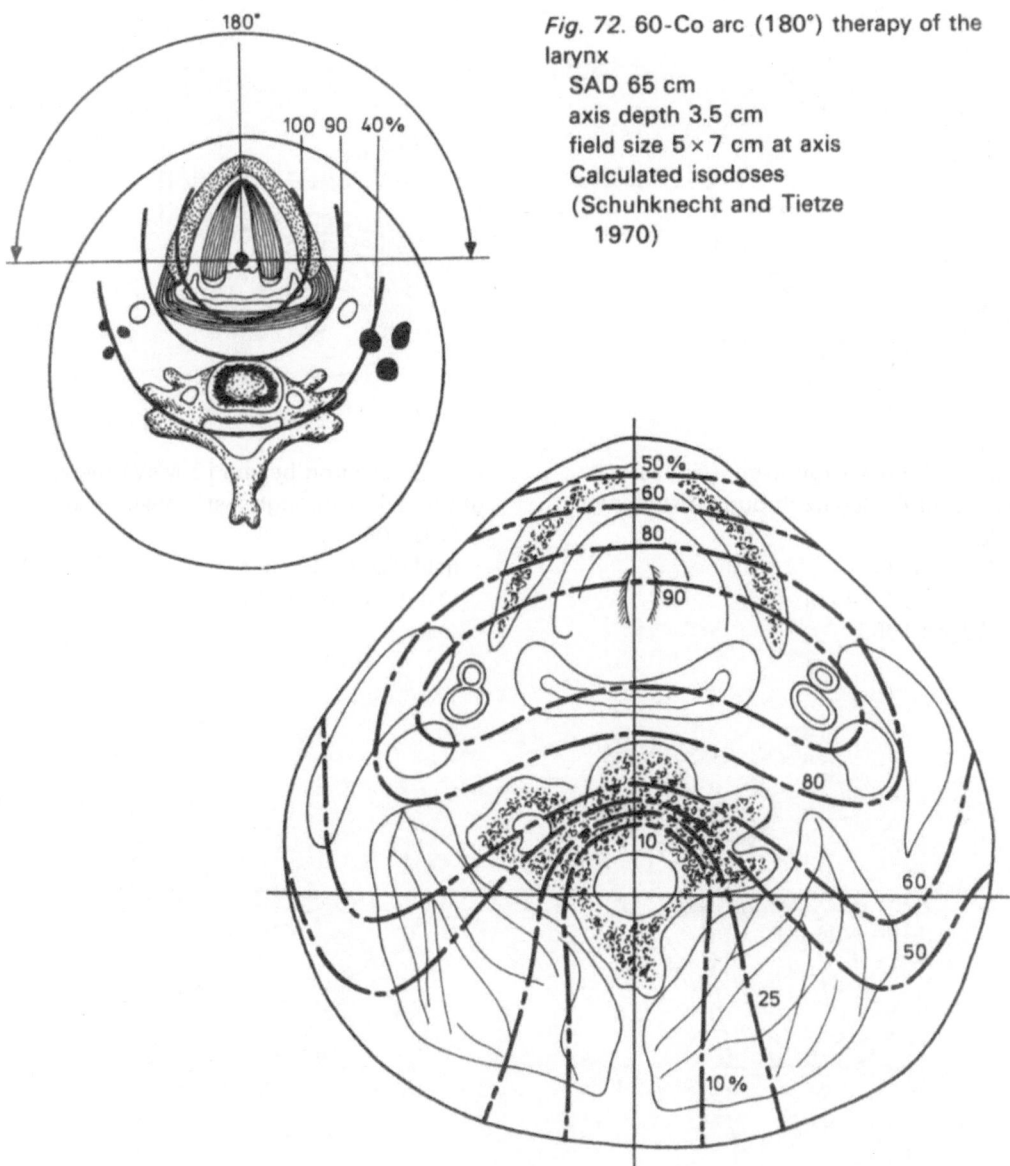

Fig. 72. 60-Co arc (180°) therapy of the larynx
  SAD 65 cm
  axis depth 3.5 cm
  field size 5 × 7 cm at axis
  Calculated isodoses
  (Schuhknecht and Tietze
    1970)

Fig. 73. Excentric 60-Co arc therapy of the larynx and regional lymph nodes
  SAD 65 cm
  axis depth in vertebral canal 4.5 cm from dorsal
  arcs: 200° on both sides
    (±20°/±180°)
  field size 3 × 6 cm at 50 cm SSD
  tilt of the central beam 3°
  Plexiglas phantom
  (Stratev and Rödel 1967)

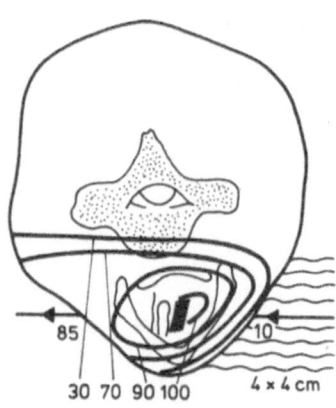

Fig. 74. High-energy X-ray (8 MV) irradiation of the larynx through a stationary field
FSD 100 cm
field size 4 × 4 cm
(Wood 1959)

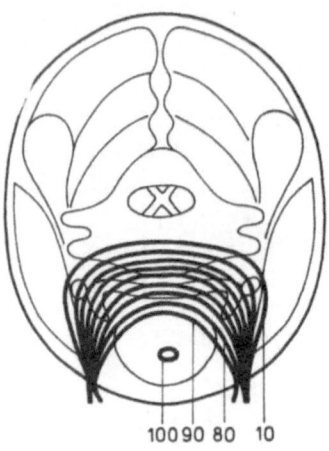

Fig. 75. Electron beam (15 MeV) therapy of the larynx through a stationary field
FSD 100 cm
field size 6 × 6 cm
(Krüger et al. 1964)

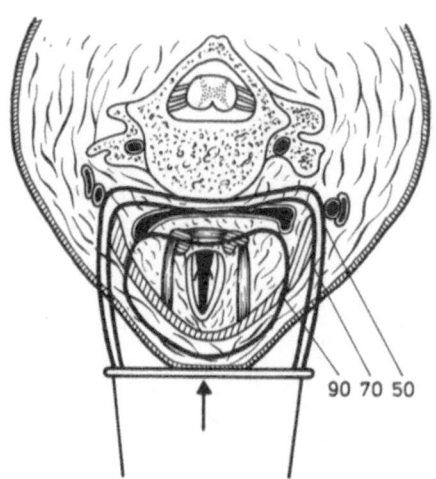

Fig. 76. Electron beam (9 MeV) therapy of the larynx with a stationary field
FSD 100 cm
field size 4.5 × 6 cm
(Becker et al. 1959)

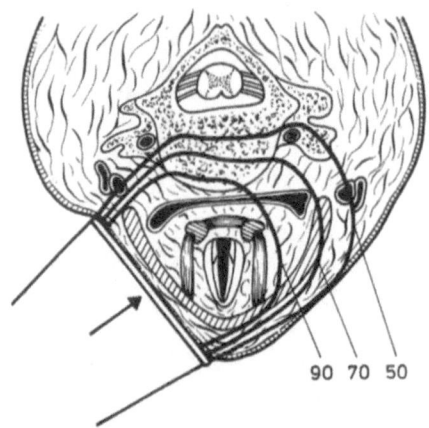

Fig. 77. Electron beam therapy (15 MeV) of the larynx with a stationary field
FSD 100 cm
field size 4.5 × 6 cm
(Becker et al. 1959)

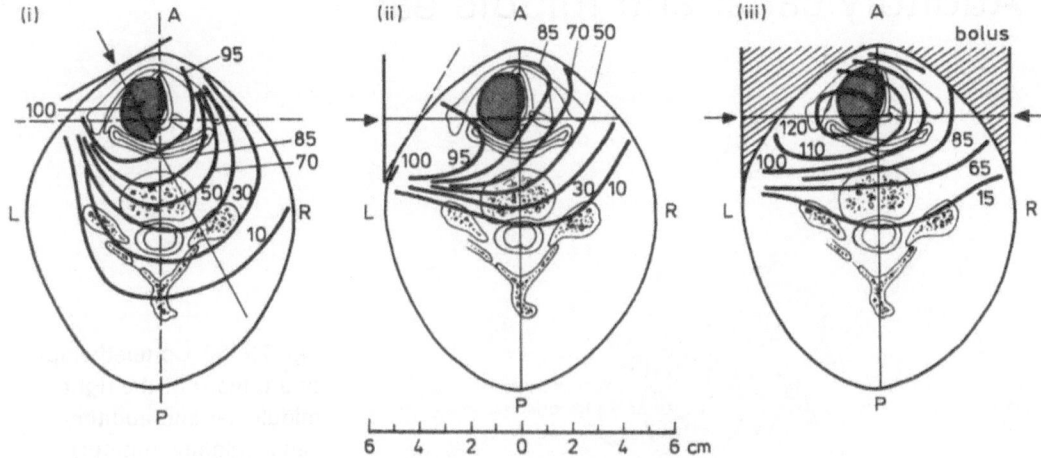

Fig. 78. Electron beam (20 MeV) therapy of a larynx tumour on the left side
FSD 90 cm
field size 5 × 4 cm each
Water phantom

(*i*)   left lateral field, central beam perpendicular to the surface
(*ii*)   left lateral field, central beam oblique to the surface
(*iii*) two opposing fields (dose delivered to the left side is twice the dose of the right portal). Irregular surface is compensated for with bolus
(Perry et al. 1962)

Auditory canal and middle ear

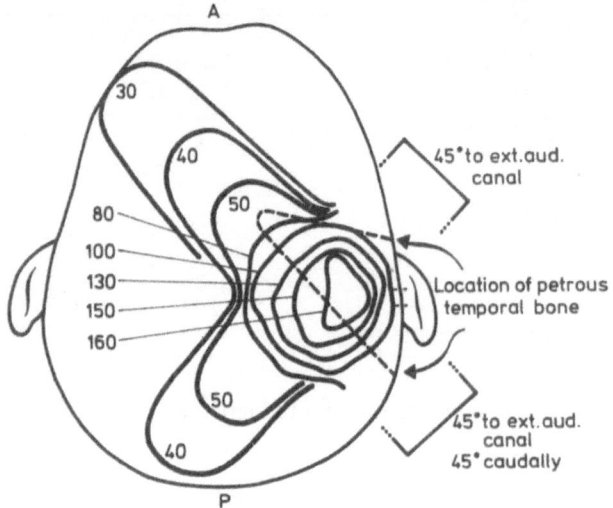

Fig. 79. 60-Co teletherapy of a tumour of the right middle ear and auditory canal (glomus tumour) through two stationary fields
　　SSD 60 cm
　　field size 4 × 6 cm each
　　(Miller 1962)

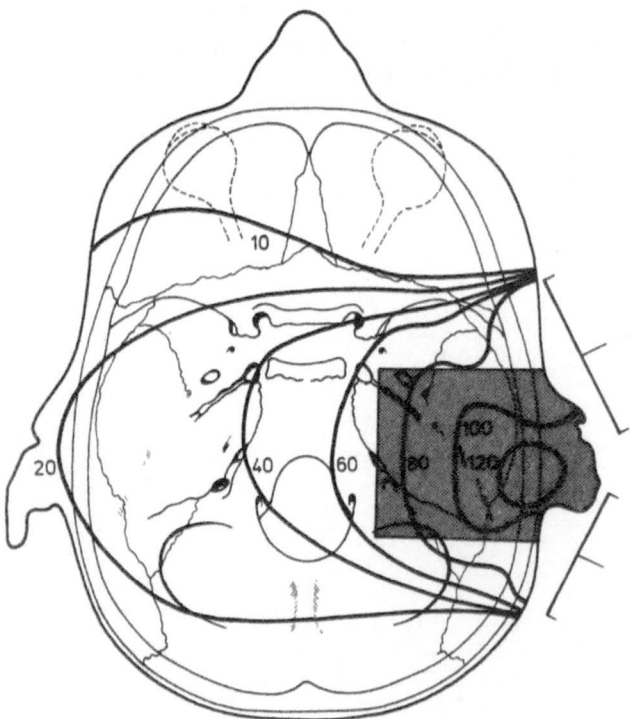

Fig. 80. 60-Co brachy-therapy of a tumour of the external auditory canal through two stationary fields
　　SSD 12 cm
　　field size 5 × 7 cm each
　　(Lederman et al. 1965)

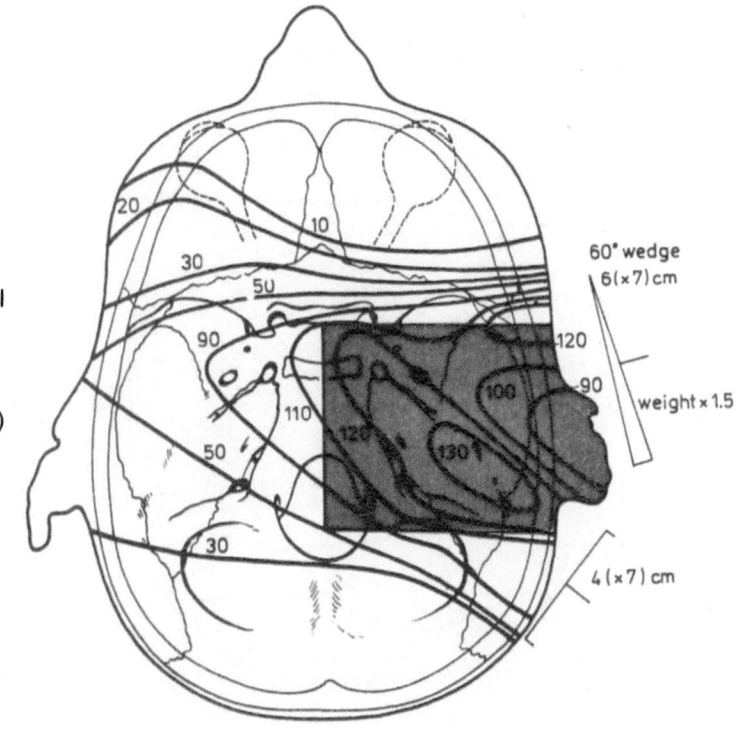

Fig. 81. 60-Co tele-
therapy of a mastoidal
tumour through
two stationary fields
Anterolateral field:
   60-Co (2500 Curie)
   SSD 70 cm
   field size 6 × 7 cm
   60° wedge
Posterolateral field:
   60-Co (150 Curie)
   SSD 30 cm
   field size 4 × 7 cm
   (Lederman et al.
    1965)

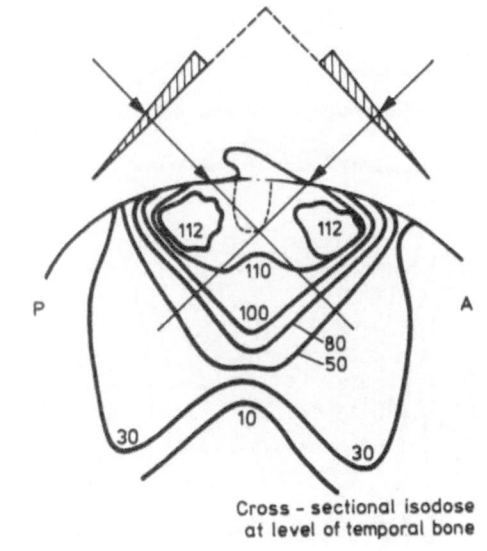

Fig. 82. 60-Co tele-
therapy of the
auditory canal and
middle ear through
two wedge fields
(in case of a
tympanojugular
chemodectoma)
   SSD 80 cm
   field size 6 × 10 cm
   (Maruyama 1972)

Cross - sectional isodose
at level of temporal bone

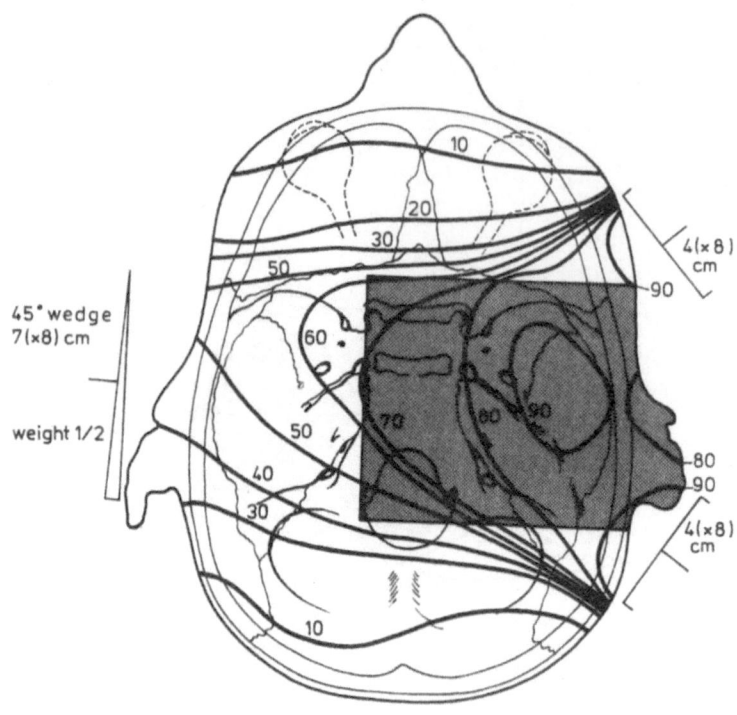

Fig. 83. 60-Co tele-
therapy of a tympa-
notubal tumour
through three
stationary fields
Right lateral fields:
  60-Co (150 Curie)
  SSD 12 cm
  field size
    4 × 8 cm each
Left lateral field:
  60-Co (2500 Curie)
  SSD 70 cm
  field size 7 × 8 cm
  45° wedge
  (Lederman et al.
  1965)

45° wedge
7 (×8) cm

weight 1/2

4 (× 8) cm

90

80
90

4 (×8) cm

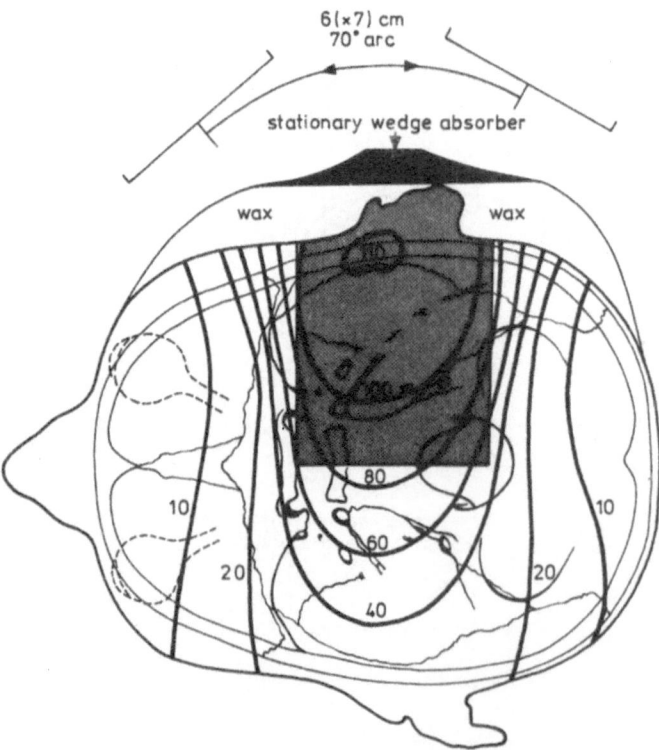

6 (×7) cm
70° arc

stationary wedge absorber

wax   wax

Fig. 84. 60-Co arc
therapy (70°) of a
petromastoid tumour
(irregular surface
compensated for with
build-up wax, irra-
diation through
wedge absorber)
  SAD 70 cm
  axis depth 4 cm
  field size 6 × 7 cm
  (Lederman et al.
  1965)

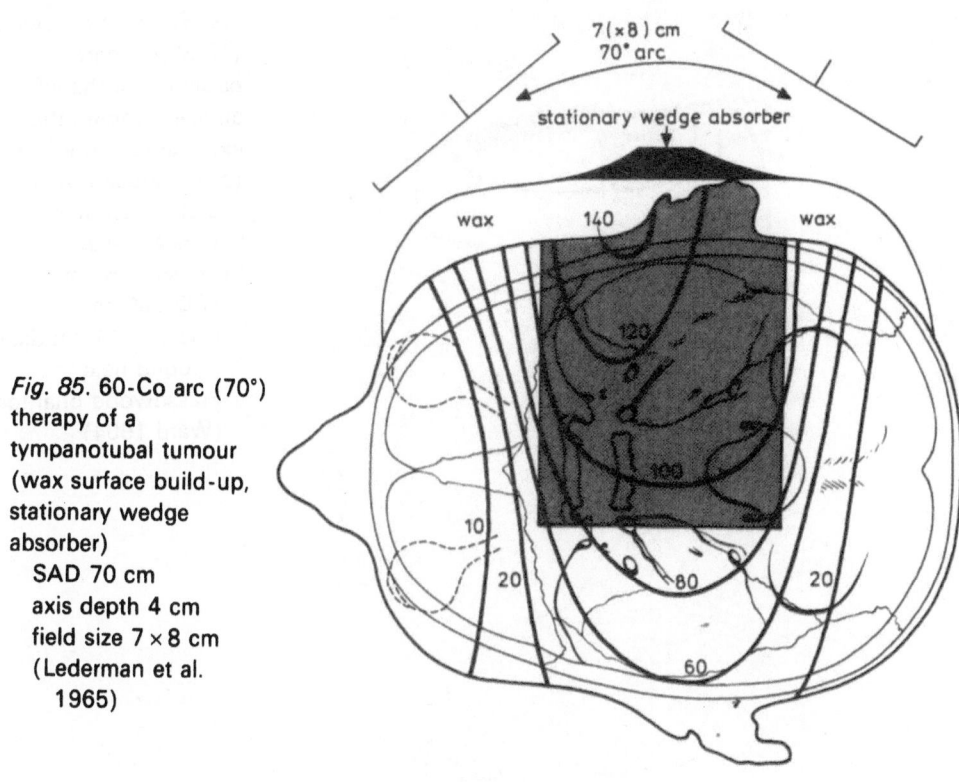

Fig. 85. 60-Co arc (70°)
therapy of a
tympanotubal tumour
(wax surface build-up,
stationary wedge
absorber)
 SAD 70 cm
 axis depth 4 cm
 field size 7 × 8 cm
 (Lederman et al.
  1965)

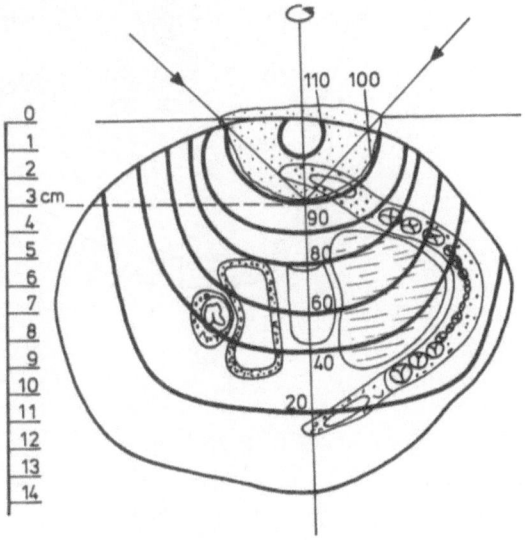

Fig. 86. 60-Co convergent beam
therapy (conical rotation)
of a tumour of the left ear
 SAD 70 cm
 axis depth 3 cm
 field size 6 × 6 cm on the surface
 angle of incidence 45°
 Pressdwood phantom
 (Castro and Whitcomb 1963)

Auditory canal and middle ear | 55

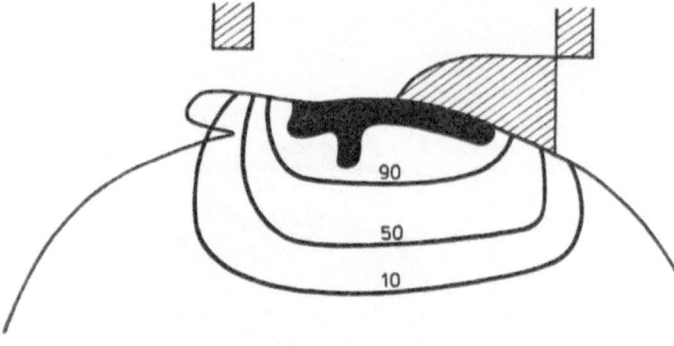

Fig. 87. Electron beam (15 MeV) therapy of basaloma of the left auricle invading the external auditory canal (dose reduced by the use of a wax block over the cheek —max. thickness 2.5 cm)
    FSD 100 cm
    field size 11 cm diam round field
    Pressdwood phantom
    (Ward 1964)

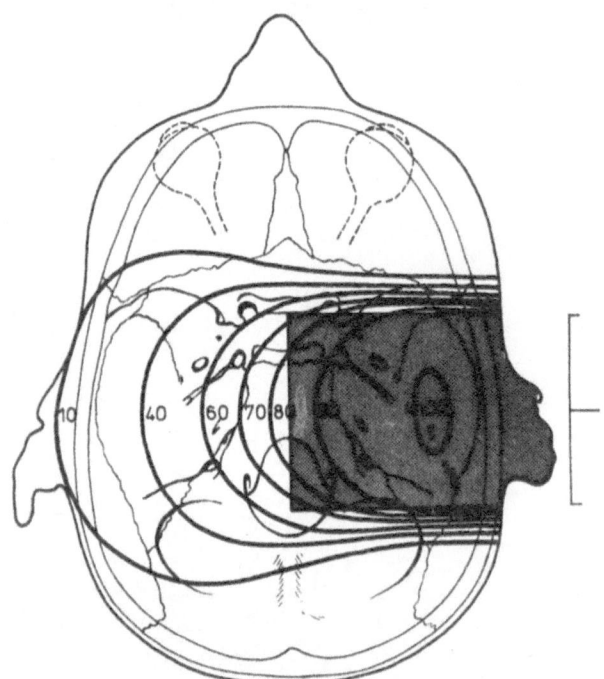

Fig. 88. Electron beam (30 MeV) therapy of a petromastoid tumour through a single stationary field
    FAD 100 cm
    field size 6 × 7 cm
    (Lederman et al. 1965)

Parotid

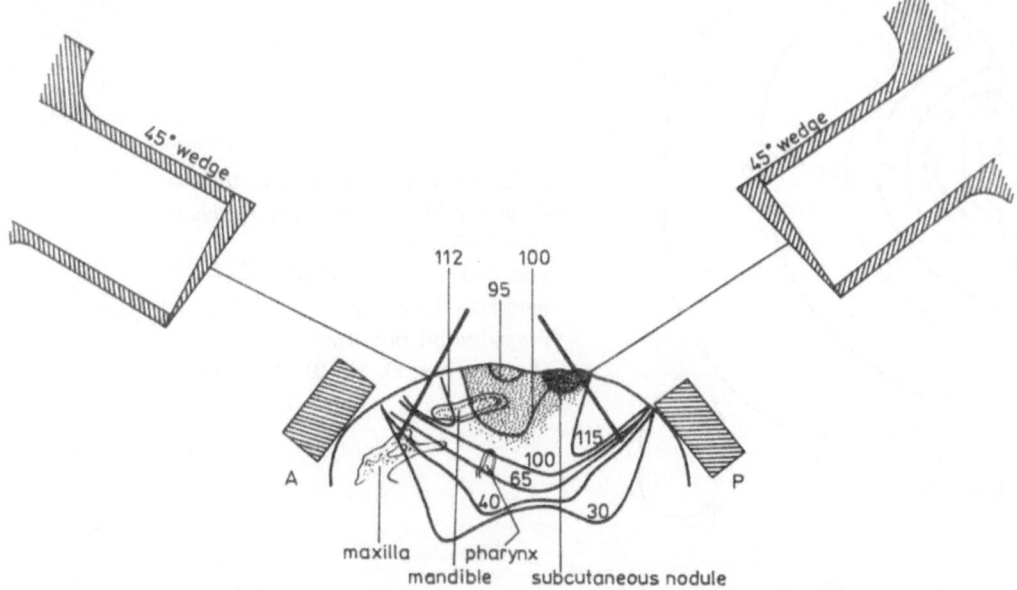

Fig. 89. 60-Co teletherapy of the parotid through two 45° wedge fields with shielding blocks
SSD 60 cm
field size 8 × 14 cm each
Water phantom
(Fletcher 1956*a*)

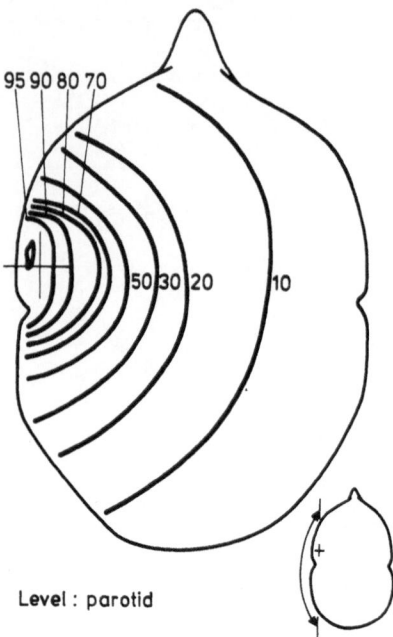

Level : parotid

Fig. 90. Arc (180°) therapy of the parotid with 2 MV high-energy X-rays
    FAD 100 cm
    axis depth 1 cm at 270°
    field size 5 × 8 cm
    Pressdwood phantom
    (Friedman et al. 1959)

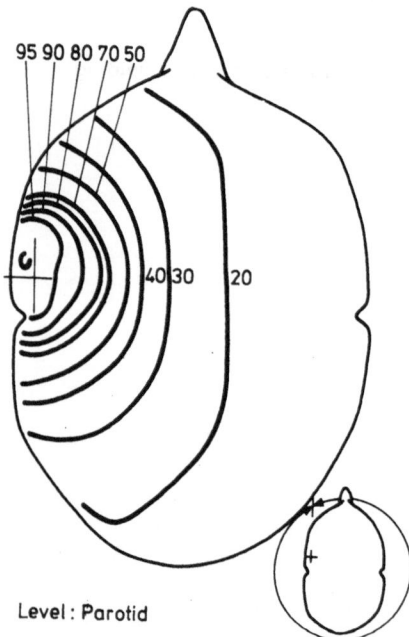

Level : Parotid

Fig. 91. Rotation (360°) therapy of the parotid with 2 MV high-energy X-rays
    FAD 100 cm
    axis depth 1 cm at 270°
    field size 5 × 8 cm
    Pressdwood phantom
    (Friedman et al. 1959)

Thyroid

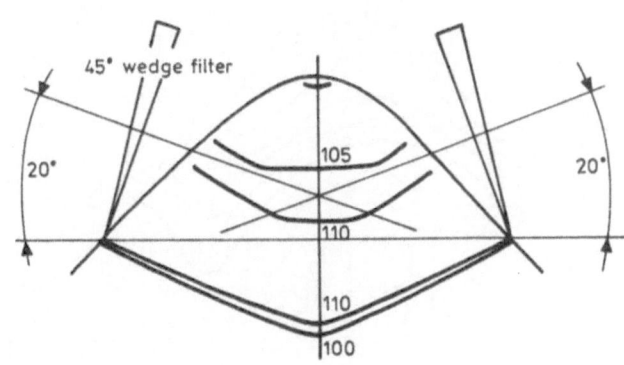

Fig. 92. 60-Co tele-
therapy of the thyroid
through two 45°
wedge fields
  SSD 70 cm
  field size 8 × 10 cm
    each
  Water phantom
  (Fletcher 1973)

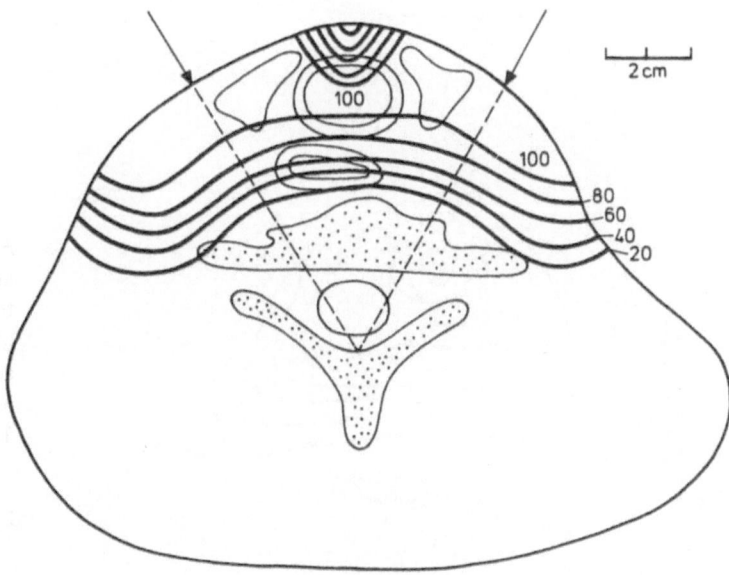

Fig. 93. Irradiation
with 7.5 MeV
electrons of the
thyroid through two
stationary fields
  FSD 100 cm
  field size 6 × 8 cm
    each
  Alderson–Rando
    phantom
  (Németh and
    Kuttig 1973)

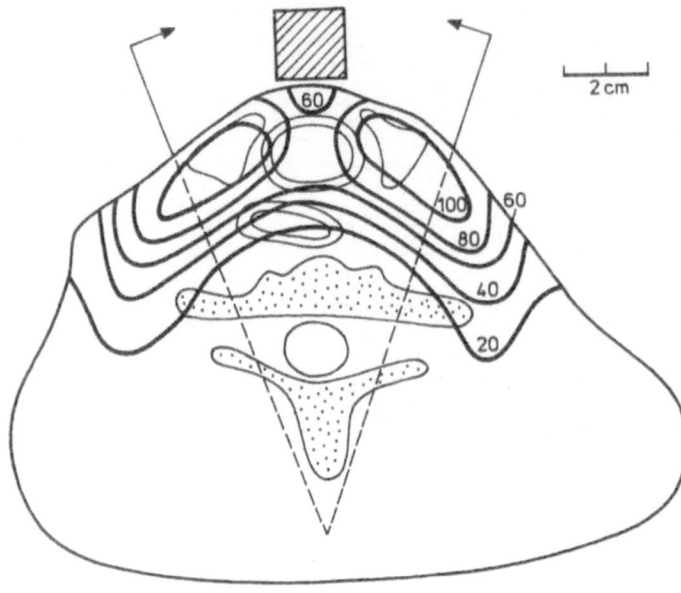

Fig. 94. Telecentric 40°
arc therapy of the
thyroid with 7.5 MeV
electrons (central
shielding with a
lead block of
15 × 15 × 90 mm)
  FAD 120 cm
  axis depth 10 cm
  field size 3 × 9 cm at
    axis
  Alderson–Rando
    phantom
  (Németh and Kuttig
    1973)

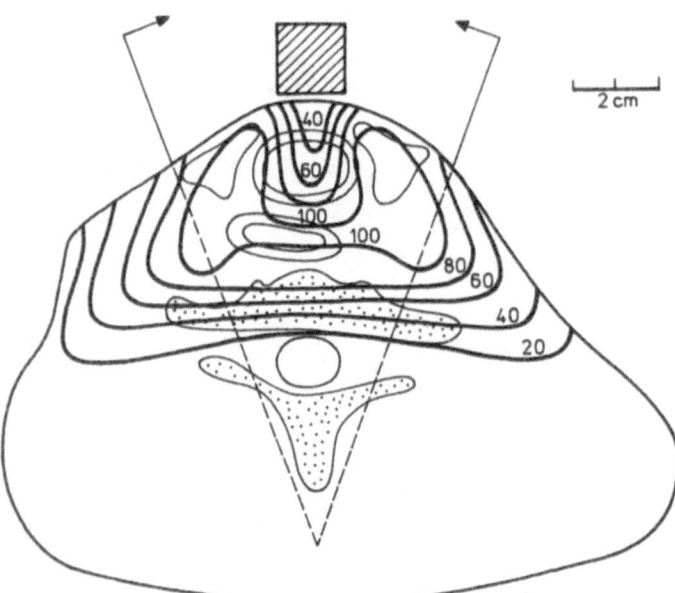

Fig. 95. Telecentric 40°
arc therapy of the
thyroid with 10 MeV
electrons (central
shielding with a
lead block of
15 × 15 × 90 mm)
  FAD 120 cm
  axis depth 10 cm
  field size 3 × 9 cm at
    axis
  Alderson–Rando
    phantom
  (Németh and Kuttig
    1973)

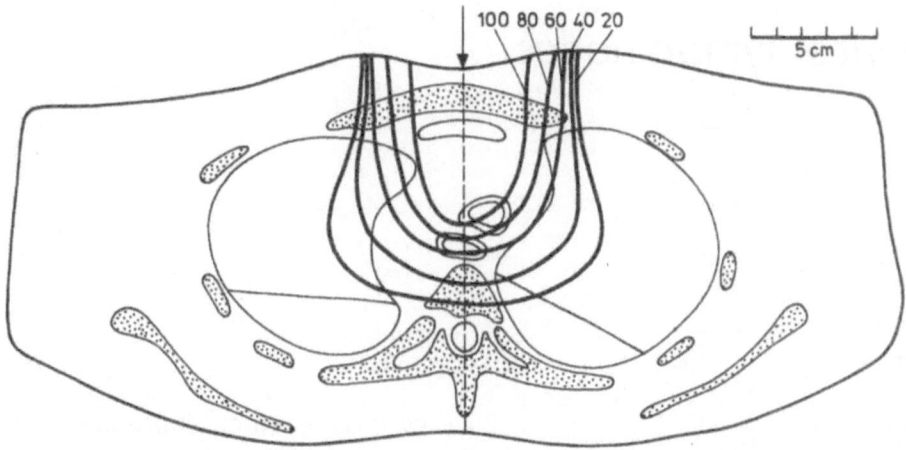

Fig. 96. Electron beam (15 MeV) therapy of the thyroid in the upper retrosternal region through a single stationary field (20° caudal tilt of the central beam)
 FSD 100 cm
 field size 8 × 12 cm
 Alderson–Rando phantom
 (Németh and Kuttig 1973)

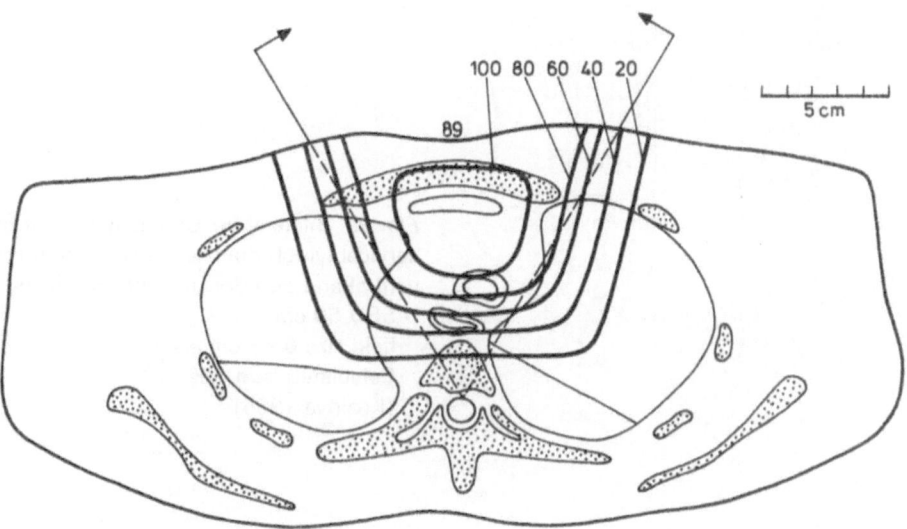

Fig. 97. Telecentric 60° arc therapy of the thyroid with 15 MeV electrons in the upper retrosternal region
 FAD 120 cm
 axis depth 10 cm
 field size 3 × 12 cm at axis
 Alderson–Rando phantom
 (Németh and Kuttig 1973)

Cervical lymph nodes

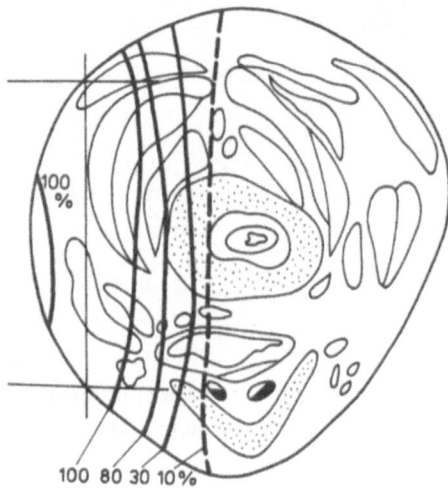

Fig. 98. Unilateral 60-Co teletherapy of the cervical lymph drainage area through a ventral and a dorsal stationary field
SSD 50 cm
field size 6 × 8 cm
Calculated isodoses
(Kozlova 1965)

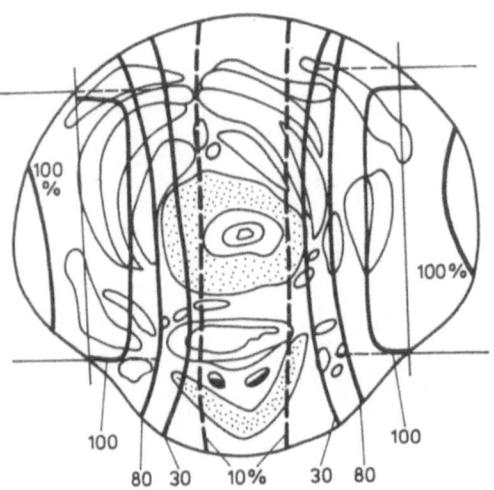

Fig. 99. Bilateral 60-Co teletherapy of the cervical lymph drainage area through two ventral and two dorsal stationary fields
SSD 50 cm
field size 6 × 8 cm each
Calculated isodoses
(Kozlova 1965)

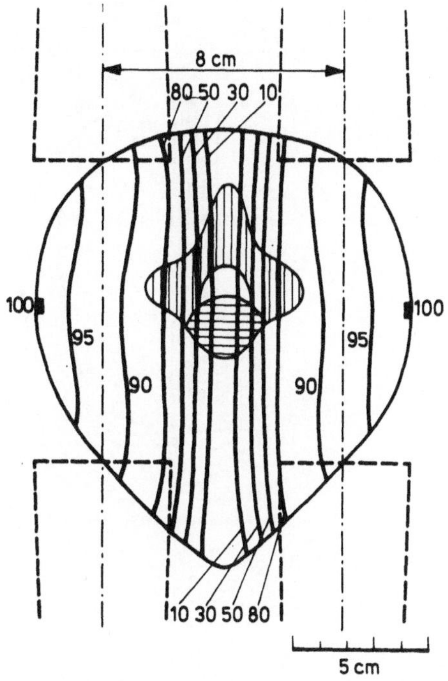

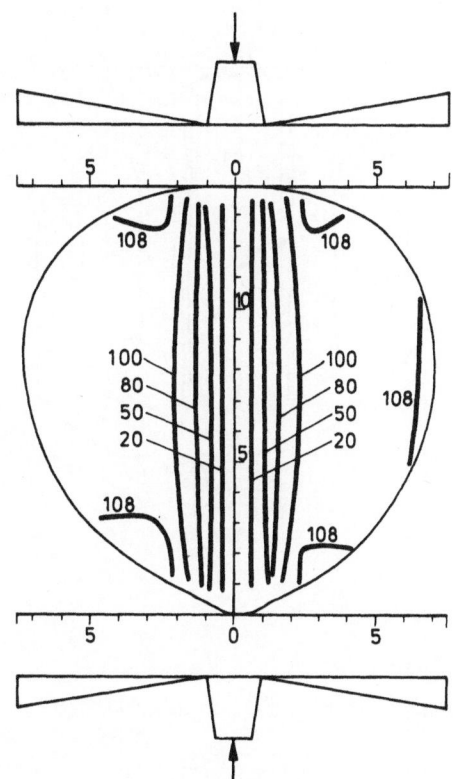

Fig. 100. Bilateral 60-Co teletherapy of the cervical lymph nodes with tangential ventral and dorsal fields
   SSD 60 cm
   field size 5 × 10 cm each
   Homogeneous cervical phantom
   (Scherer and Rassow 1971)

Fig. 101. Bilateral 60-Co teletherapy of the cervical lymph drainage area through a ventral and a dorsal stationary field (with tissue compensating filters). Centre of the field shielded by a lead bridge measuring 55 × 100 mm in height and length, respectively, and being 11 mm wide above and 144 mm wide below
   SSD 60 cm
   field size 15 × 15 cm each
   M-3 phantom
   (Kuhn and Gyüdi 1972)

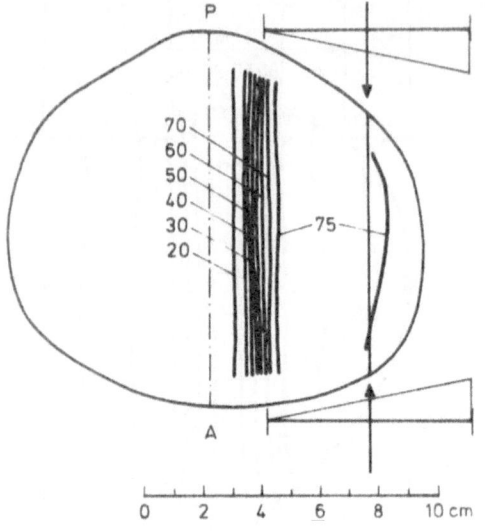

Fig. 102. Unilateral high-energy X-ray (4.8 MV) therapy of the cervical lymph nodes through 35° ventral and dorsal wedge fields
 FSD 100 cm
 field size 7 × 16 cm each
 (Hanks et al. 1969)

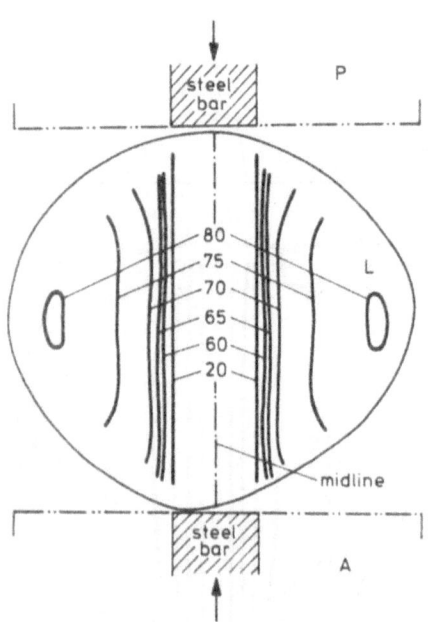

Fig. 103. High-energy X-ray (4.8 MV) irradiation of bilateral cervical lymph nodes through a ventral and a dorsal field. (Larynx shielded with two steel bars 2 cm wide and 5 cm high)
 FSD 100 cm
 field size 10 × 15 cm each
 (Hanks et al. 1969)

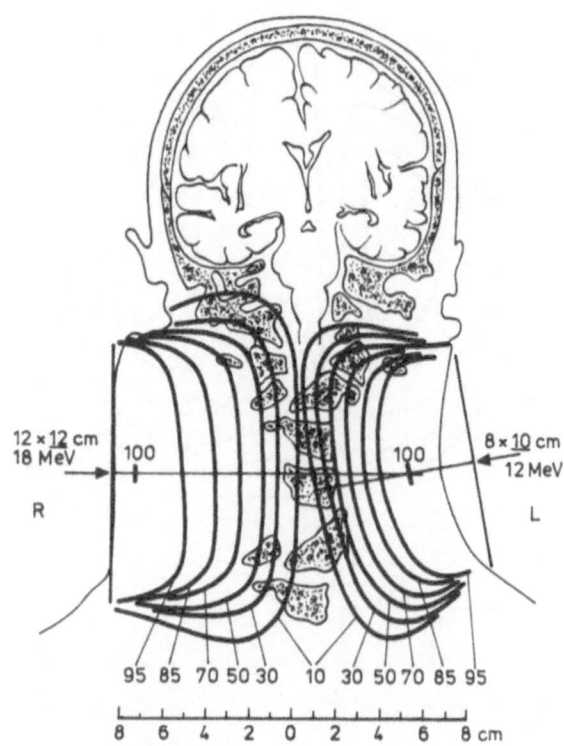

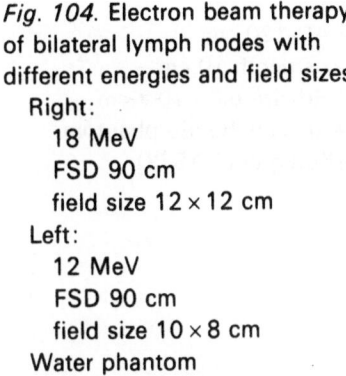

Fig. 104. Electron beam therapy of bilateral lymph nodes with different energies and field sizes
    Right:
       18 MeV
       FSD 90 cm
       field size 12 × 12 cm
    Left:
       12 MeV
       FSD 90 cm
       field size 10 × 8 cm
    Water phantom
    (Perry et al. 1962)

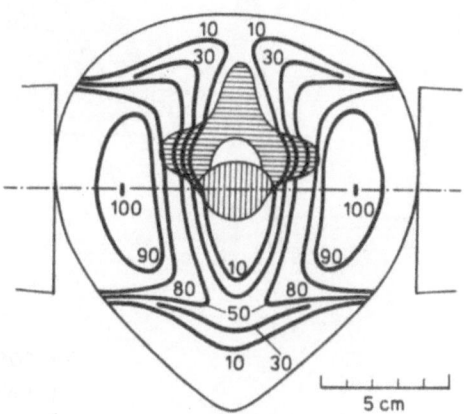

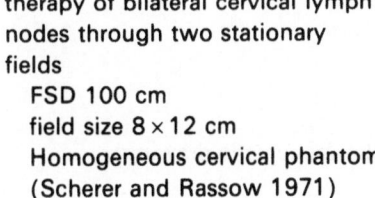

Fig. 105. Electron beam (10 MeV) therapy of bilateral cervical lymph nodes through two stationary fields
    FSD 100 cm
    field size 8 × 12 cm
    Homogeneous cervical phantom
    (Scherer and Rassow 1971)

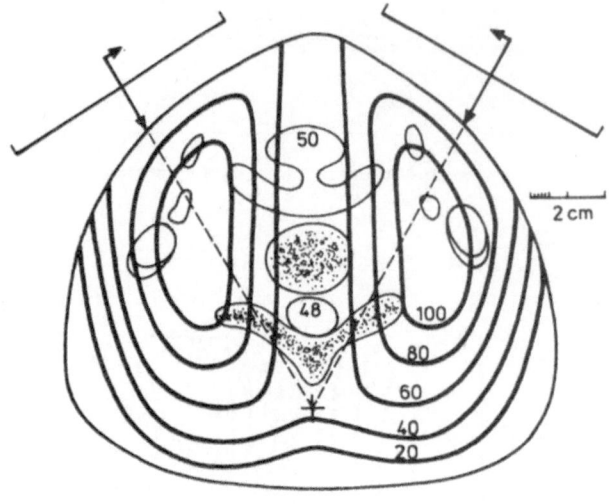

Fig. 106a. 60° arc therapy of bilateral cervical lymph drainage areas with 20 MeV electrons using a shutter tube (see Fig. 106*b*)
    FAD 120 cm
    axis depth 10 cm
    field size 6.6 × 10.7 cm
    Alderson–Rando phantom
    (Kuttig et al. 1973)

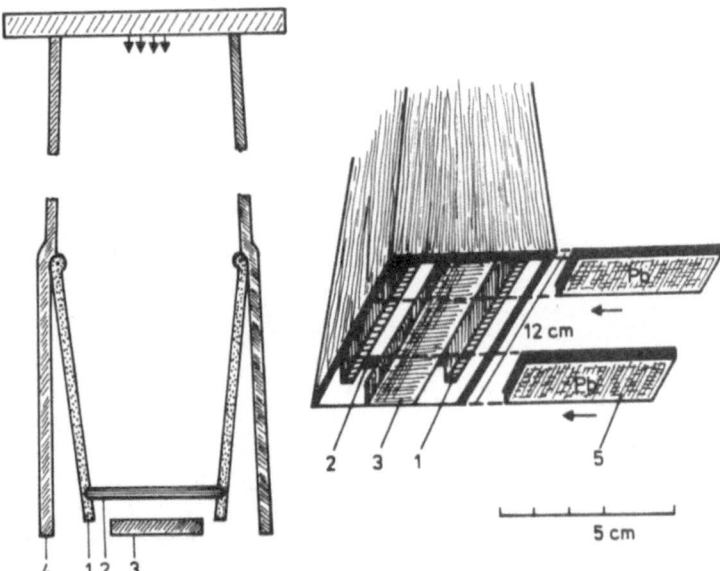

Fig. 106b. Shutter tube (schematic drawing)
   1. metal plates
   2. metal bow for synchronous guiding of the plates
   3. lead block
   4. wall of the tube
   5. lead plates for limiting the field length
   (Kuttig et al. 1973)

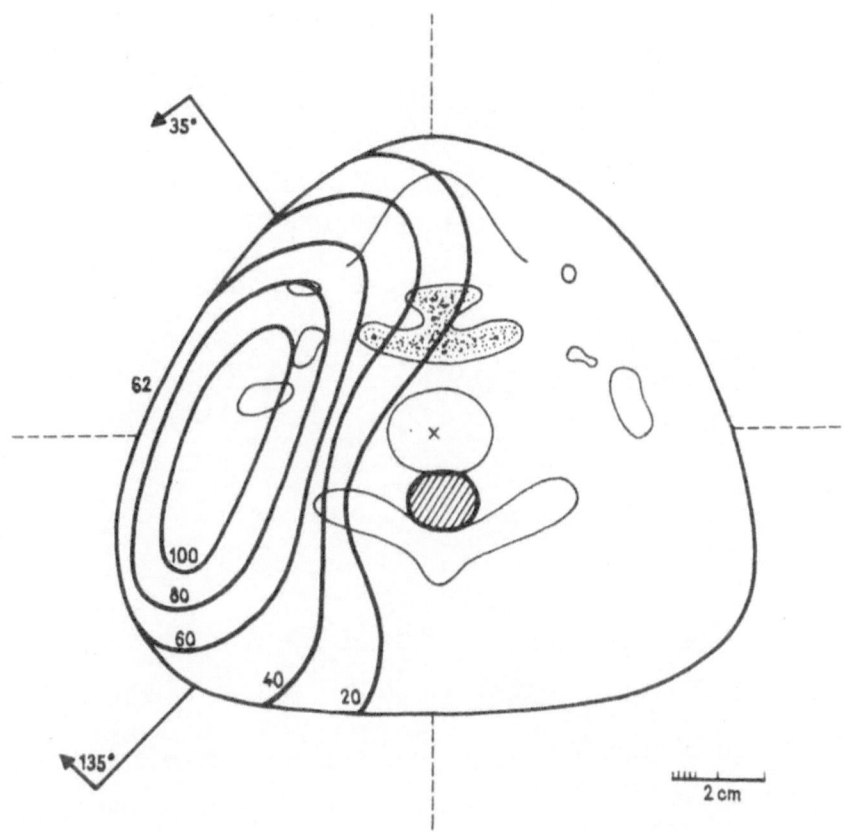

Fig. 107. Telecentric 100° arc therapy of unilateral lymph nodes with 10 MeV electrons
 FAD 120
 axis depth 6 cm
 field size 3 × 8 cm
 Alderson–Rando phantom
 (Poser et al. 1973*a*)

Thorax

Lung

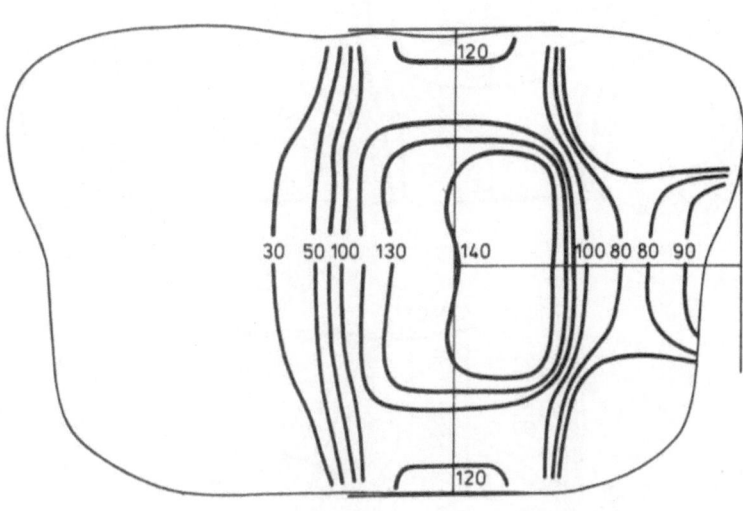

Fig. 108. 60-Co
teletherapy of left
lobe bronchial
tumour through three
stationary fields
   SSD 50 cm
   field size 10 × 15 cm
     each
   (Baštecký and
     Chvojka 1964)

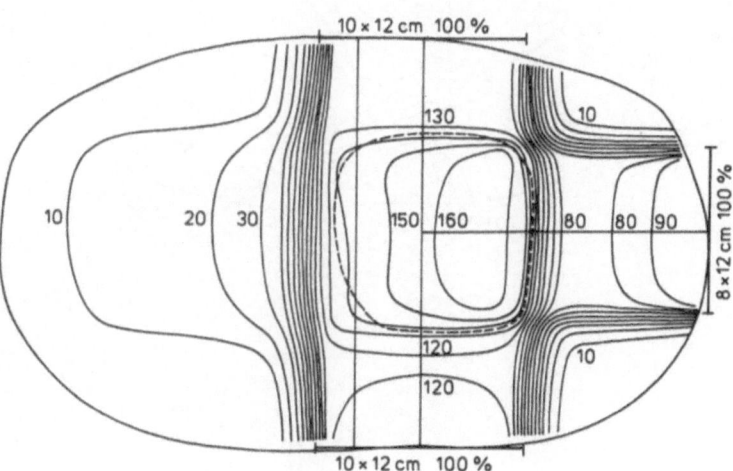

Fig. 109. 60-Co
teletherapy of left
lobe bronchial
tumour through three
stationary fields
   SSD 80 cm
   field size
     10 × 12 cm
     ventral and
     dorsal
     8 × 10 cm lateral
   Calculated isodoses
   (Starzynska 1968)

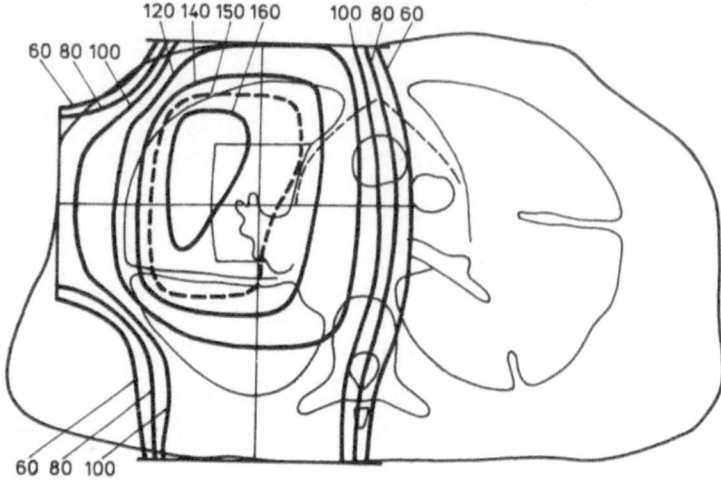

Fig. 110. 60-Co teletherapy of left lobe bronchial tumour through three stationary fields
  SSD 50 cm
  field size 8 × 10 cm each
  Calculated isodoses
  (Gyenes 1972)

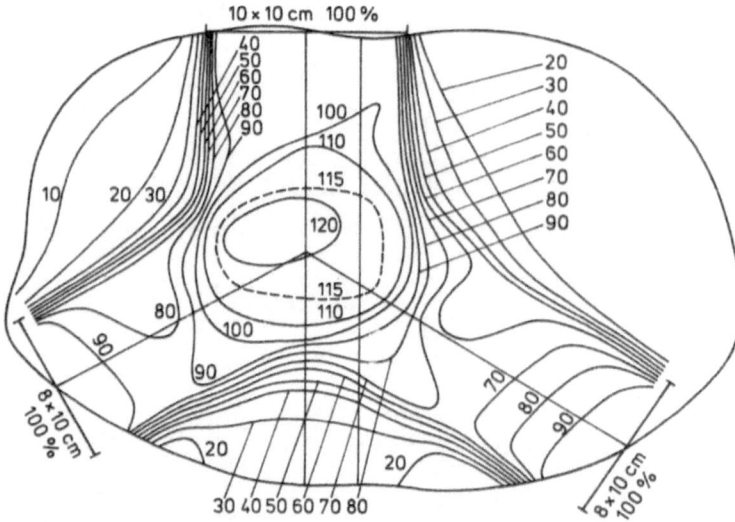

Fig. 111. 60-Co teletherapy of left lobe bronchial tumour through three stationary fields
  SSD 80 cm
  field size
    10 × 10 cm ventral
    8 × 10 cm each dorsolateral
  Calculated isodoses
  (Starzynska 1968)

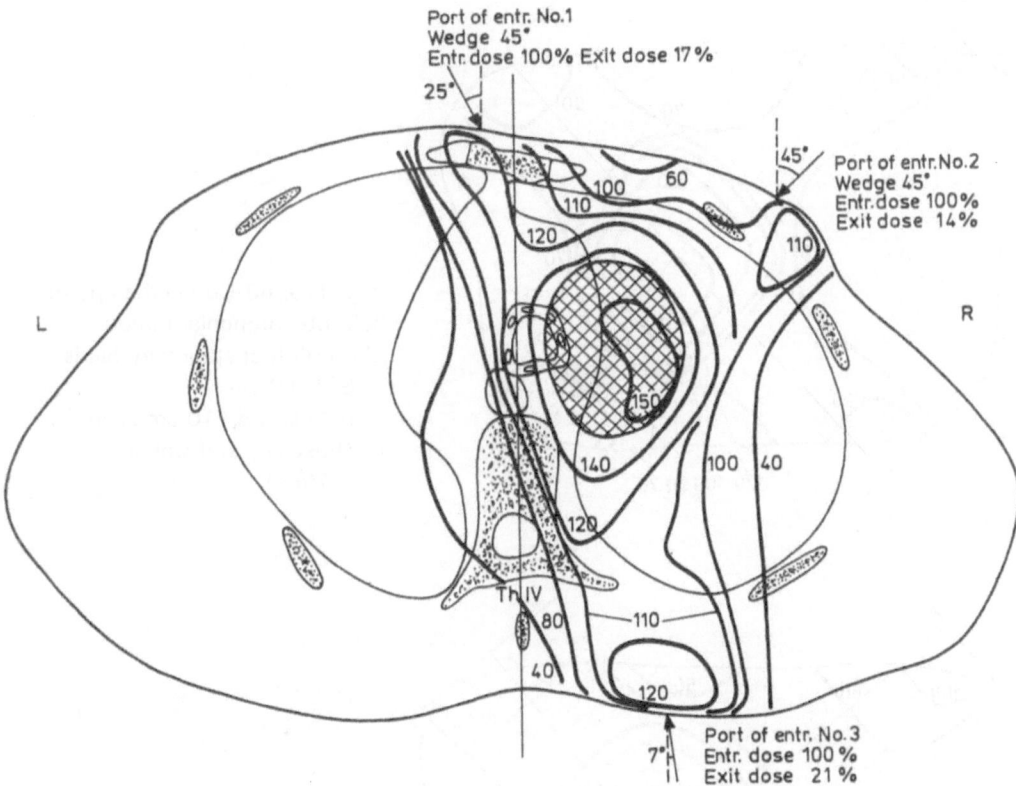

Fig. 112. 60-Co teletherapy of right lobe bronchial tumour through three stationary fields
(two 45° wedge fields)
  SSD 70 cm
  field size 7 × 11 cm each
  (Lindgren and Nordberg 1965)

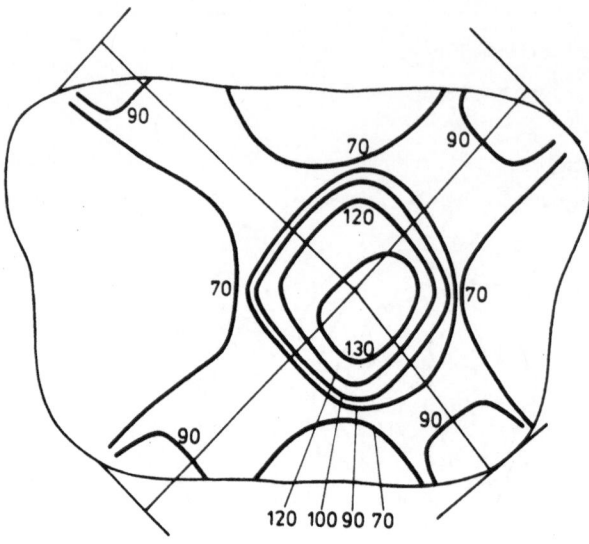

Fig. 113. 60-Co teletherapy of
left lobe bronchial tumour
through four stationary fields
　SSD 50 cm
　field size 8 × 10 cm each
　(Baštecký and Chvojka
　　1964)

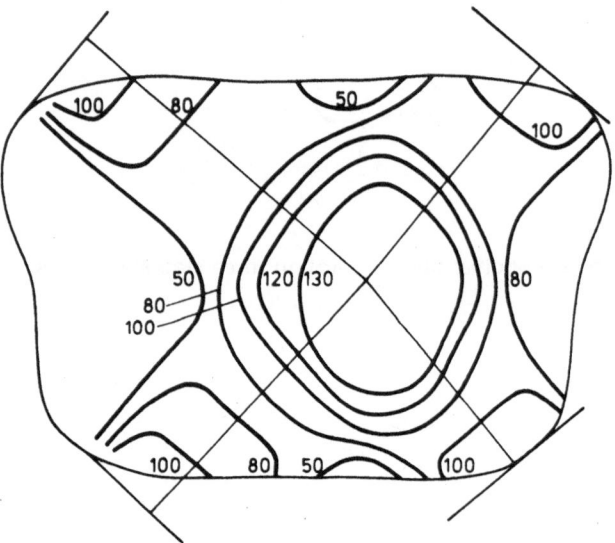

Fig. 114. 60-Co teletherapy of
a left lobe bronchial tumour
through four stationary fields
　SSD 50 cm
　field size 10 × 15 cm each
　(Baštecký and Chvojka
　　1964)

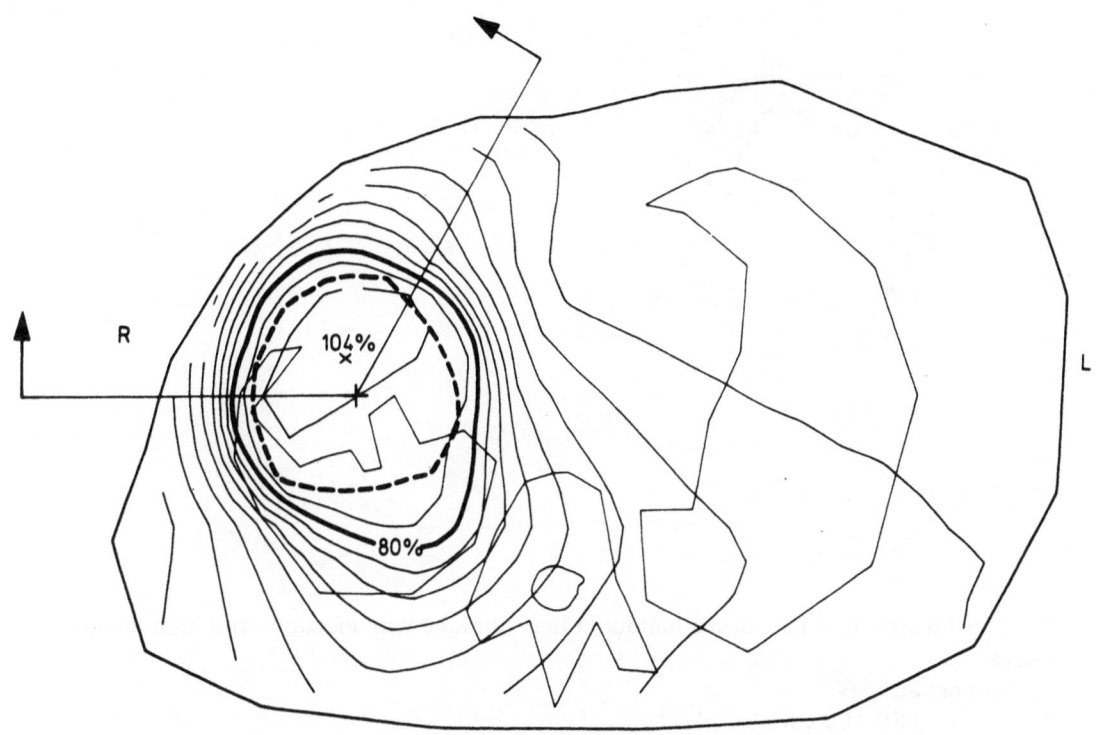

Fig. 115. Arc therapy (120° — 30°/90°) of a right lobe bronchial tumour with 42 MV high-energy X-rays
    FAD 120 cm
    axis depth 10 cm
    field size 8 × 10 cm
    Computer calculated isodoses

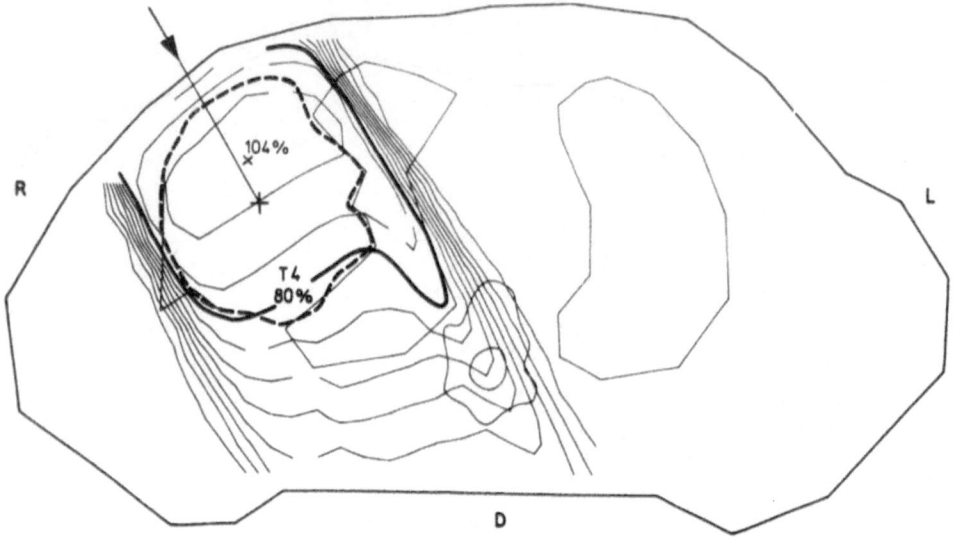

Fig. 116. Irradiation of Pancoast's tumour in the right lobe with electrons and high-energy X-rays
  Electrons: 35 MeV
            FSD 100 cm
            field size 10 × 12 cm
  High-energy X-rays: 42 MV
                FSD 100 cm
                field size 10 × 12 cm
  Computer calculated isodoses

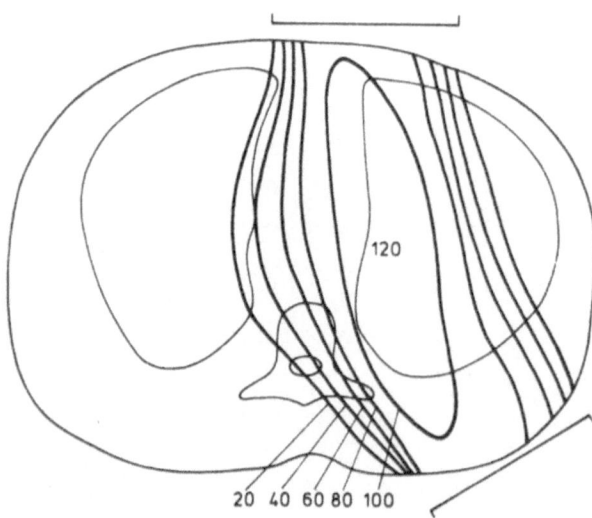

Fig. 117. Electron beam (43 MeV) therapy of right lobe bronchial tumour through two stationary fields (30° tilt of dorsal field)
  FSD 100 cm
  field size 10 × 14 cm each
  Alderson–Rando phantom
  (Heuss and Hoeffken 1969)

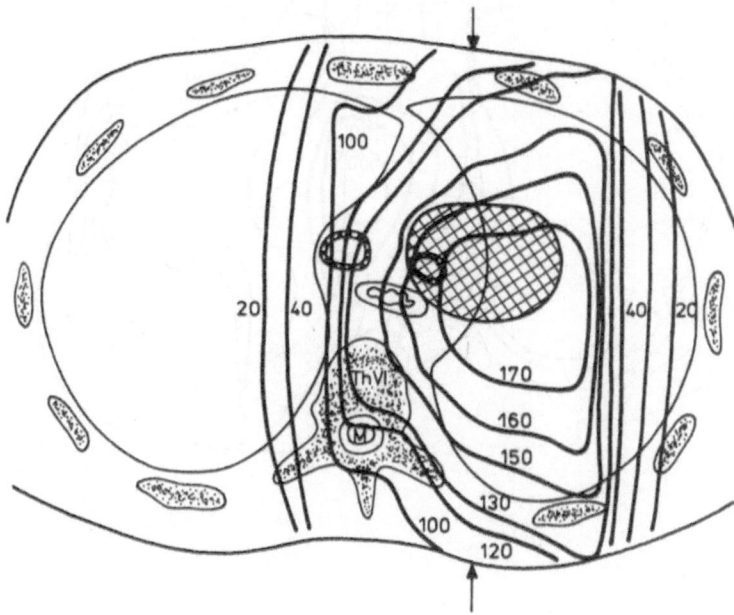

Fig. 118. Electron
beam (35 MeV)
therapy of a left lobe
bronchial tumour
through two
opposing fields
   FSD 110 cm
   field size 14 × 14 cm
    each (a–p diam.
    18.3 cm)
  Anatomical thorax
    phantom
  (Landberg et al.
    1972)

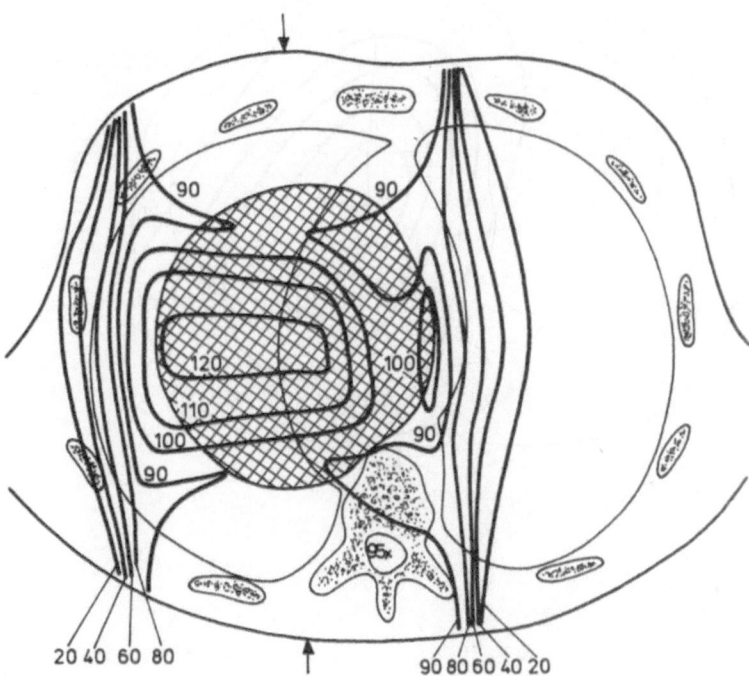

Fig. 119. Electron
beam (35 MeV)
therapy of a left lobe
bronchial tumour
through two
opposing fields
   FSD 110 cm
   field size 14 × 14 cm
    each (a–p diam.
    23.8 cm)
  Anatomical thorax
    phantom
  (Landberg et al.
    1972)

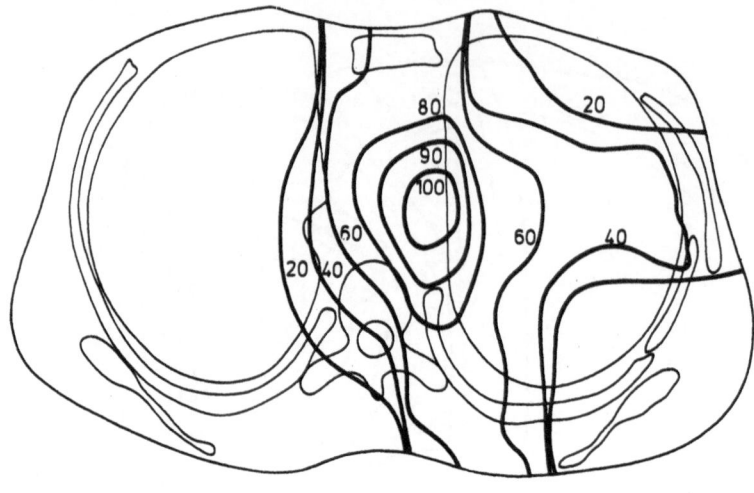

Fig. 120. Electron beam (30 MeV) therapy of left hilar tumour through three stationary fields (ventral field in the midline, lateral field perpendicular to the ventral field, dorsal field shifted 4 cm to the left from the midline)

FSD 100 cm
field size 6 × 8 cm each
Alderson–Rando phantom
(Kuttig et al. 1971)

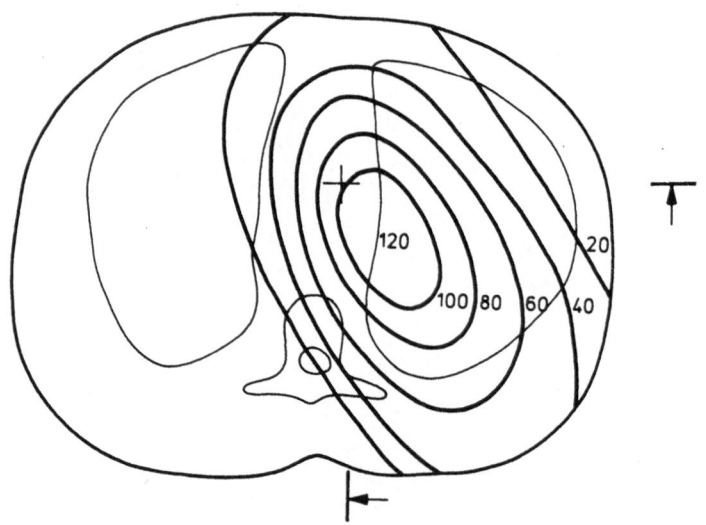

Fig. 121. 43 MeV electron beam 90° arc therapy of a left lobe bronchial tumour
FAD 120 cm
axis depth 14 cm
field size 6 × 12 cm
Alderson–Rando phantom
(Heuss and Hoeffken 1972)

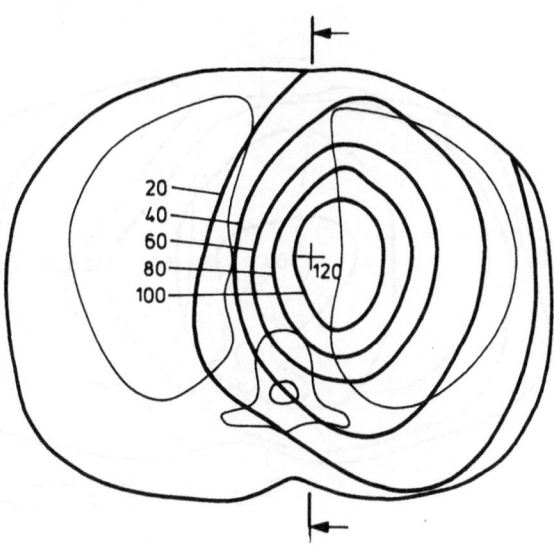

Fig. 122. 35 MeV electron beam arc
(180°) therapy of a left lobe
bronchial tumour
    FAD 120 cm
    axis depth 10 cm from ventral
      surface
    field size 7 × 14 cm
    Alderson–Rando phantom
    (Heuss and Hoeffken 1972)

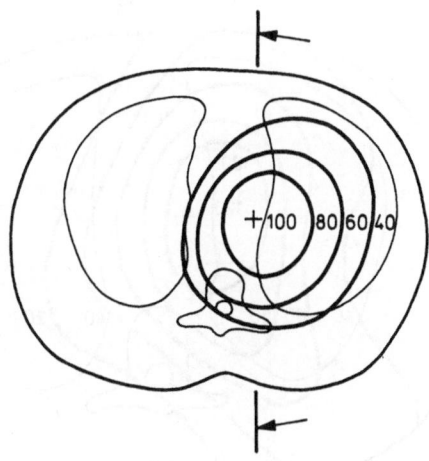

Fig. 123. 43 MeV electron beam arc
(180°) therapy of a left lobe
bronchial tumour
    FAD 120 cm
    axis depth 11.2 cm from ventral
      surface
      3 cm from lateral surface
    field size 7 × 16 cm
    Alderson–Rando phantom
    (Heuss 1971)

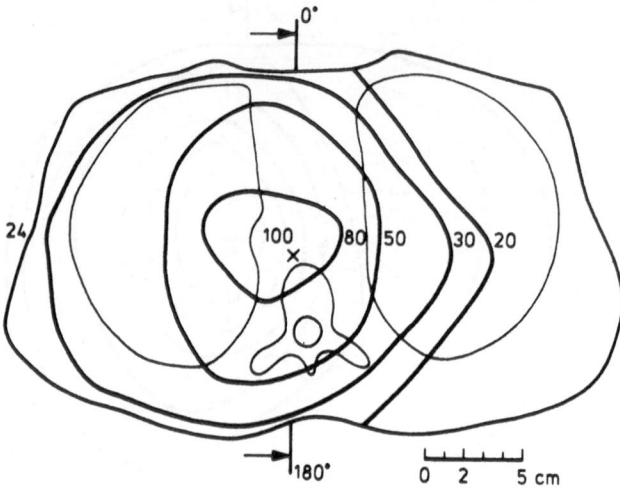

Fig. 124. Arc (180°) therapy of a right lobe bronchial tumour with 42 MeV electrons
    FAD 120 cm
    axis depth 14 cm in the midline
    field size 8 × 12 cm at axis
    Alderson–Rando phantom
    (Fehrentz et al. 1969)

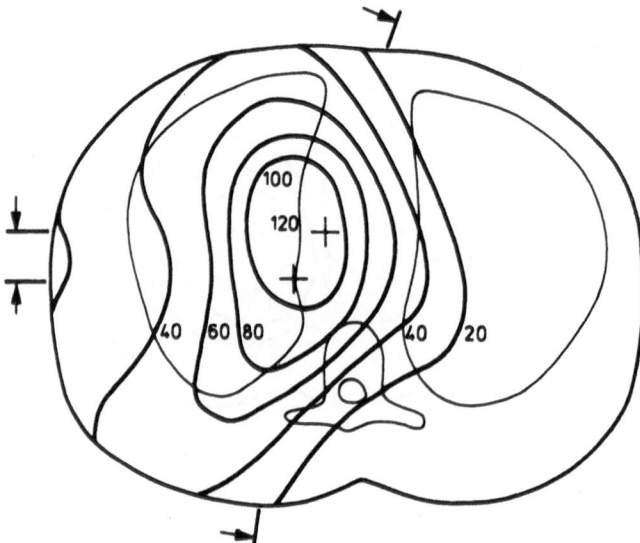

Fig. 125. Two-centre, two-arc irradiation of left lobe bronchial tumour with 35 MeV electrons
    FAD 120 cm
    Ventral arc: 110°
       axis depth 10 cm
       field size 5 × 12 cm
    Dorsal arc: 80°
       axis depth 11 cm
       field size 5 × 12 cm
    Alderson–Rando phantom
    (Heuss and Hoeffken 1969)

Mediastinum

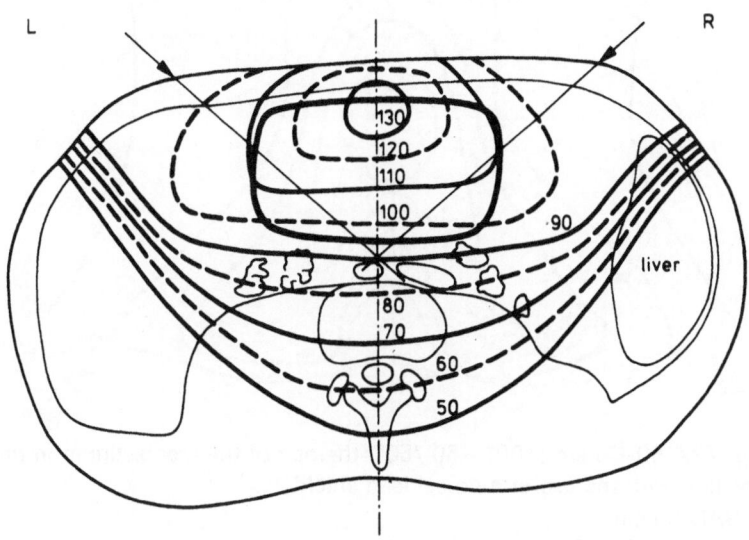

Fig. 126. 60-Co teletherapy of the mediastinum through two ventral stationary fields
  SSD 60 cm
  field size 10 × 15 cm
  Calculated isodoses
  (Gyenes, personal communication)

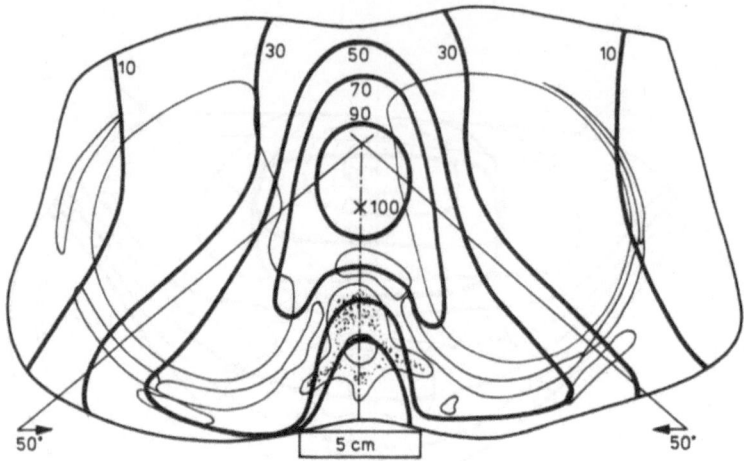

Fig. 127. 60-Co arc (100°—50°/50°) therapy of the mediastinum in prone
position with the use of a dorsal lead shield
    SAD 80 cm
    field size 6 × 18 cm
    Alderson–Rando phantom
    (Kärcher 1976)

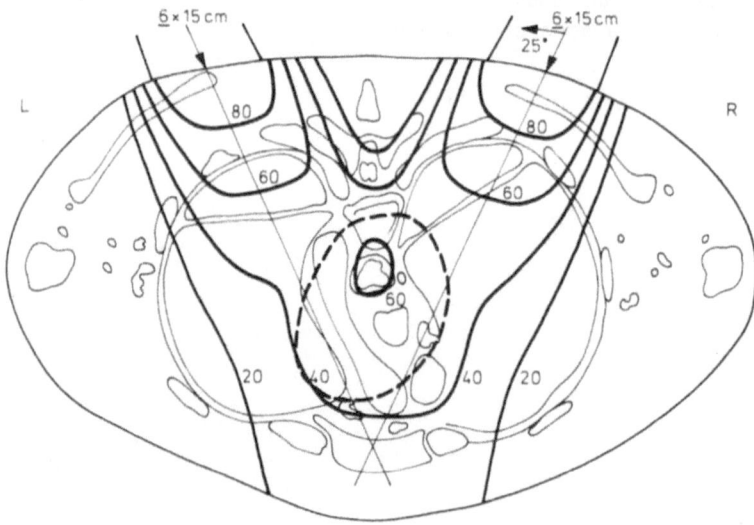

Fig. 128. 60-Co teletherapy of the mediastinum through two dorsal stationary fields
    SSD 60 cm
    field size 6 × 15 cm each
    Calculated isodoses
    (Gyenes, personal communication)

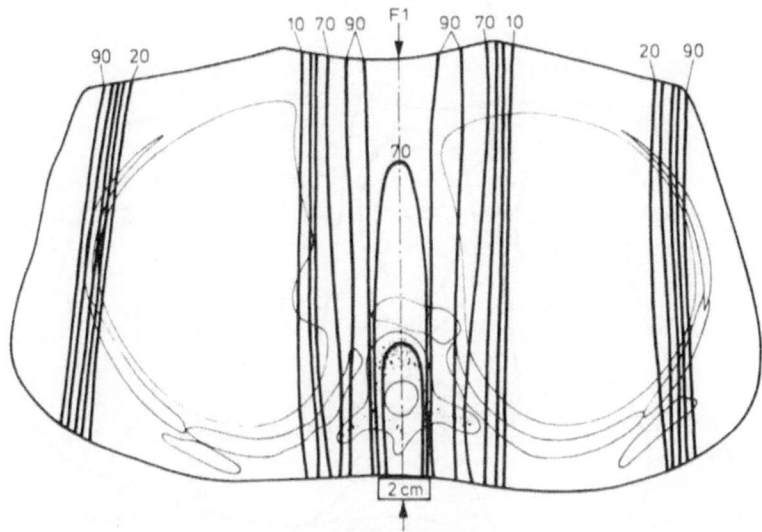

Fig. 129. 60-Co teletherapy of the mediastinum by use of the satellite method. Combination of two stationary fields with 180° arc therapy. (Application of additional lead shield to protect the spinal cord)

    SSD 130 cm each

    Alderson–Rando phantom

    (Kärcher 1976)

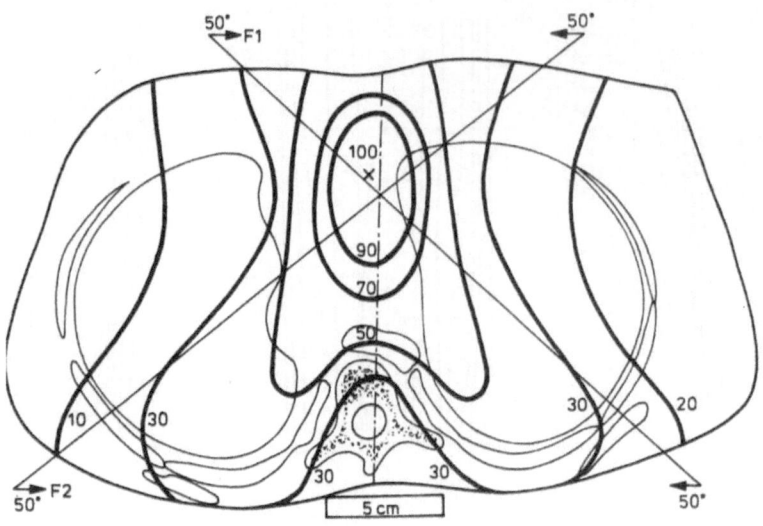

Fig. 130. One-centre, two-arc 60-Co therapy of the mediastinum with
two 100° (50°/50°) arcs
  SAD 80 cm
  field size 6 × 18 cm
  Alderson–Rando phantom
  (Kärcher 1976)

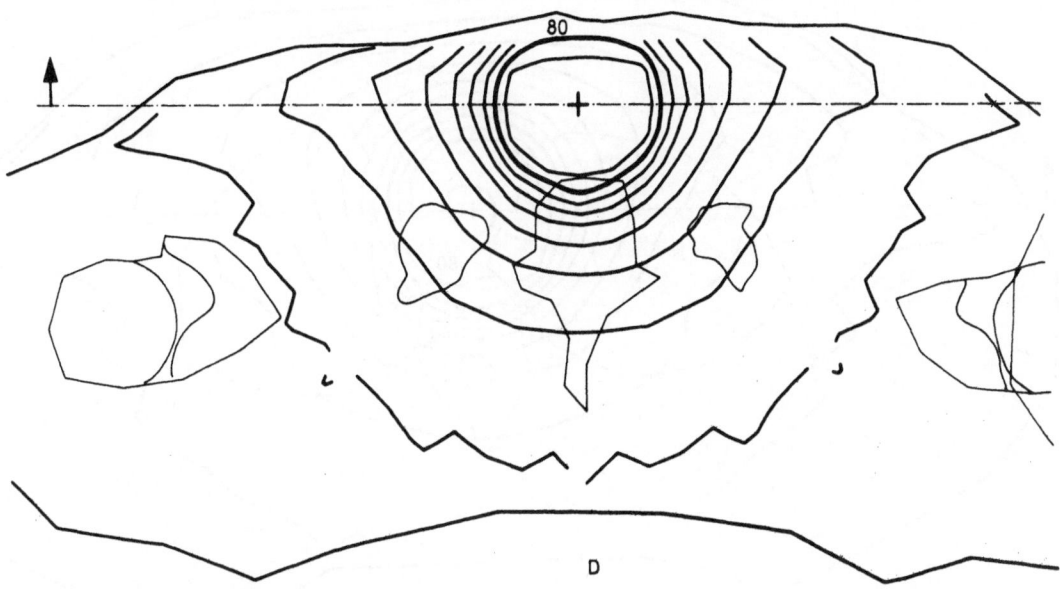

Fig. 131. Arc therapy (180° — 90°/90°) of the upper mediastinum with high-energy
X-rays (42 MV)
    FAD 120 cm
    axis depth 6 cm
    field size 6 × 10 cm
    Computer calculated isodoses

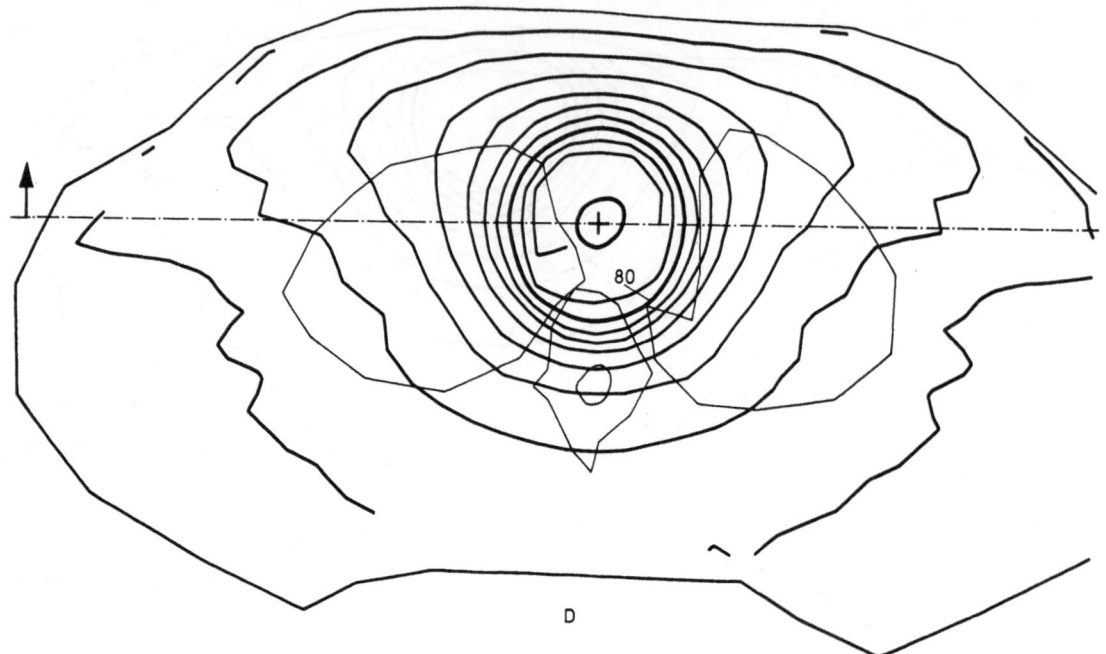

Fig. 132. Arc therapy (180° — 90°/90°) of the mediastinum with high-energy X-rays
(42 MV)
   FAD 120 cm
   axis depth 10 cm
   field size 6 × 10 cm
   Computer calculated isodoses

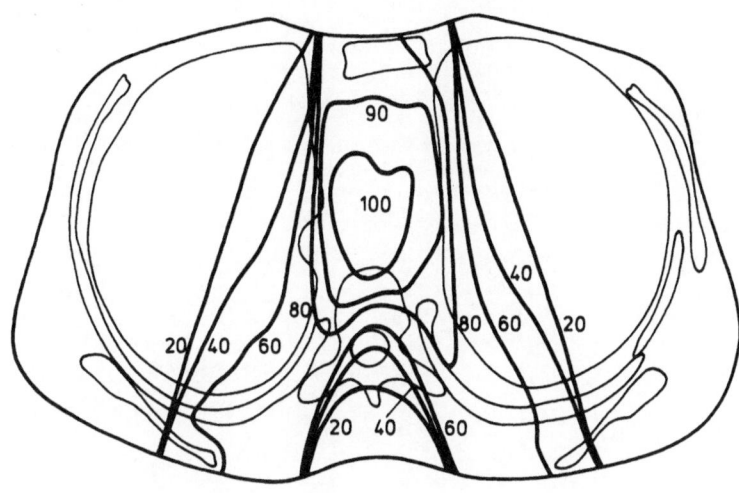

Fig. 133. Electron beam (30 MeV) therapy of the mediastinum through three stationary fields (ventral field in the midline, two dorsal fields shifted to the left and right by 5 cm each and a 20° tilt of the central beam)
    FSD 100 cm
    field size
      6 × 8 cm each
    Alderson–Rando
      phantom
    (Kuttig et al. 1971)

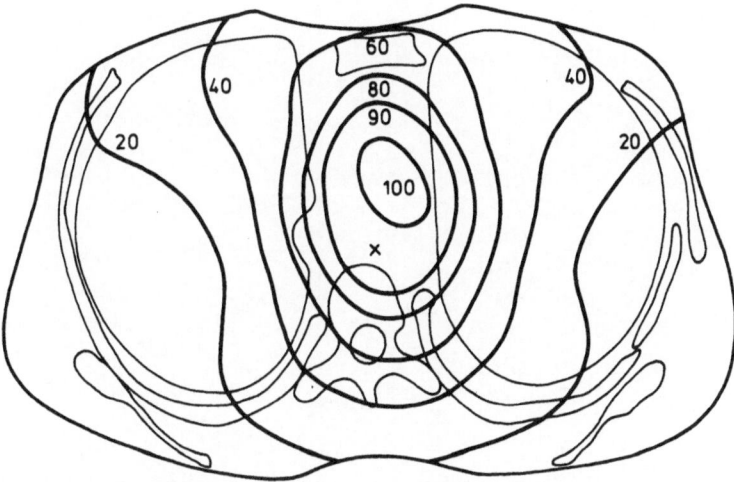

Fig. 134. Arc therapy (180° — 90°/90°) of the mediastinum with 42 MeV electrons
    FAD 120 cm
    axis depth 9 cm
    field size 6 × 8 cm
      at axis
    Alderson–Rando
      phantom
    (Kuttig et al. 1971)

Breast

Breast and chest wall

Fig. 135. 60-Co
teletherapy of the
chest wall with two
flanking tangential
stationary fields with
rice bolus
    SSD 80 cm
    field size 10 × 15 cm
      each (length of
      bolus 26 cm)
    Calculated isodoses
    (Koeck et al. 1964)

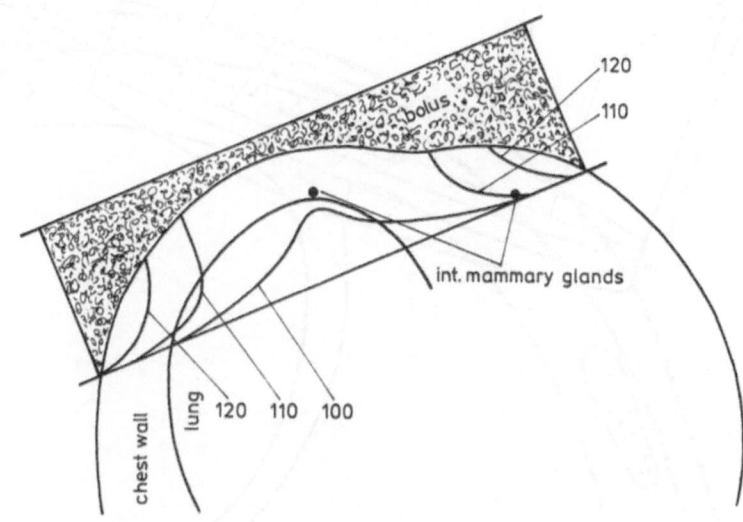

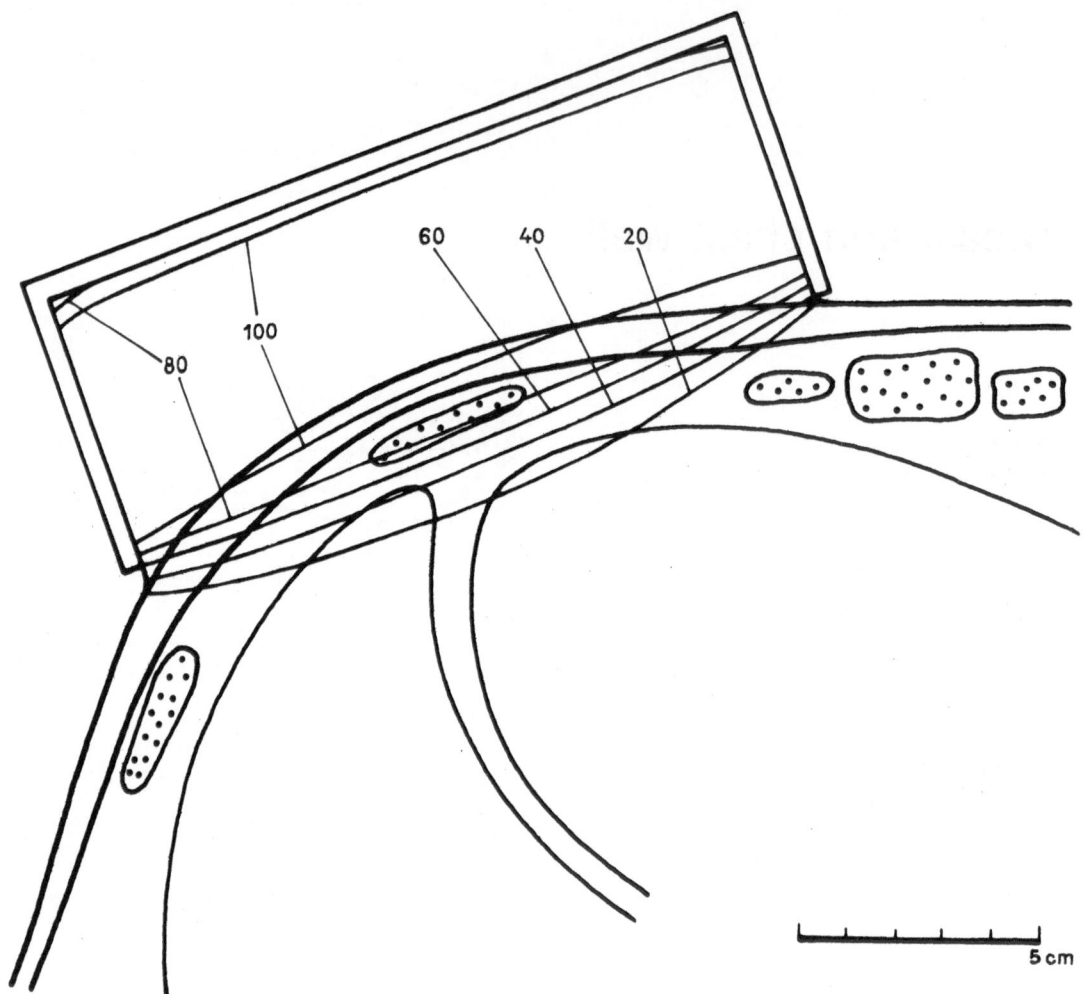

Fig. 136. 60-Co teletherapy of a breast tumour through two opposing stationary fields (the breast is compressed by use of a plastic box having adjustable walls)
    SSD 50 cm
    field size 6 × 15 cm each
    Wax phantom

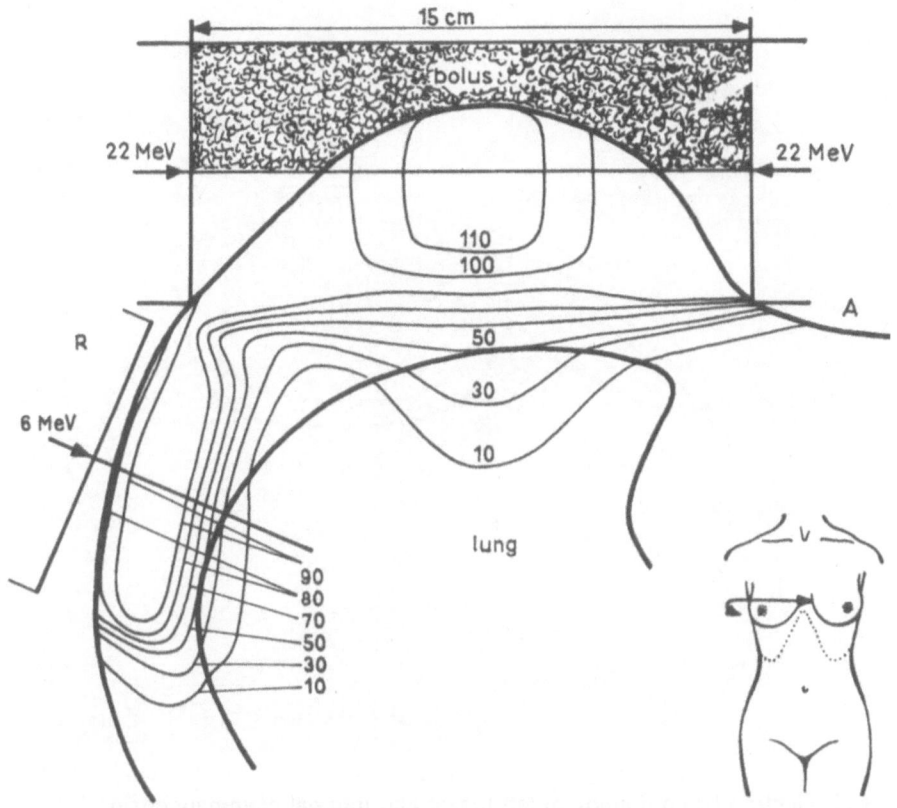

Fig. 137. Electron beam therapy of the right breast and chest wall through three stationary fields

    Breast: 22 MeV

             FSD 90 cm

             field size 7 × 18 cm each (with bolus)

    Chest wall: 6 MeV

              FSD 90 cm

              field size 8 × 20 cm

Inhomogeneous phantom with skeleton

(Laughlin 1967)

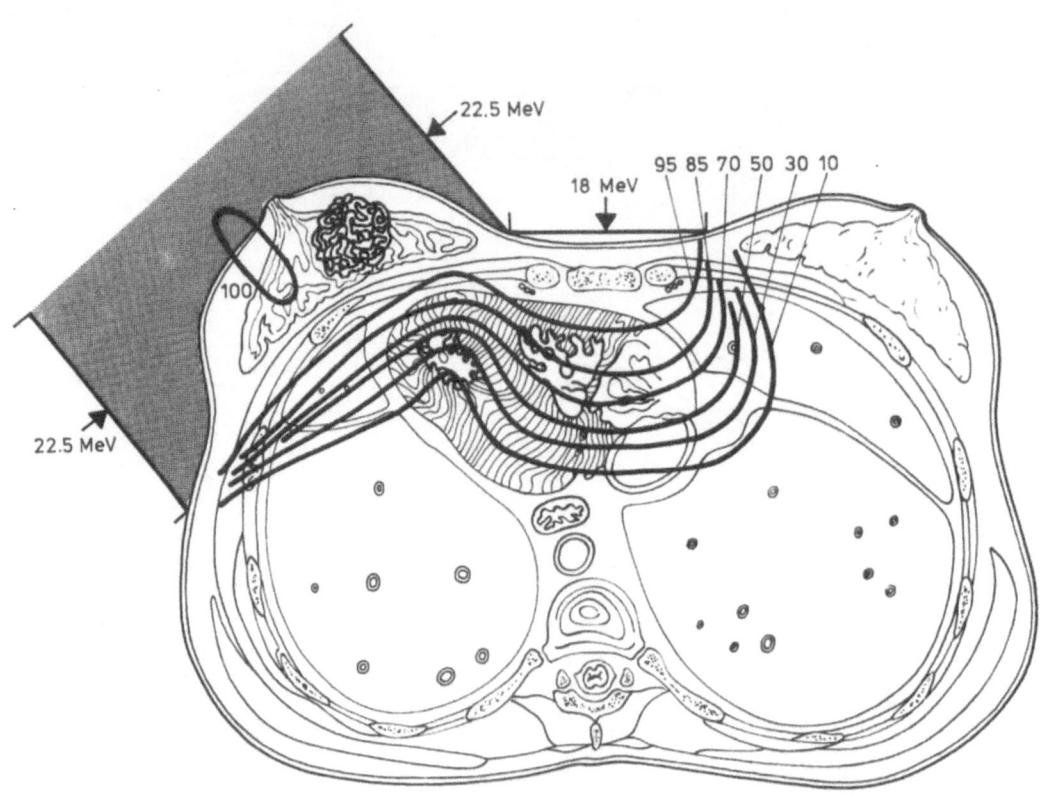

Fig. 138. Electron beam therapy of left breast and internal mammary chain

    Breast: two tangential stationary fields with bolus

        22.5 MeV

        FSD 90 cm

        field size 9×15 cm each

    Internal mammary chain: 18 MeV

                FSD 90 cm

                field size 7×15 cm

(Chu et al. 1960)

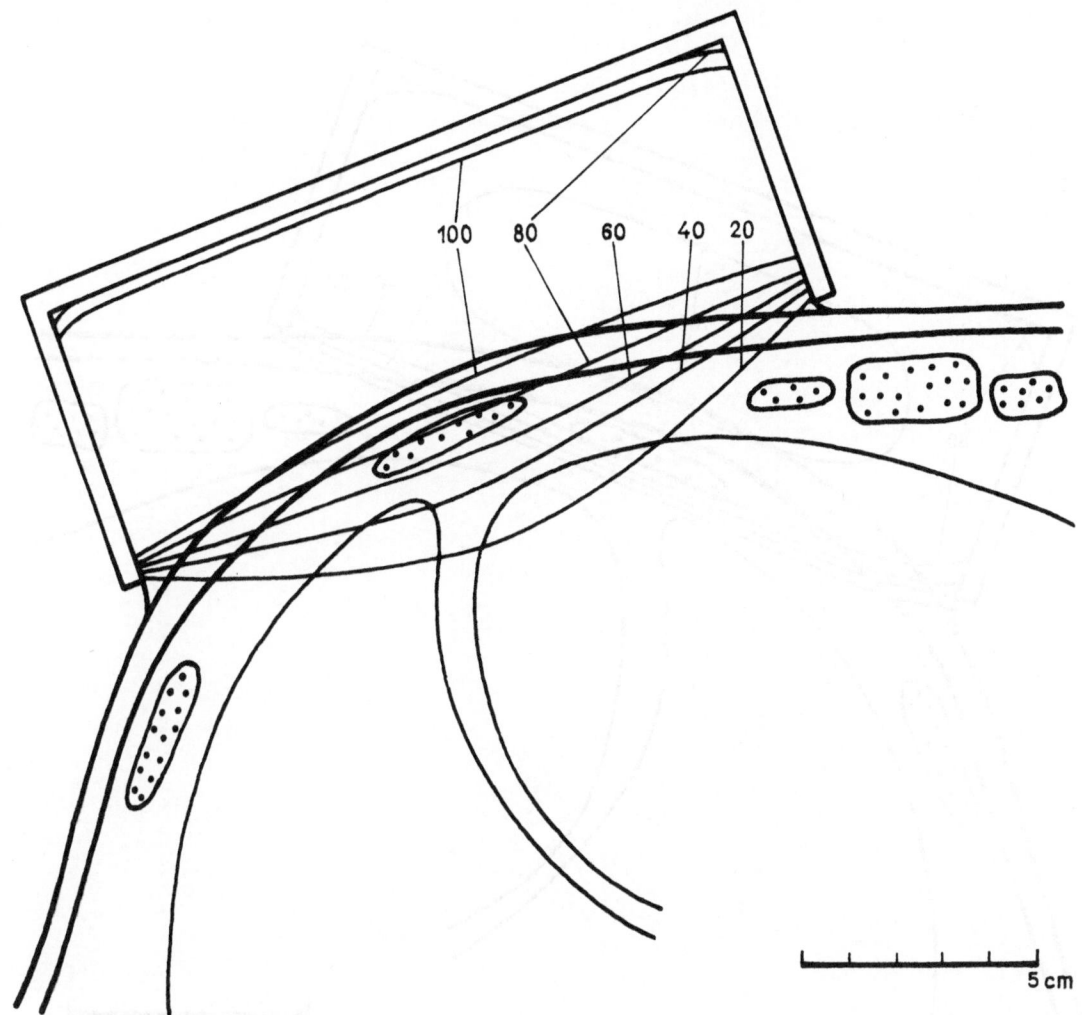

Fig. 139. Electron beam therapy (17 MeV) of a breast tumour through two opposing stationary fields (breast compressed by means of a plastic box with adjustable walls)
  FSD 100 cm
  field size 6 × 15 cm each
  Wax phantom

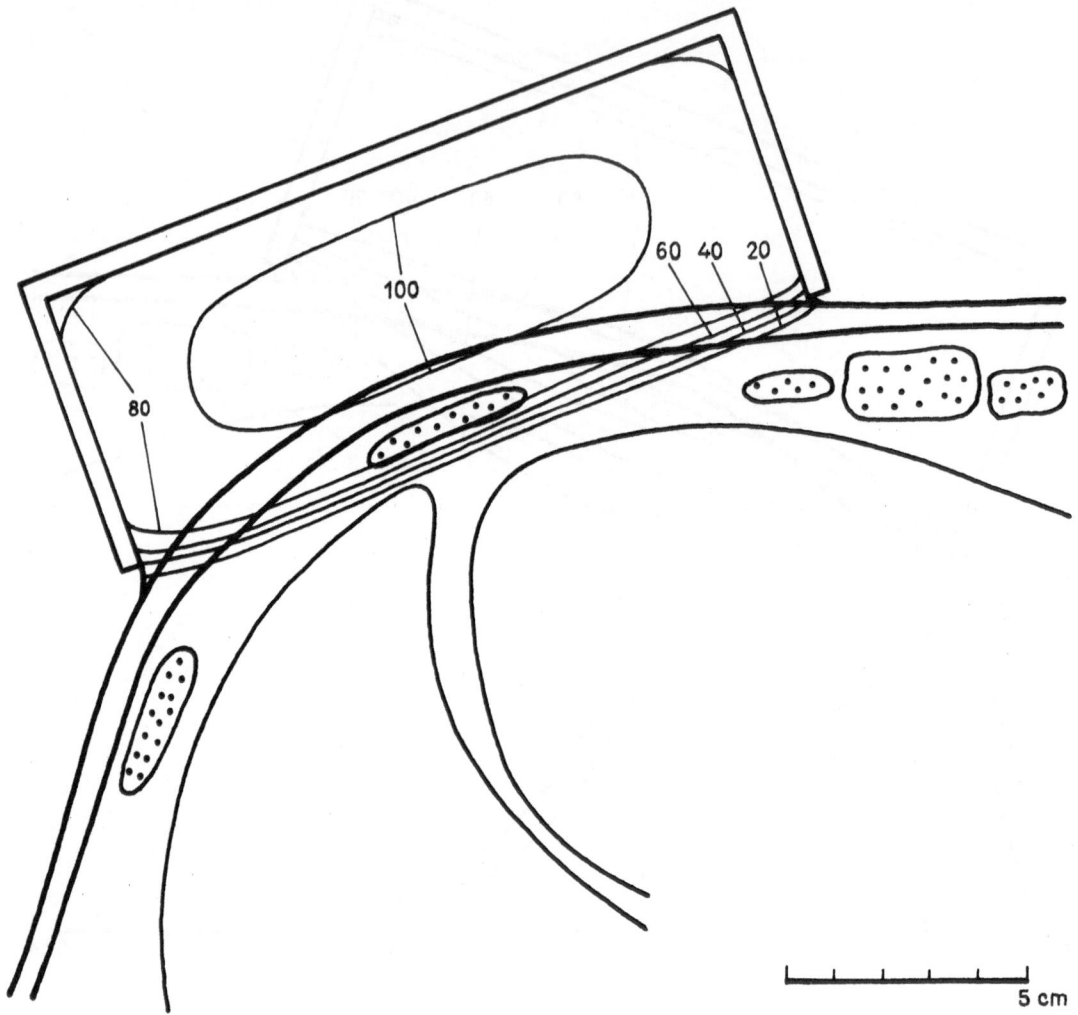

Fig. 140. Irradiation of breast tumour with 42 MV high-energy X-rays through two opposing stationary fields (breast compressed by means of a plastic box with adjustable walls)
  FSD 100 cm
  field size 6 × 15 cm
  Wax phantom

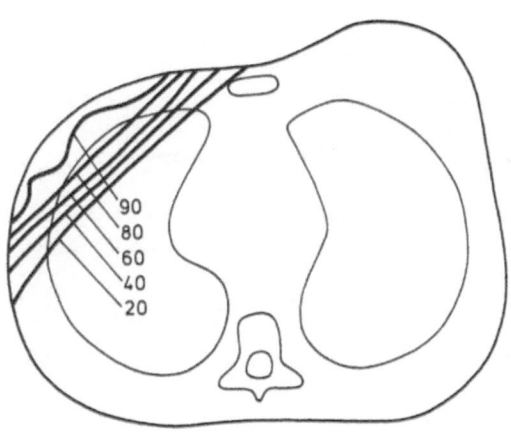

Fig. 141. 60-Co teletherapy of
the chest wall through two
tangential stationary fields
  SSD 50 cm
  field size 8 × 15 cm each
  the beams form an obtuse
      angle (40°/155°)
  boundaries of field:
    ipsilateral sternal
        border
    posterior axillary line
  Plexiglas–water phantom
  (Frischbier and Kuttig 1963)

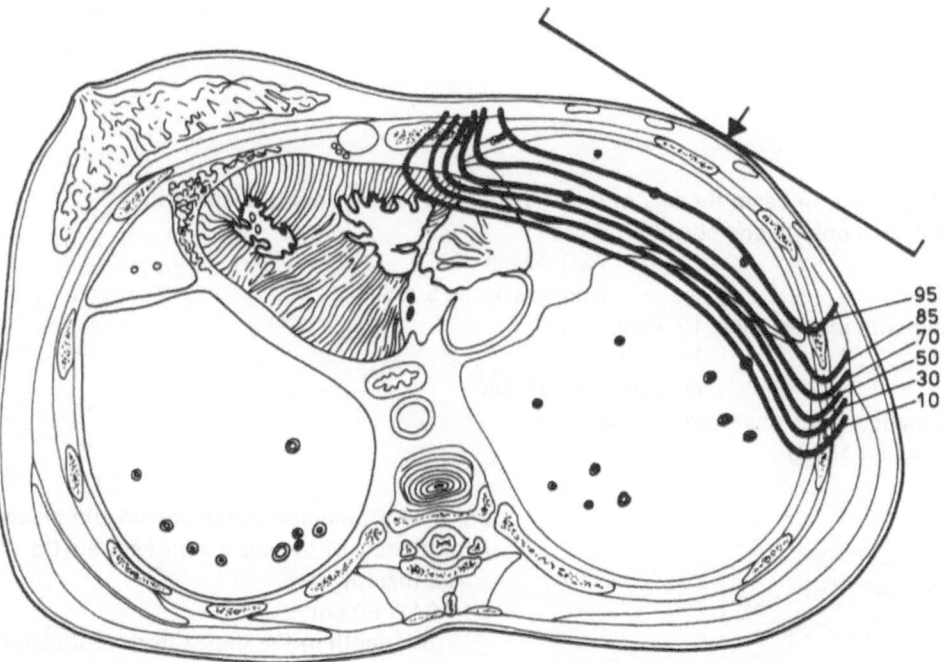

Fig. 142. Irradiation with 10.4 MeV electrons of a thoracic skin recurrence following
radical mastectomy
  FSD 90 cm
  field size 15 × 15 cm
  Inhomogeneous phantom
  (Chu et al. 1960)

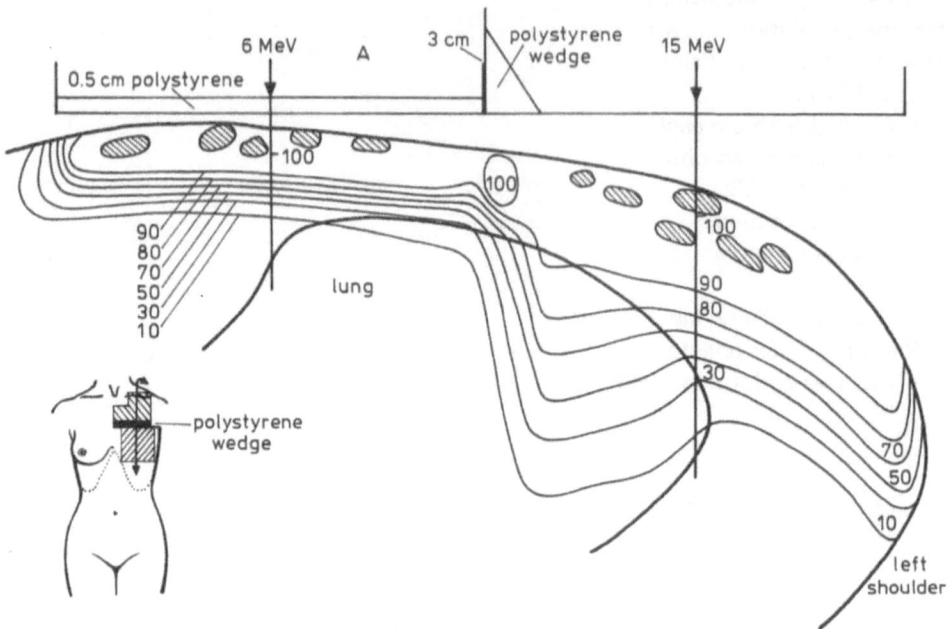

Fig. 143. Electron beam therapy of the chest wall following radical mastectomy
Field with polystyrene absorber: 6 MeV
       FSD 90 cm
       field size 15 × 15 cm
Field with wedge filter: 15 MeV
      FSD 90 cm
      field size 15 × 15 cm
Inhomogeneous phantom with skeleton
(Laughlin 1967)

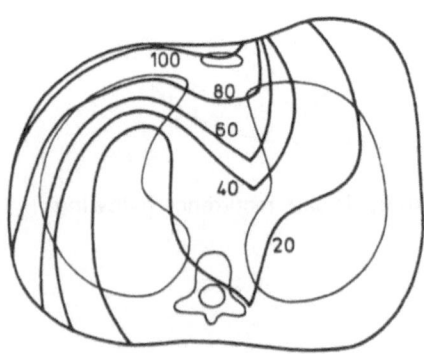

Fig. 144. Combined tangential arc and wedge field therapy of the chest wall with 60-Co
 Arc therapy:
  SAD 60 cm
  axis depth in the thorax from ventral and lateral corresponds to half the a–p diameter of the thorax phantom
  arc 150° (40°/190°)
  field size 6 × 18 cm at axis
  at 150° the beam is tilted to extend approx. 2 cm beyond the chest wall
 Internal mammary field:
  SSD 50 cm
  field size 6 × 12 cm
  wedge 15°
 Plexiglas–water phantom
 (Frischbier and Kuttig 1963)

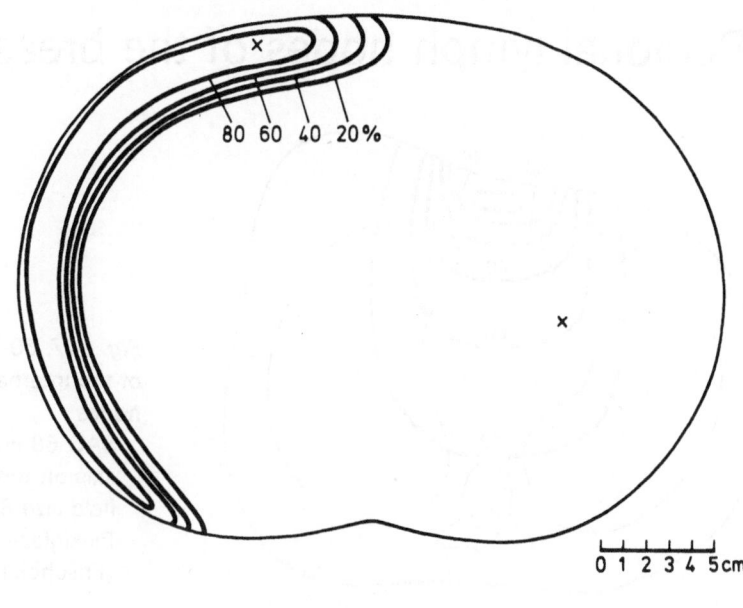

Fig. 145. Arc therapy of the chest wall with 7.5 MeV electrons
FAD 120 cm
axis depth 10% of the a–p diameter to dorsal
30% of the transversal diameter to the contralateral side
arc –20°/–95°
field size 3 × 14 cm
tilt of the central beam 3°
Alderson–Rando phantom
(Fournier et al. 1972)

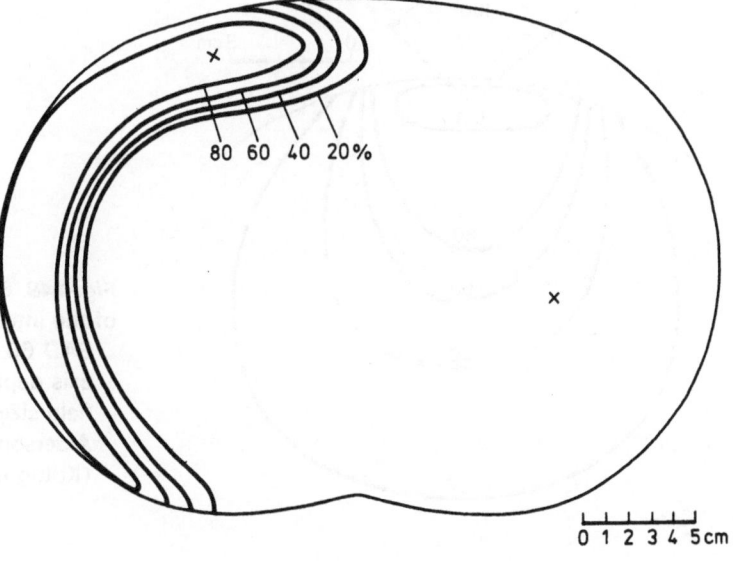

Fig. 146. Arc therapy of the chest wall with 10 MeV electrons
FAD 120 cm
axis depth 10% of the a–p diameter to dorsal
30% of the transversal diameter to the contralateral side
arc –20°/–95°
field size 3 × 14 cm
tilt of the central beam 3°
Alderson–Rando phantom
(Fournier et al. 1972)

Regional lymph nodes of the breast

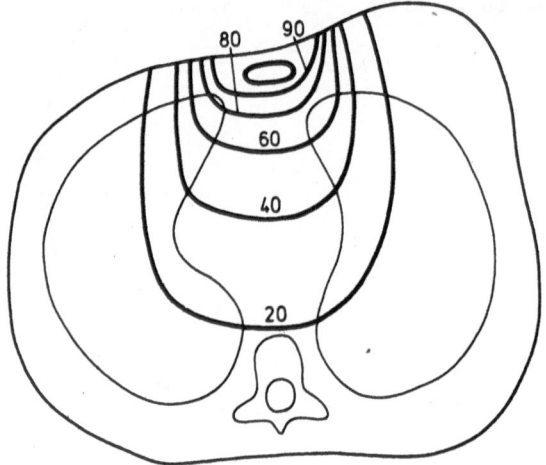

Fig. 147. 60-Co arc (100°) therapy
of the internal mammary lymph
nodes
   SAD 60 cm
   axis on the surface
   field size 8 × 12 cm
   Plexiglas–water phantom
   (Frischbier and Kuttig 1963)

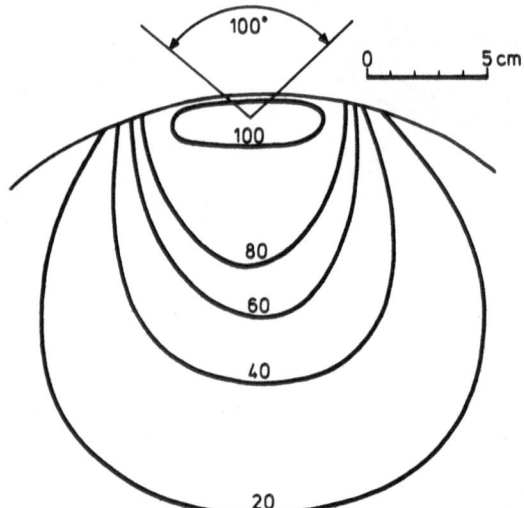

Fig. 148. 60-Co arc (100°) therapy
of the internal mammary chain
   SAD 60 cm
   axis depth 1 cm
   field size 8 × 12 cm
   Alderson–Rando phantom
   (Kuttig et al. 1970)

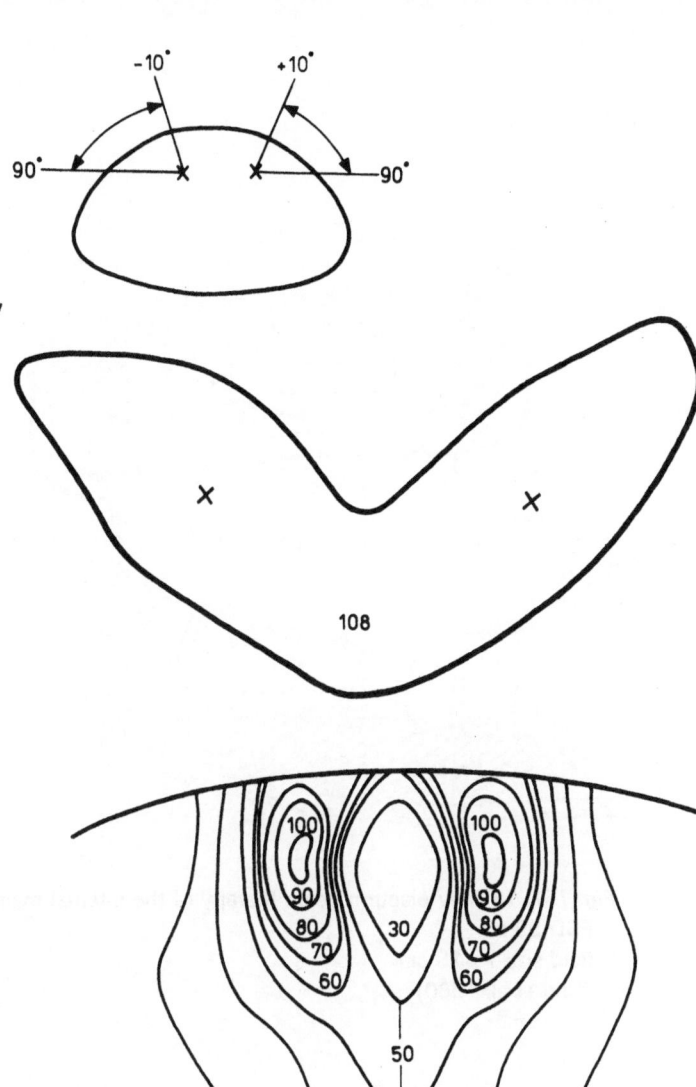

Fig. 149. Biaxial arc therapy
of the internal mammary
chain with 60-Co
  SAD 60 cm
  axis depth 3 cm
  arcs 80° (10°/90°) each
  distance of axes 6 cm
  field size 4 × 10 cm
  Computer calculated
    isodoses

Fig. 150. 100° arc therapy
of the internal mammary
lymph nodes with 60-Co.
(Field is divided by a lead
block measuring
2.9 × 7.2 × 12 cm mounted
on the radiation source)
  SAD 50 cm
  axis depth 3 cm
  field size 8 × 12 cm
  Alderson–Rando phantom
  (Kutting et al. 1970)

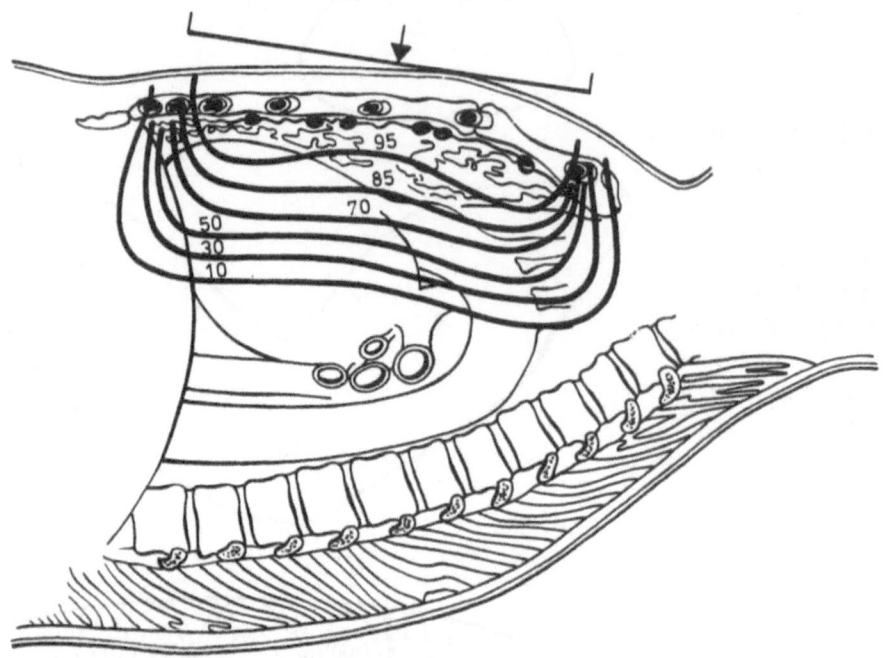

Fig. 151. 18 MeV electron beam therapy of the internal mammary lymph nodes
FSD 90 cm
field size 7 × 15 cm
(Chu et al. 1960)

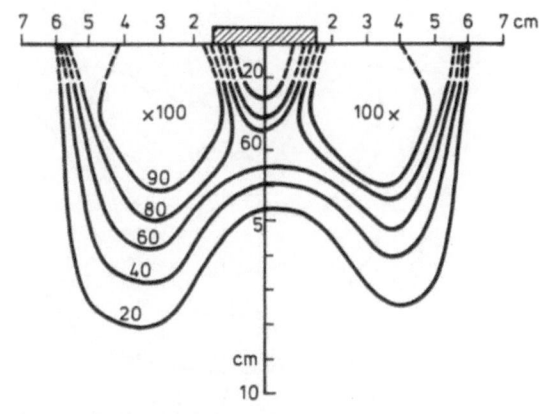

Fig. 152. 10 MeV electron beam therapy of the internal mammary lymph nodes through two oblique stationary fields
(sternum protected with lead blocks 3.4 cm wide and 1.5 cm thick)
FSD 100 cm
field size 6 × 12 cm
angle of incidence 20° for both beams
Alderson–Rando phantom
(Kuttig et al. 1972)

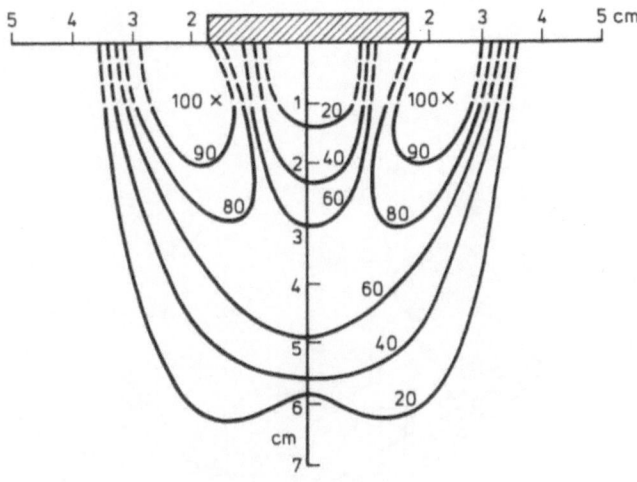

Fig. 153. 15 MeV electron beam therapy of the internal mammary nodes through two oblique stationary fields
(sternum protected with lead blocks 3.4 cm wide and 1.5 cm thick)
FSD 100 cm
field size 4 × 12 cm
angle of incidence 20° for both beams
Alderson–Rando phantom
(Kuttig et al. 1972)

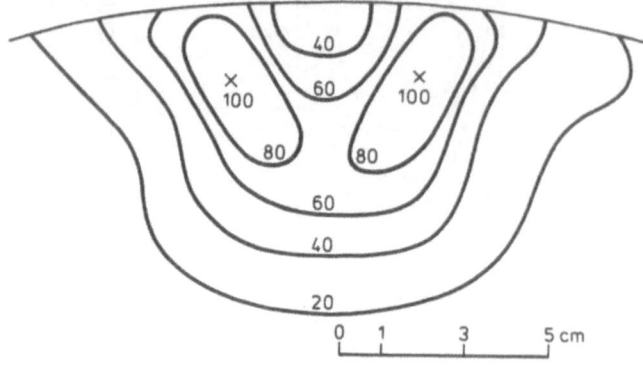

0 1   3   5 cm

Fig. 154. Arc therapy (120°) of the internal mammary chain with 15 MeV electrons using a shutter tube (see Fig. 106*b*)
    FAD 120 cm
    axis depth 3 cm
    Alderson–Rando phantom
    (Kuttig et al. 1972)

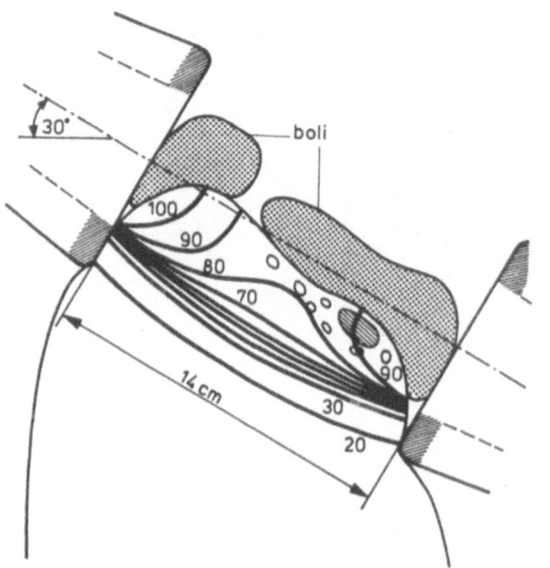

Fig. 155. X-ray therapy (300 kV, 10 mA) of the supraclavicular lymph nodes through two opposing stationary fields
    HVL 44 mm Cu (filter
       5 mm Cu)
    FSD 30 cm
    field size 6 × 15 cm
    Polystyrene phantom
    (Sack and Scherer 1972)

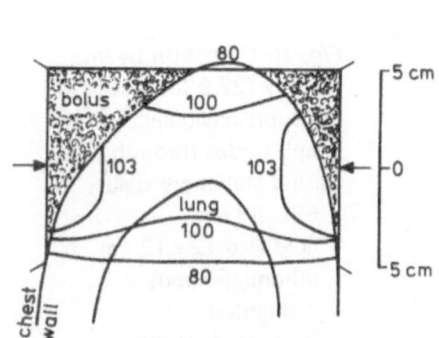

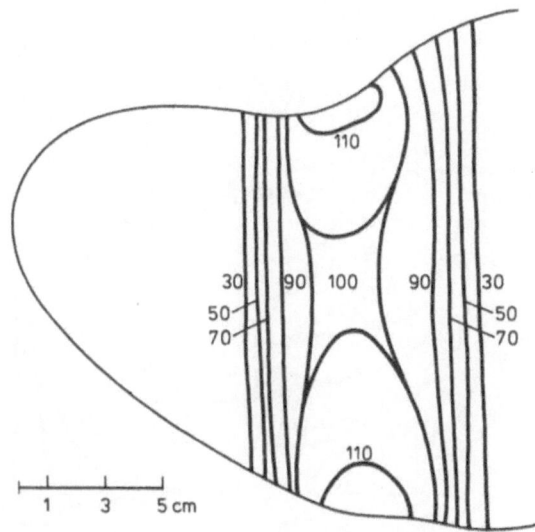

Fig. 156. 60-Co teletherapy of the supra- and subclavicular as well as axillary lymph nodes through a ventral and a dorsal field
SSD 80 cm
field size 10 × 25 cm
(Koeck et al. 1964)

Fig. 157. 60-Co teletherapy of the supra- and subclavicular as well as axillary lymph nodes through a ventral and a dorsal field (2/3 of the total dose to the ventral portal, while 1/3 to the dorsal one)
SSD 50 cm
field size 6 × 14 cm
(Kuttig et al. 1970)

Fig. 158. Electron beam therapy (18 MeV) of a supraclavicular metastasis
FSD 90 cm
field size 8 × 10 cm
Inhomogeneous
  phantom with
  skeleton
(Laughlin 1967)

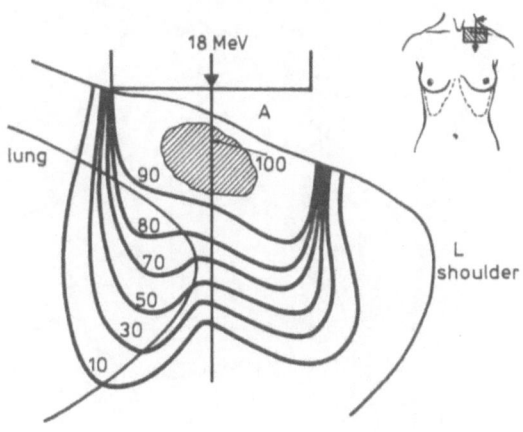

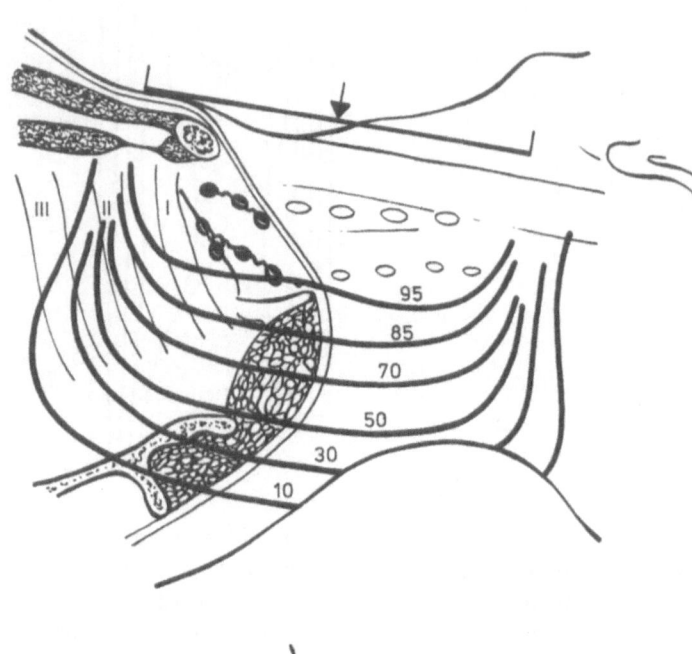

Fig. 159. Electron beam therapy (22.5 MeV) of the supraclavicular lymph nodes through a ventral stationary field
FSD 90 cm
field size 12 × 12 cm
Inhomogeneous phantom
(Chu et al. 1960)

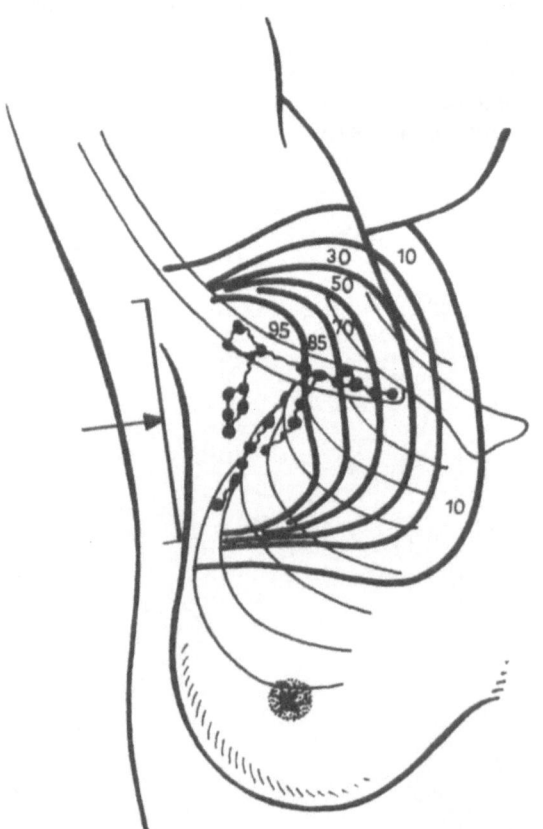

Fig. 160. Electron beam therapy (20 MeV) of the axillary lymph nodes through a stationary field
FSD 90 cm
field size 8 × 8 cm
Inhomogeneous phantom
(Chu et al. 1960)

Gastrointestinal tract and extraintestinal abdominal organs

Esophagus

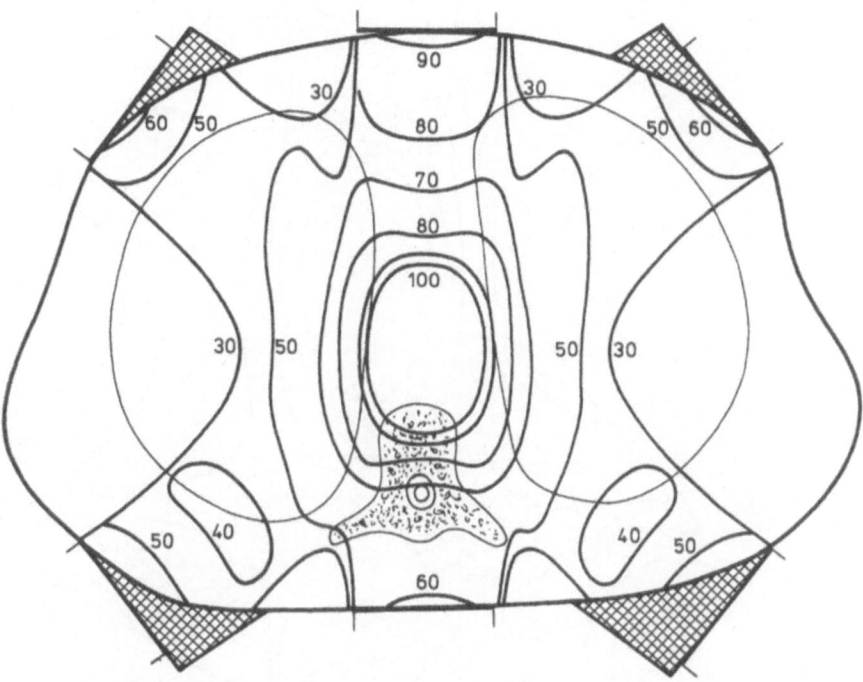

Fig. 161. X-ray therapy (250 kV, 20 mA) of the esophagus through six
stationary fields
   HVT 1.5 mm Cu
   FSD 50 cm
   field size
      5 × 12 cm each
   Water phantom
   (Chance 1958)

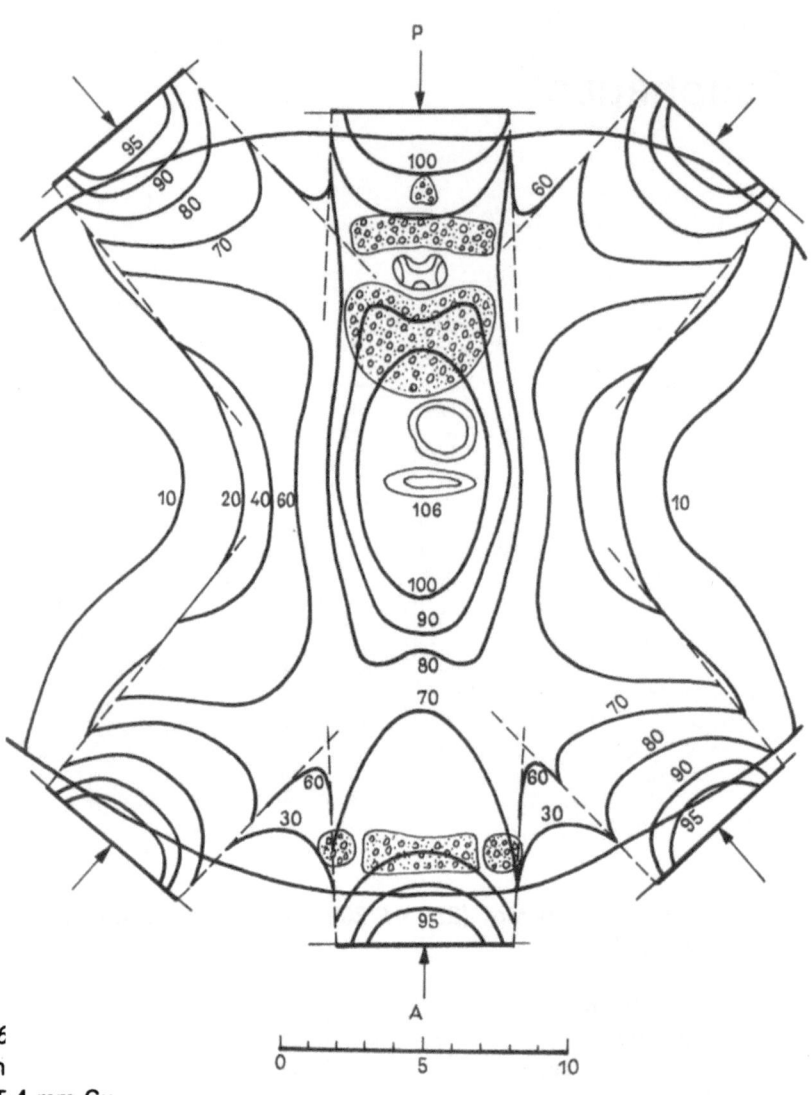

Fig. 16
station
  HVT 4 mm Cu
  FSD 80 cm
  field size 6 × 15 cm each
  Water phantom
  (Johns et al. 1950)

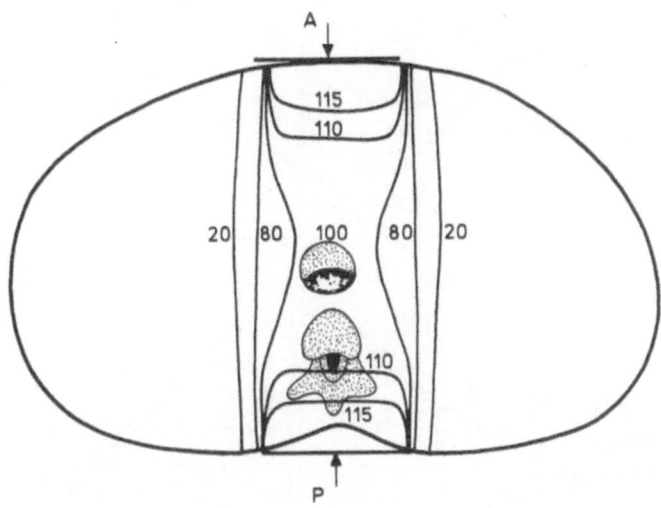

Fig. 163. 60-Co teletherapy of the esophagus through two opposing fields
   SSD 70 cm
   field size 8 × 12 cm each
   Water phantom
   (Fletcher 1956a)

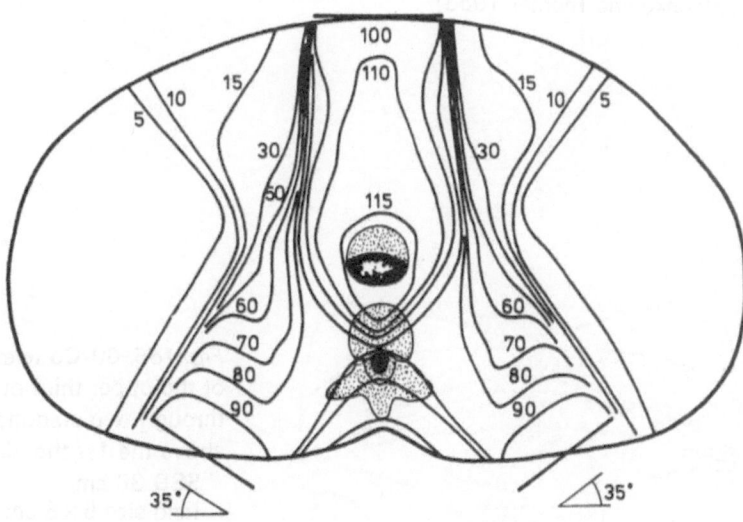

Fig. 164. 60-Co teletherapy of the esophagus through three stationary fields
   SSD 50 cm
   field size 6 × 12 cm each
   (Fletcher 1956a)

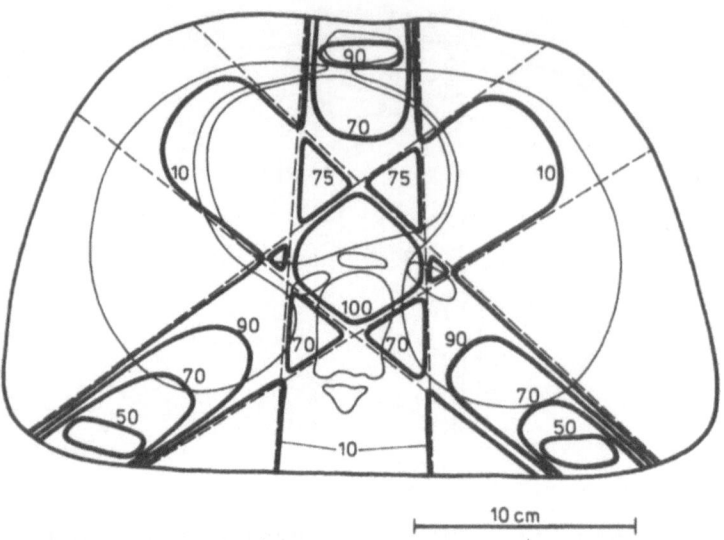

Fig. 165. 60-Co teletherapy of the esophagus through three
stationary fields
    SSD 50 cm
    field size 5 × 15 cm ventral
              4 × 15 cm each dorsal
    Calculated isodoses
    (Matschke and Richter 1963)

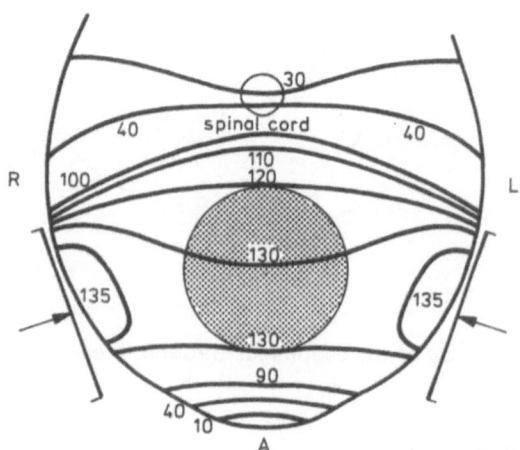

Fig. 166. 60-Co teletherapy (150 Curie)
of the upper third of the esophagus
through two stationary fields (tumour
above the 1st thoraic vertebra)
    SSD 30 cm
    field size 5 × 8 cm each
    Temex phantom
    (Lederman et al.
        1966)

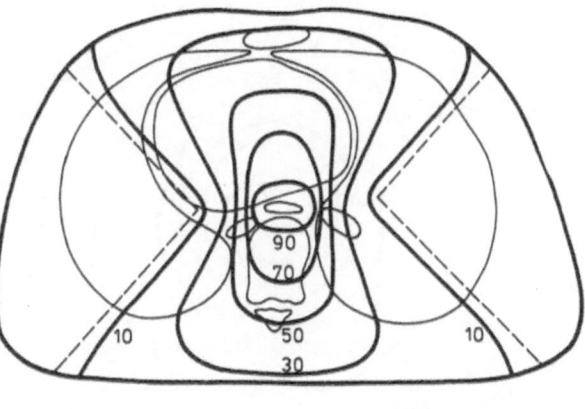

Fig. 167. One-centre two-arc irradiation of the esophagus with 60-Co
  SAD 52 cm
  axis depth 10 cm in the midline
  arcs: +90°/−90° ventral and
    dorsal
  field size 4 × 15 cm at axis
  Calculated isodoses
  (Matschke and Richter 1963)

10 cm

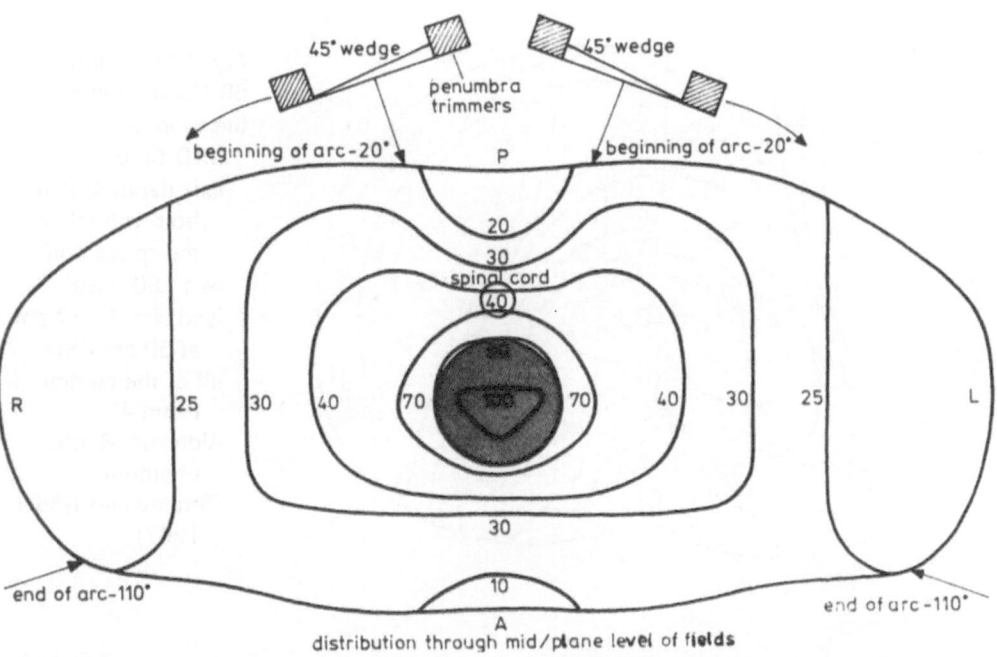

Fig. 168. One-centre two-arc (90°) irradiation of the upper third of the esophagus with 60-Co wedge fields
  SAD 80 cm
  axis depth 10 cm in the midline
  field size 5 × 15 cm each
  45° wedges
  Temex phantom
  (Lederman et al. 1966)

Esophagus | 113

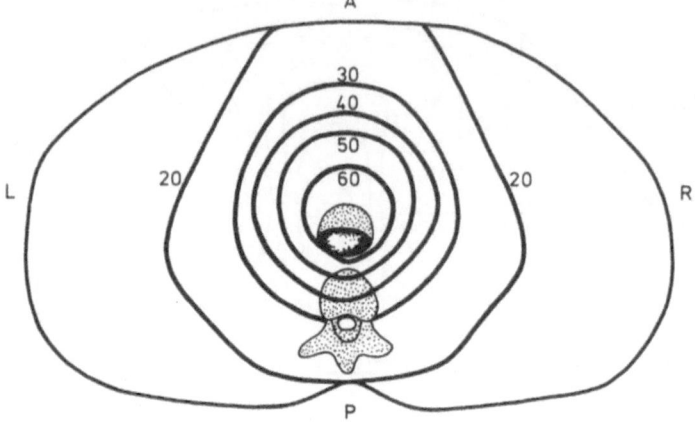

Fig. 169. 60-Co
rotation (360°) ther-
apy of the esophagus
SAD 80 cm
axis depth
10 cm in
the midline
field size 6 × 12 cm
Water phantom
(Fletcher 1956*a*)

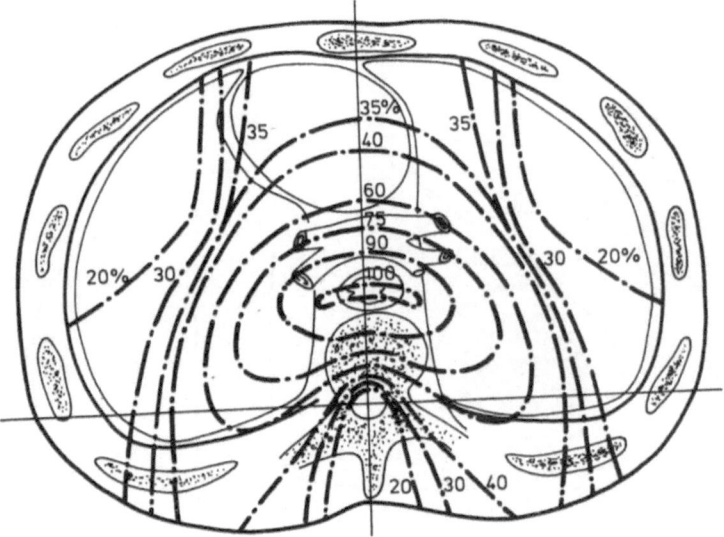

Fig. 170. Eccentric
60-Co arc therapy of
the esophagus
SAD 65 cm
axis depth 4.5 cm
from ventral (in
the spinal cord)
two 180° arcs
field size 3 × 12 cm
at 50 cm SSD
tilt of the central
beam 4°
Alderson–Rando
phantom
(Stratev and Rödel
1967)

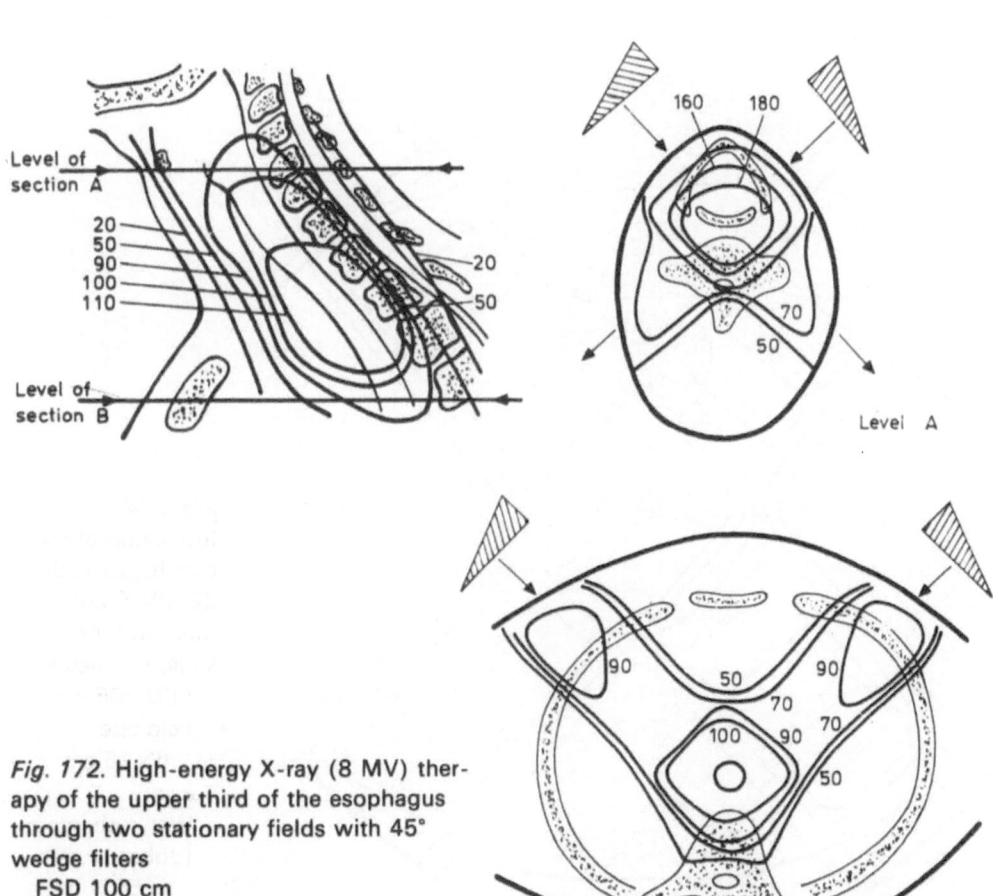

Fig. 171. Irradiation of the esophagus with 22 MV high-energy X-rays through two opposing fields
   FSD 80 cm
   field size 8 × 12 cm
   Water phatom
   (Fletcher 1956*b*)

Fig. 172. High-energy X-ray (8 MV) therapy of the upper third of the esophagus through two stationary fields with 45° wedge filters
   FSD 100 cm
   field size 5 × 10 cm each
   (Wood 1959)

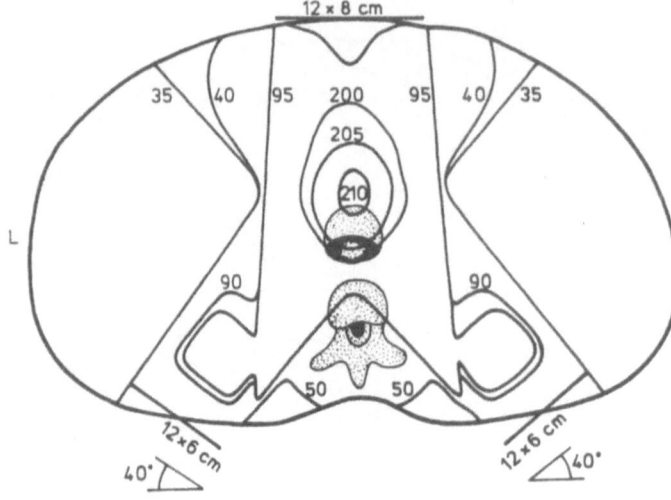

Fig. 173. Treatment of the esophagus with high-energy X-rays (22 MV) through three stationary fields
   FSD 80 cm
   field size
      8 × 12 cm ventral
      6 × 12 cm dorsal
   Water phantom
   (Fletcher 1956*b*)

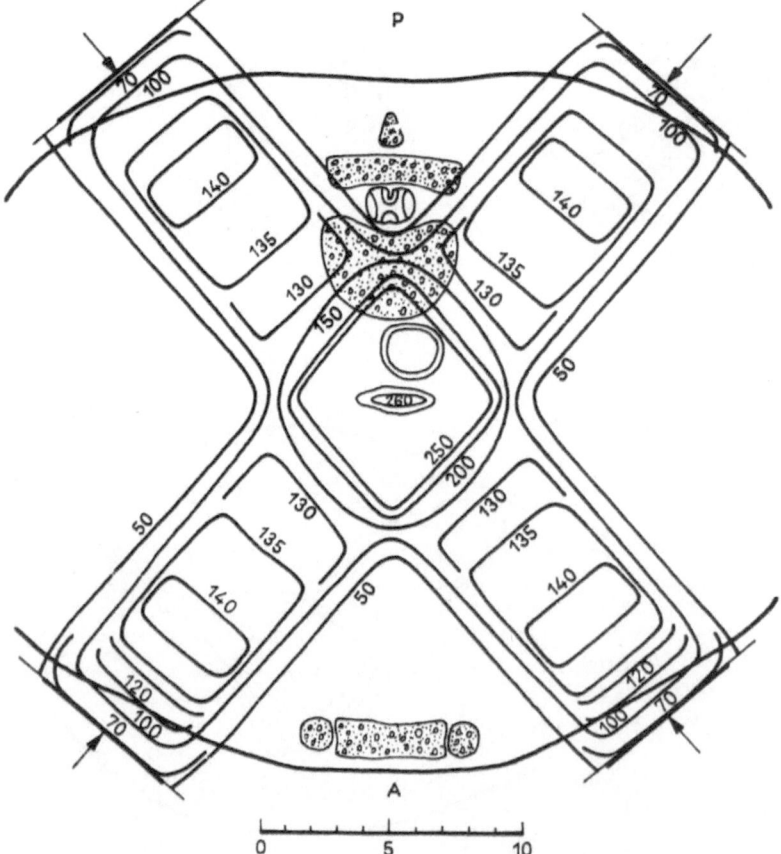

Fig. 174. Irradiation of the esophagus with 22 MV X-rays through four stationary fields
   FSD 105 cm
   field size
      6 × 15 cm each
   Water phantom
   (Johns et al. 1950)

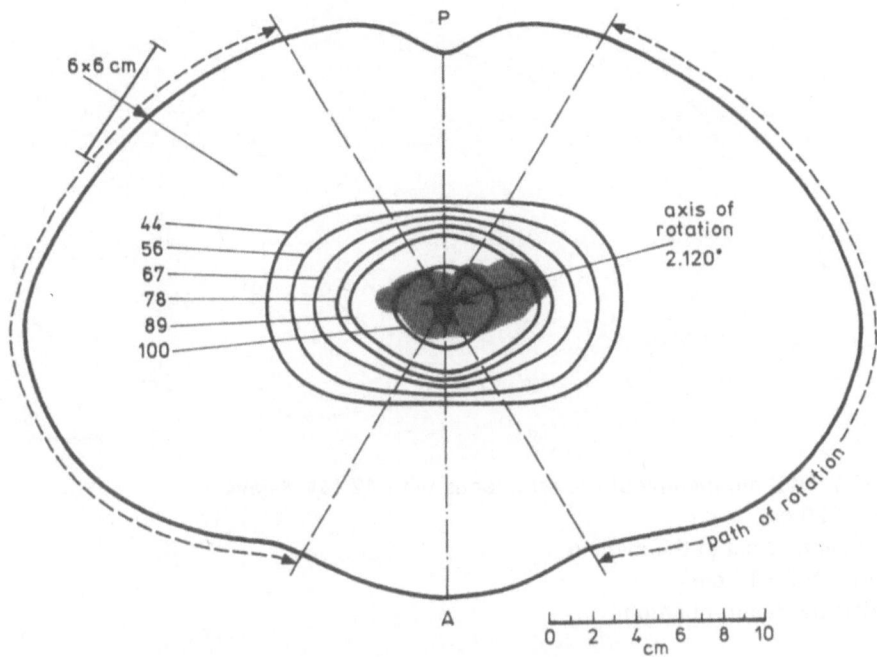

Fig. 175. One-centre two-arc treatment of the esophagus with 4.7 MV X-rays
FAD 100 cm
axis depth 14 cm from ventral in the midline
two 120° arcs
field size 6 × 6 cm
Pressdwood phantom
(Bagshaw et al. 1965)

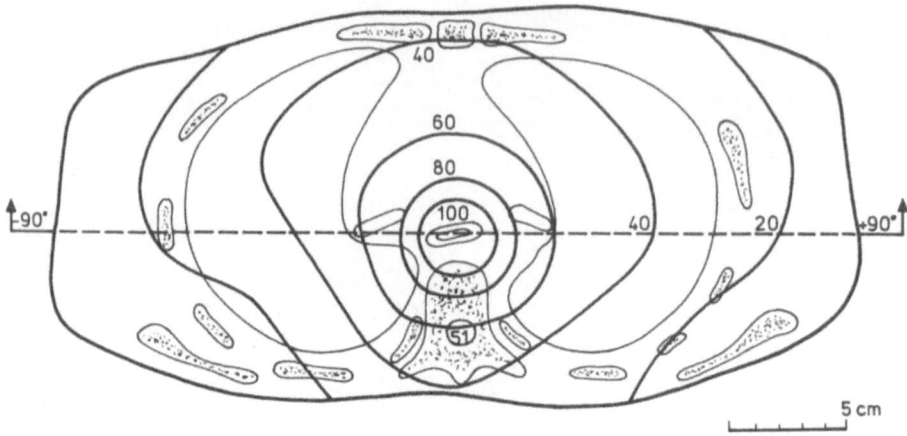

Fig. 176. 180° arc therapy of the esophagus with 42 MV X-rays
FAD 120 cm
axis depth 9 cm in the midline
field size 3 × 12 cm
Alderson–Rando phantom

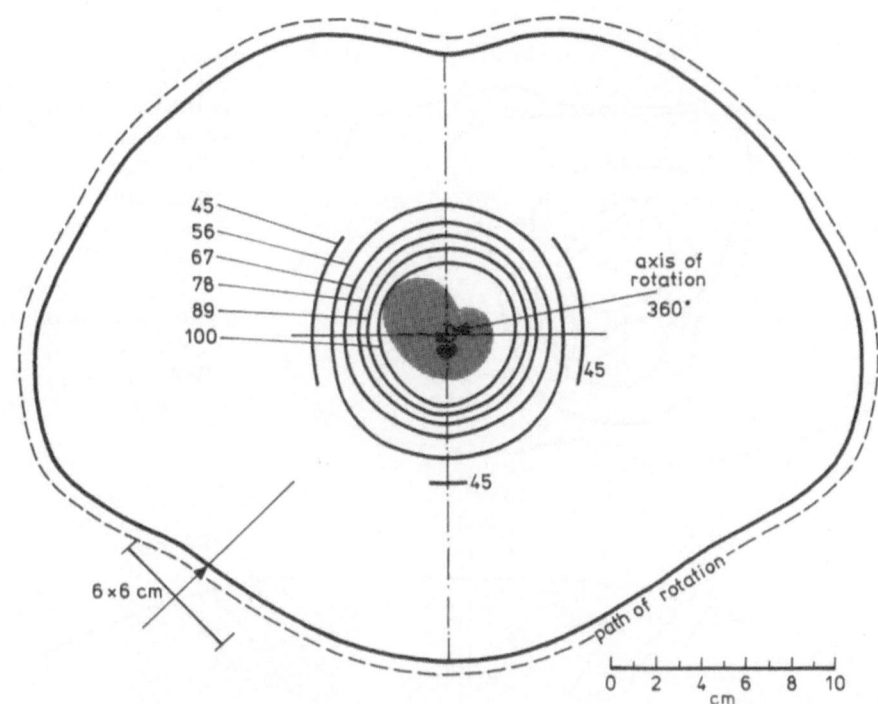

Fig. 177. Megavoltage X-ray therapy (4.7 MV) of the esophagus with 360°
rotation
    FAD 100 cm
    axis depth 14 cm from ventral in the midline
    field size 6 × 6 cm
    Pressdwood phantom
    (Bagshaw et al. 1965)

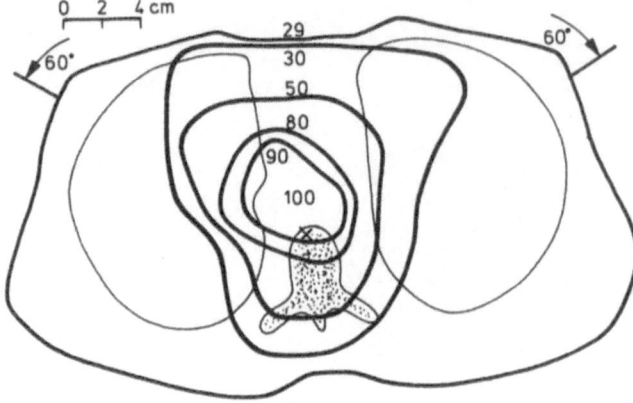

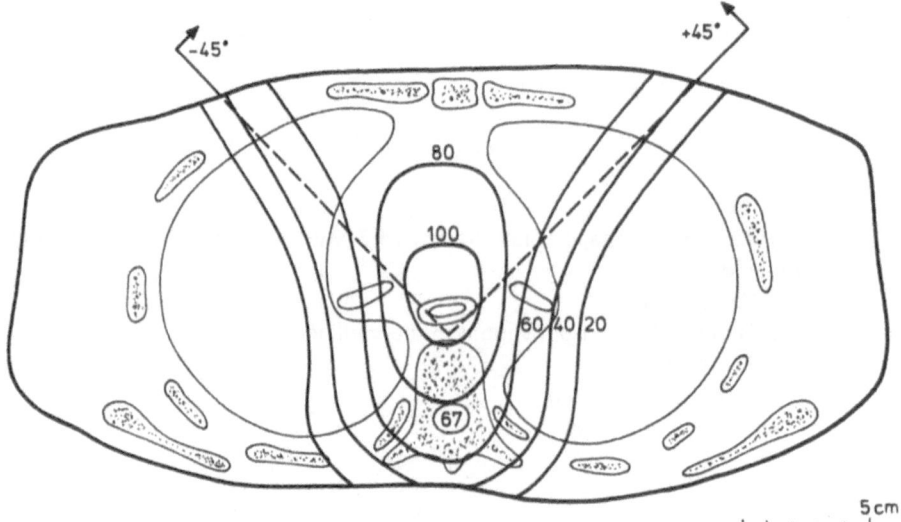

Fig. 178. Arc therapy (120°)
of the esophagus with
42 MeV electron beam
FAD 120 cm
 axis depth 10 cm
  in the midline
 field size
  6 × 12 cm at axis
Alderson–Rando
 phantom
(Fehrentz et al.
 1969)

Fig. 179. Arc therapy (90°) of the esophagus with 30 MeV electron beam
FAD 120 cm
axis depth 10 cm in the midline
field size 3 × 12 cm
Alderson–Rando phantom

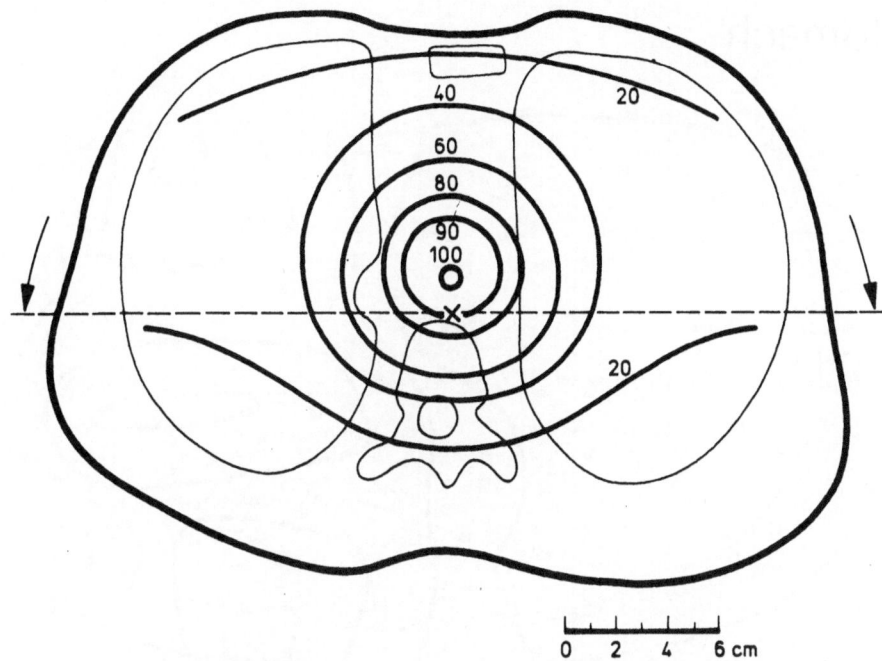

Fig. 180. Arc therapy (180°) of the esophagus with 25 MeV electrons
FAD 120 cm
axis depth 10 cm in the midline
field size 6 × 8 cm at axis
Alderson–Rando phantom
(Schnabel et al. 1972)

Stomach

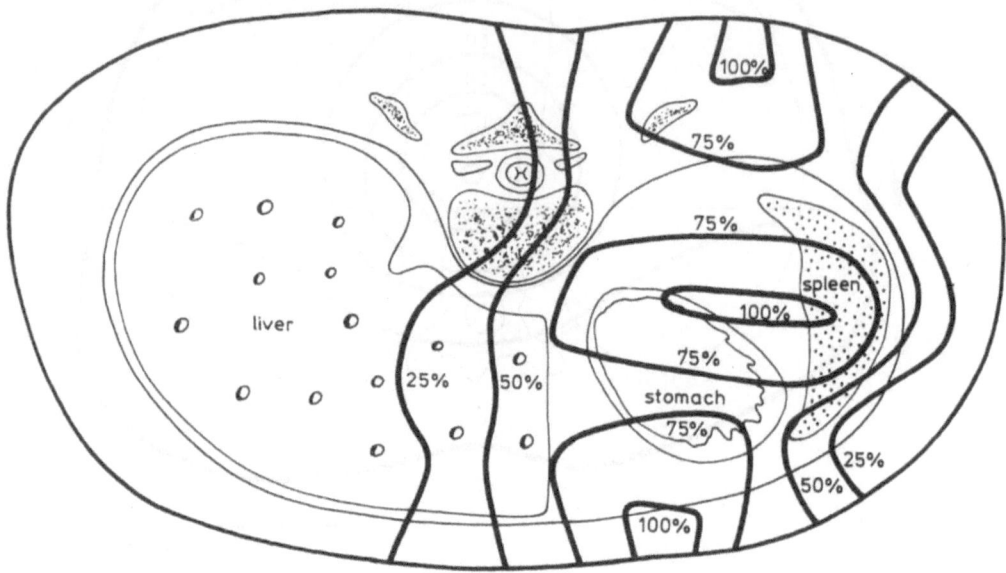

Fig. 181. X-ray therapy (200 kV, 20 mA) of the stomach through two opposing fields
HVT 0.95 mm Cu, filter 0.5 mm Cu
FSD 40 cm
field size 10 × 15 cm each
Human cadaver
(Barth et al. 1954)

Fig. 182. Rotation (360°) therapy of the stomach with X-rays (200 kV, 20 mA). *a* dose distribution on the abdominal wall; *b, c* and *d* dose distribution at different sections
HVT 0.96 mm Cu, filter 0.5 mm Cu
FAD 50 cm
axis depth at the anterolateral border of the spine
field size 3 × 8 cm at focus
Human cadaver
(Barth et al. 1954)

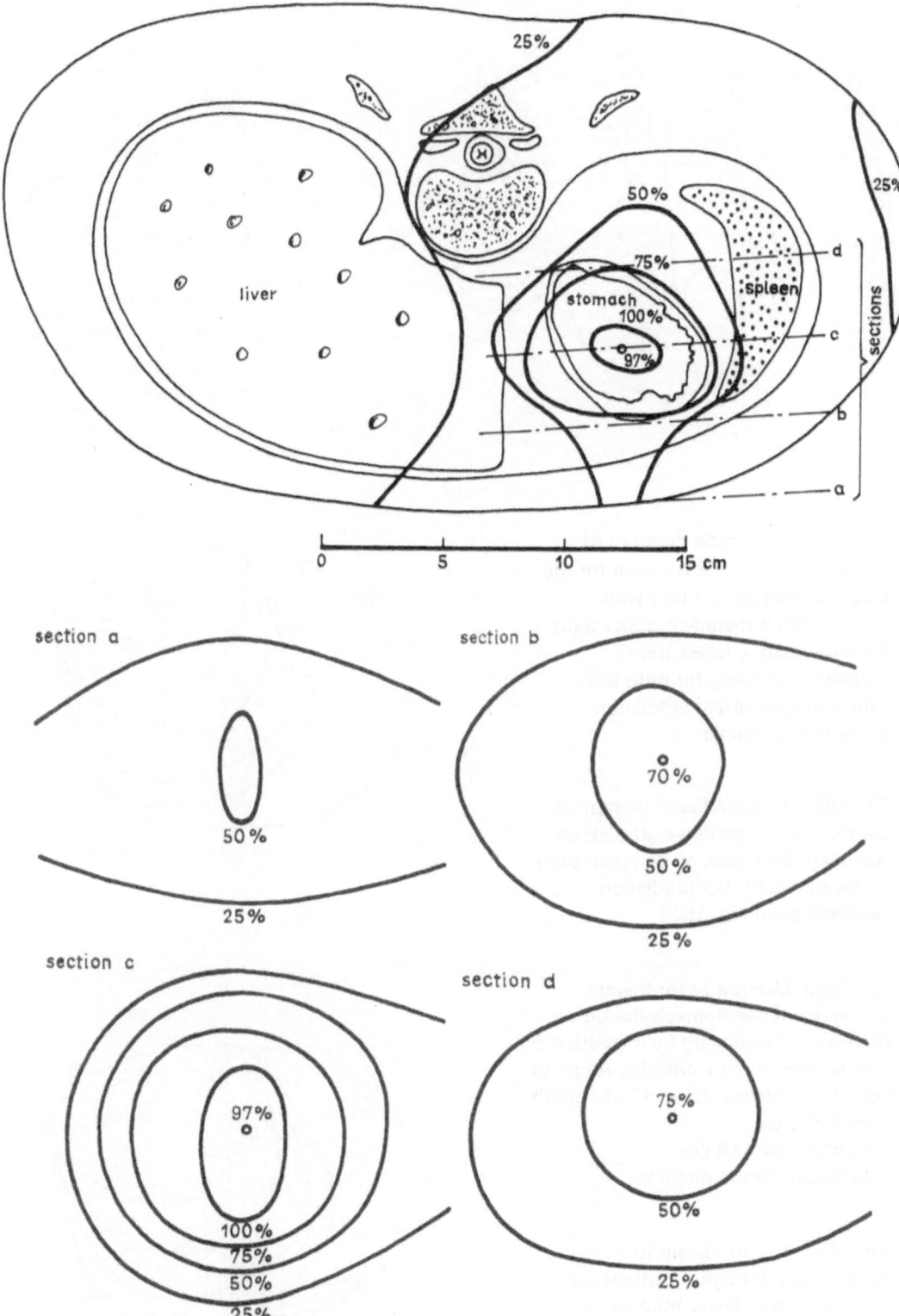

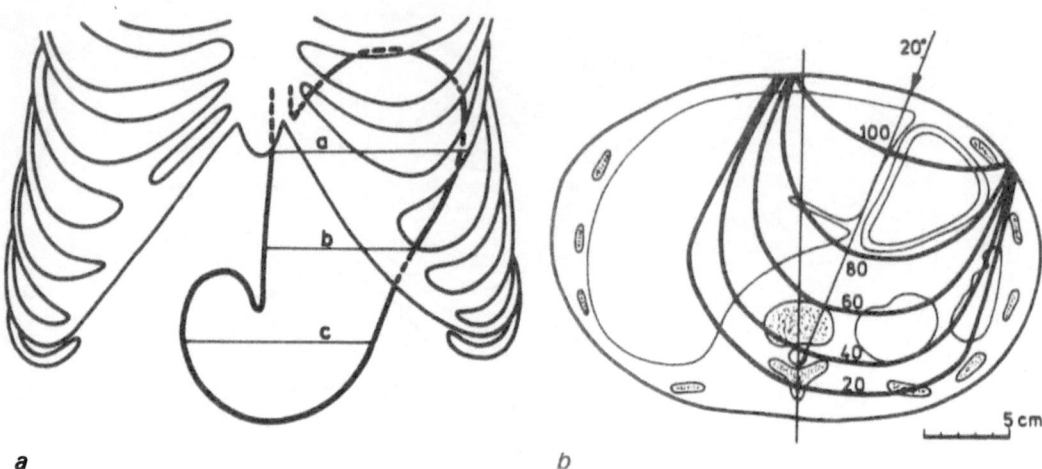

a

b

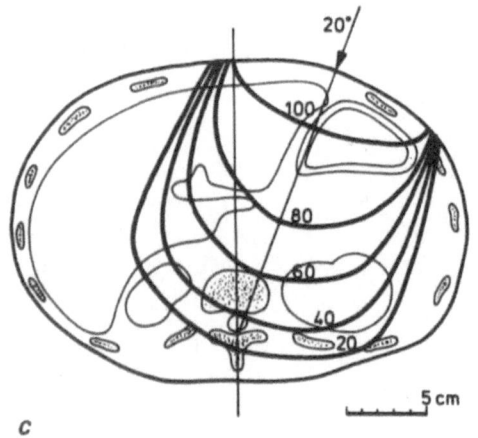

c

Fig. 183a. Schematic drawing of
sections through the stomach for the
study of dose distribution with
electron beam therapy *a* upper third,
b middle third, *c* lower third.
Treatment planning for both telecentric and small-arc irradiation
at the level of section *b*

Fig. 183b. Electron beam therapy of
the stomach through a ventrolateral
stationary field (section *a:* upper third
of the stomach). For irradiation
parameters see Fig. 183c

Fig. 183c. Electron beam therapy
(42 MeV) of the stomach through a
ventrolateral stationary field (section *b*:
middle third of the stomach). Angle of
axis to the midline 20° at 17 cm depth
   FSD 120 cm
   field size 14 × 16 cm
   Alderson–Rando phantom

Fig. 183d. Electron beam therapy of
the stomach through a ventrolateral
field (section *c*: lower third of the
stomach). For irradiation parameters
see Fig. 183c

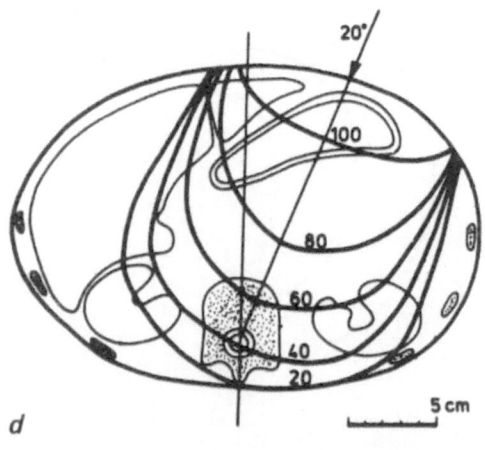

d

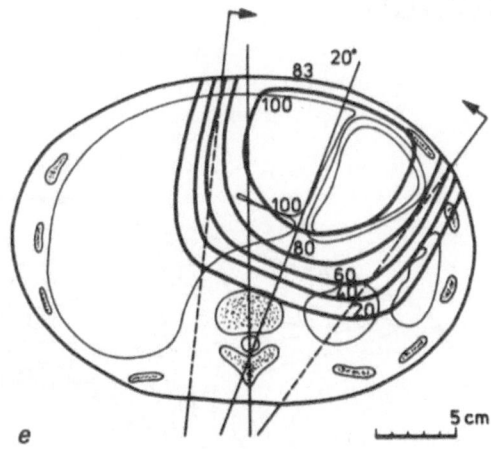

e

Fig. 183e. Telecentric small-arc irradiation of the stomach with high-energy electrons (section *a*: upper third of the stomach). For irradiation parameters see Fig. 183c

Fig. 183f. Telecentric small-arc (30°) irradiation of the stomach with high-energy electrons (25 MeV) (section *b*: middle third of the stomach). Axis adjusted to form a 20° angle with the midline at 17 cm depth in the middle third of the stomach is subsequently transferred to 30 cm depth
  FAD 120 cm
  axis depth 30 cm
  field size 3 × 16 cm
  Alderson–Rando phantom

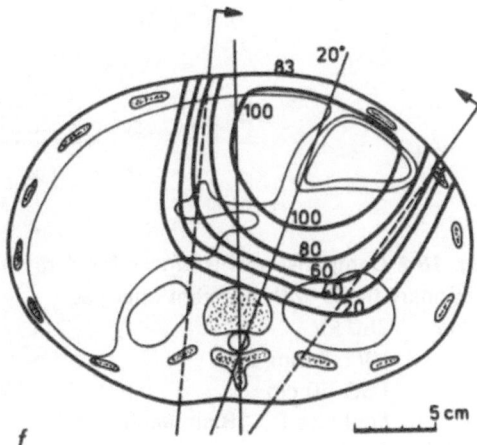

f

Fig. 183g. Telecentric small-arc irradiation of the stomach with high-energy electrons (section *c*: lower third of the stomach). For irradiation parameters see Fig. 183f

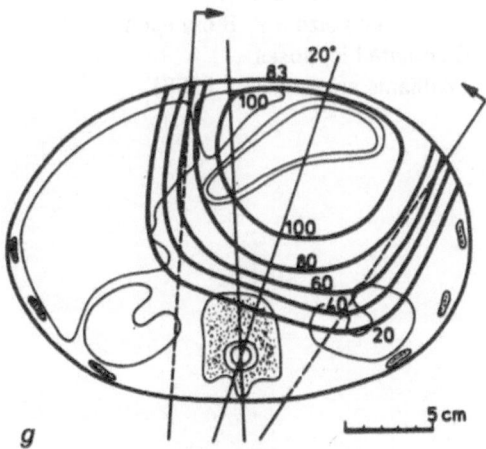

g

Stomach | 125

Rectum

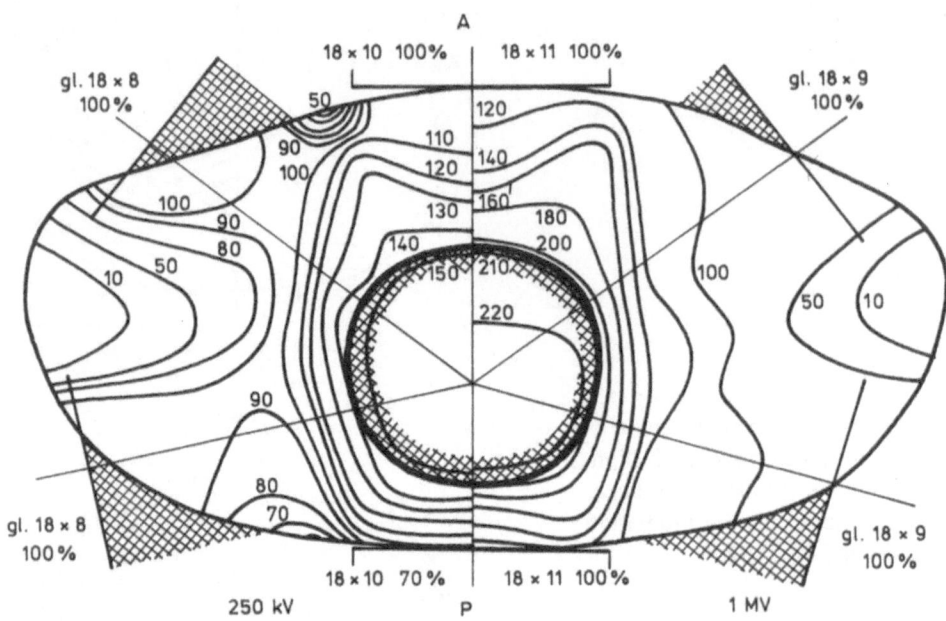

Fig. 184. Comparison of isodoses for X-ray irradiation of the rectum through four stationary fields with different energies

Left: 250 kV
       HVT 2 mm Cu
       FSD 50 cm
       field size 8 × 18 cm each

Right: 1 MV
       HVT 9.3 mm Cu
       FSD 100 cm
       field size 9 × 18 cm each

Calculated isodoses
(Williams and Horwitz 1956)

Fig. 185. Comparison of the isodose curves for the X-ray therapy of an extensive rectum carcinoma with different energies through four stationary fields
Left:
　250 kV
　HVT 2 mm Cu
　FSD 50 cm
　field size
　　10 × 18 cm each
Right:
　1 MV
　HVT 9.3 mm Cu
　FSD 100 cm
　field size
　　10 × 18 cm each
Calculated isodoses
(Williams and
　Horwitz 1956)

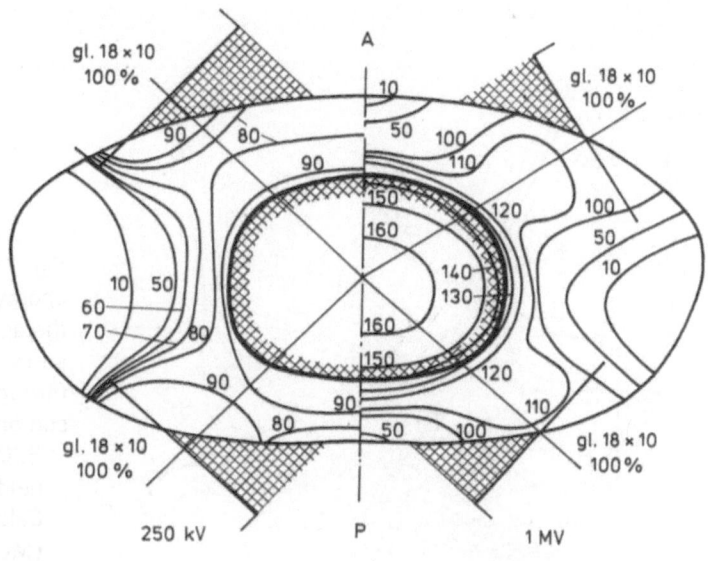

Fig. 186. One-centre two-arc (160°) 60-Co irradiation of the rectum
　SAD 75 cm
　axis depth 13 cm
　　from ventral
　　in the midline
　field size 8 × 15 cm
　(Gough 1962)

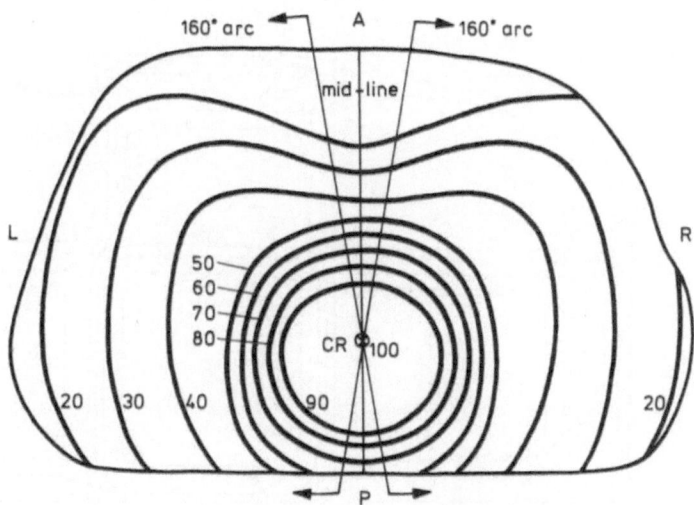

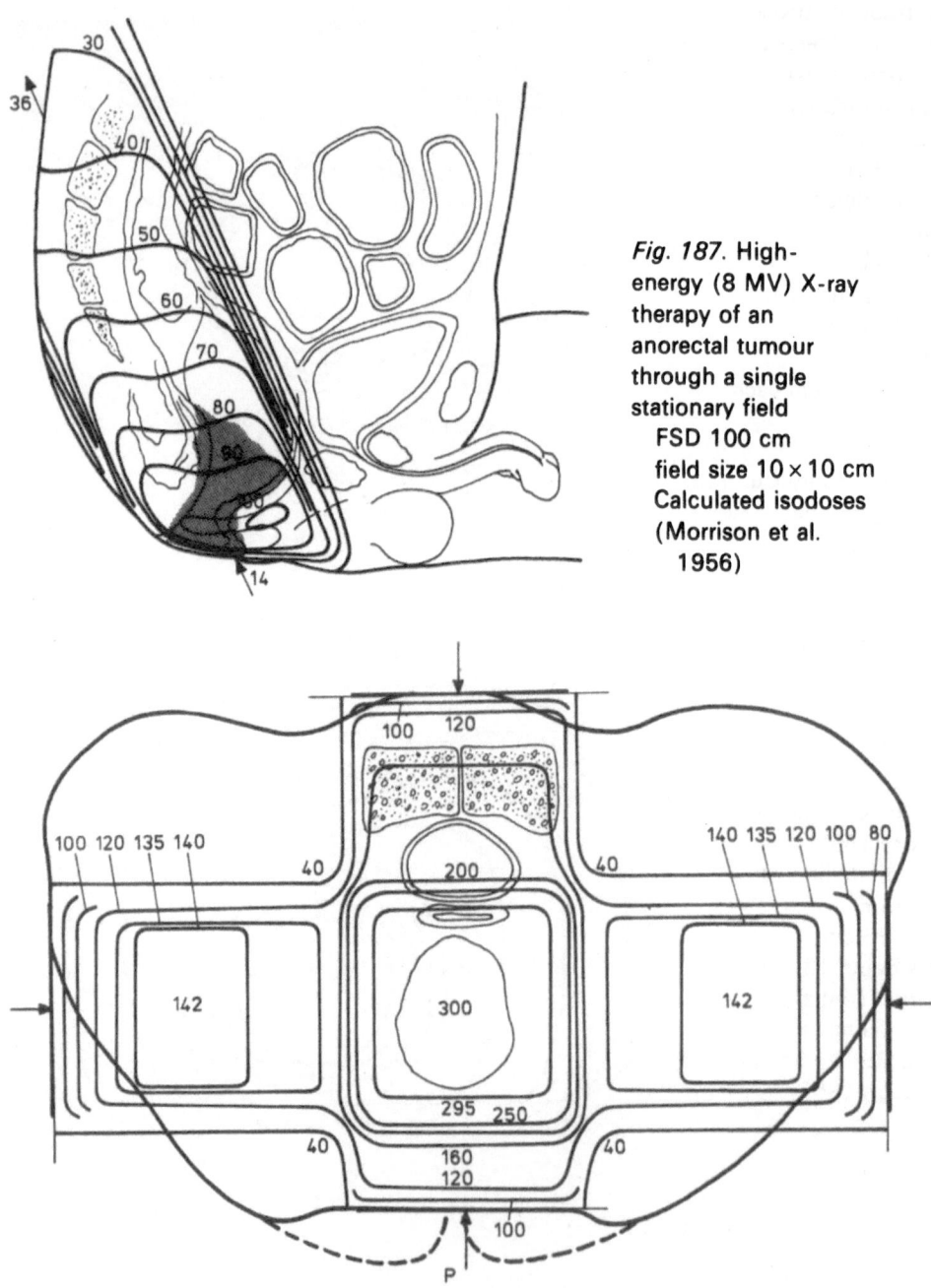

Fig. 187. High-energy (8 MV) X-ray therapy of an anorectal tumour through a single stationary field
  FSD 100 cm
  field size 10 × 10 cm
  Calculated isodoses
  (Morrison et al. 1956)

Fig. 188. Irradiation of the rectum with 22 MV X-rays through four stationary fields
  FSD 105 cm
  field size 8 × 12 cm
  Water phantom
  (Johns et al. 1950)

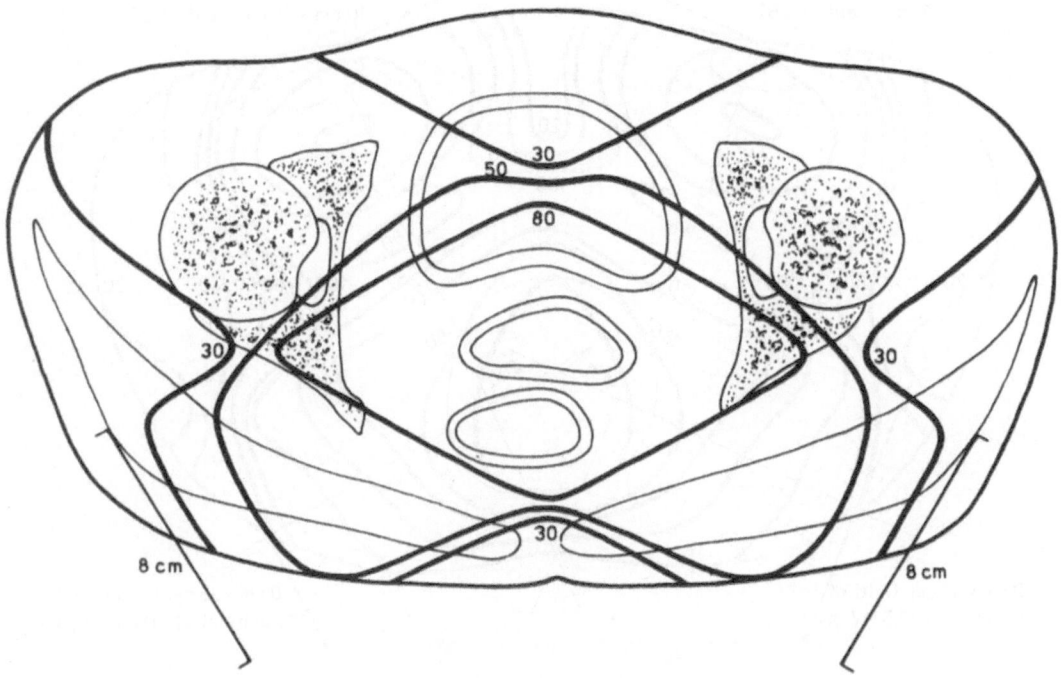

Fig. 189. Irradiation of the rectum with 42 MV X-rays through two stationary fields
FSD 100 cm
field size 8 × 14 cm each
angles of incidence 60° from dorsal
Alderson–Rando phantom
(Hellriegel 1973)

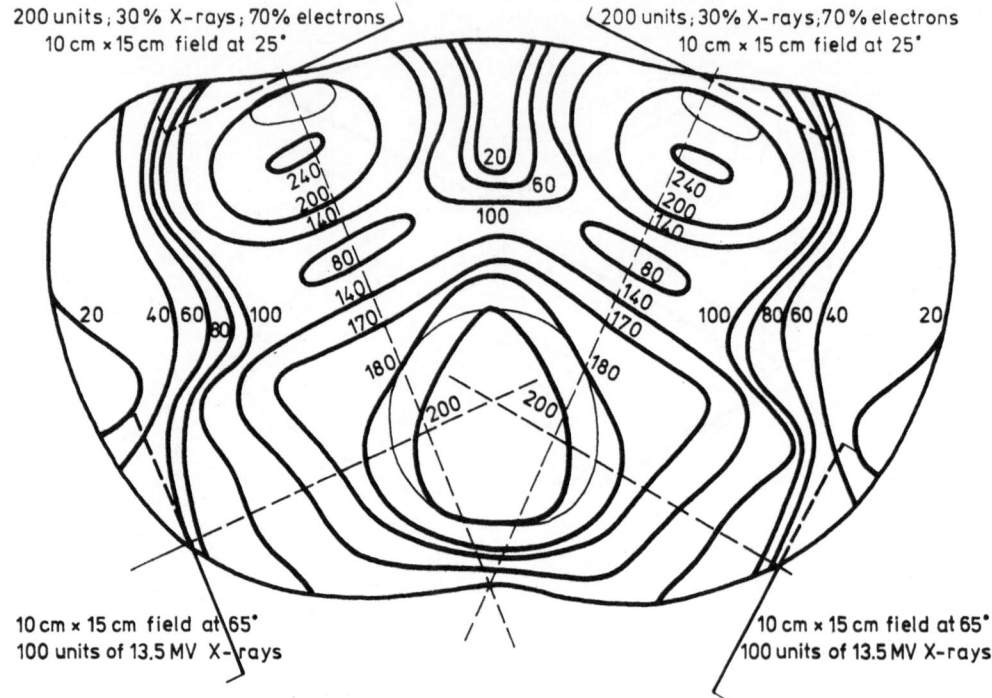

200 units; 30% X-rays; 70% electrons
10 cm × 15 cm field at 25°

200 units; 30% X-rays; 70% electrons
10 cm × 15 cm field at 25°

10 cm × 15 cm field at 65°
100 units of 13.5 MV X-rays

10 cm × 15 cm field at 65°
100 units of 13.5 MV X-rays

Fig. 190. Combined high-energy X-ray and electron beam therapy of the rectum and bilat eral inguinal lymph nodes through four stationary fields
    13.5 MV X-rays: FSD 100 cm
    13.5 MeV electrons: FSD 100 cm
    Ventral fields: 30% X-rays, 70% electrons
                field size 10 × 15 cm each
    Dorsal fields: 100% X-rays
                field size 10 × 15 cm each
Water phantom
(Gale and Innes 1960)

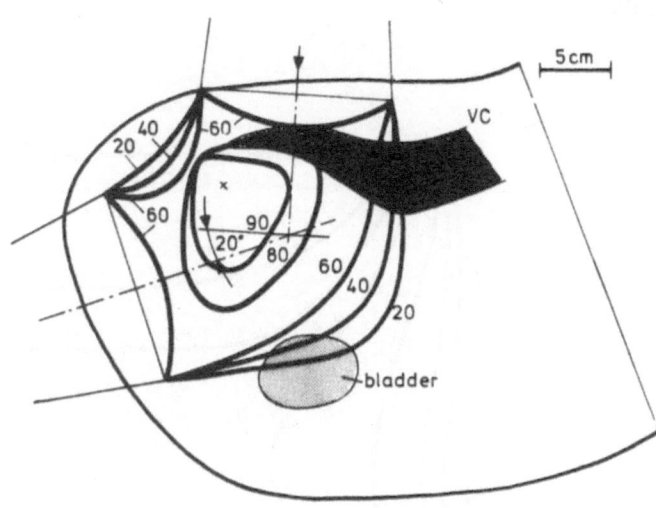

Fig. 191. Electron beam therapy (43 MeV) of the rectum through two stationary fields
    FSD 120 cm
    field size 14 × 10 cm each
    Polystyrene phantom
    (Scherer et al. 1972)

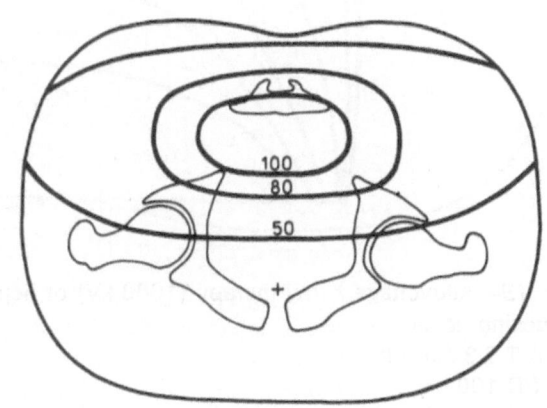

Fig. 192. One-centre two-arc eccentric irradiation of the rectum with 35 MeV electrons
    FAD 120 cm
    axis depth 16 cm in the
        midline
    arcs 60° (±30°/±90°)
    tilt of central beam
      ±5 cm on the surface
    field size 8 × 16 cm
    Alderson–Rando phantom
    (Heuss and Hoeffken
      1972)

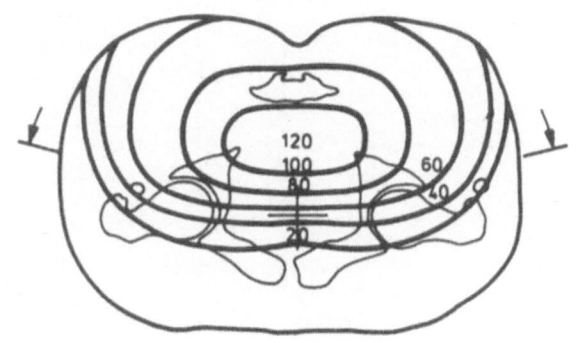

Fig. 193. Arc therapy of the rectum with 35 MeV electrons
    FAD 120 cm
    axis depth 12 cm
    arc: 150° (+75°/−75°)
    field size 5 × 14 cm at axis
    Alderson–Rando phantom
    (Klein et al. 1971)

Liver

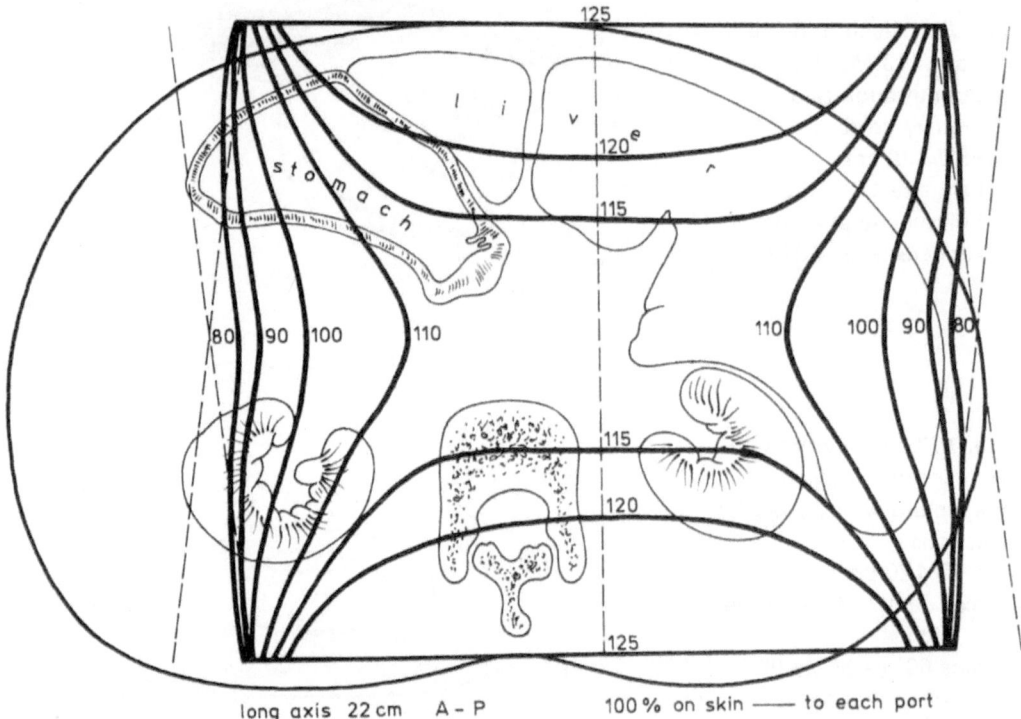

Fig. 194. Kilovoltage X-ray therapy (1000 kV) of hepatic metastases through two opposing fields
   HVT 3.8 mm Pb
   FSD 100 cm
   field size 20 × 24 cm each
   (Phillips et al. 1954)

Female genital organs

Uterine cervix

Parametrium

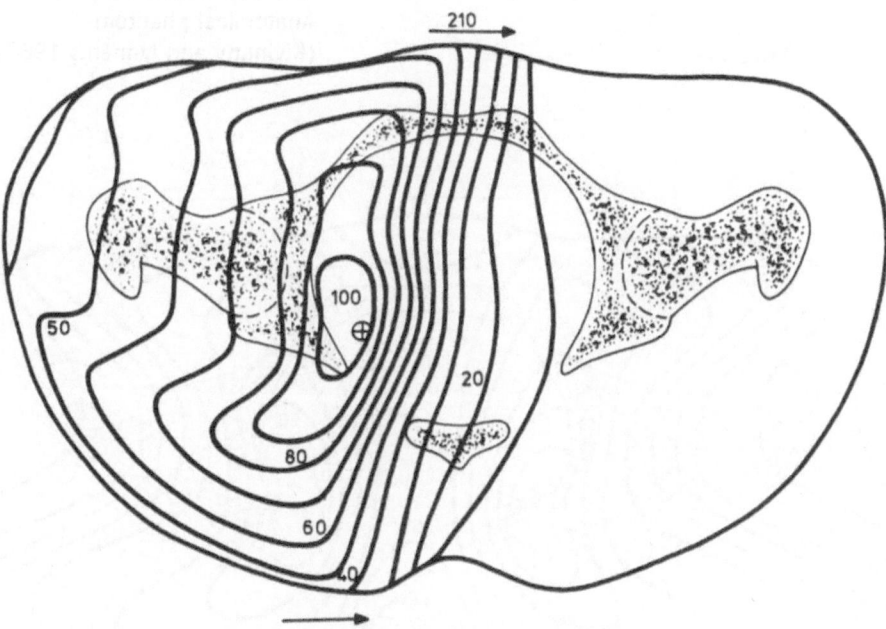

Fig. 195. Convergent beam arc (210°) therapy of the left parametrium with kilovoltage X-rays (200 kV)
   Filter 2 mm Cu
   FAD 50 cm
   axis depth 4 cm laterally from the median
   angle of convergence 60°
   field size 3.5 × 7 cm
   Plexiglas–water–bone phantom
   (Spechter 1962)

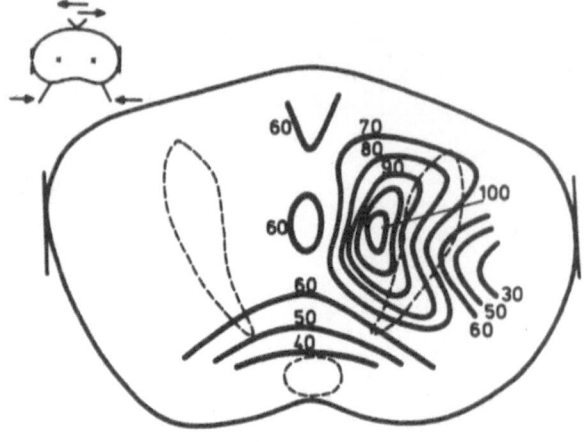

Fig. 196. Two-arc (200° each) irradiation of the parametrium with kilovoltage X-rays (250 kV)
  HVT 1.2 mm Cu
  FAD 50 cm
  axis depth 4.5 cm laterally from the midline
  angle of convergence 60°
  field size 3.5 × 7 cm
  Anatomical phantom
  (Kiviniitty and Unnérus 1968)

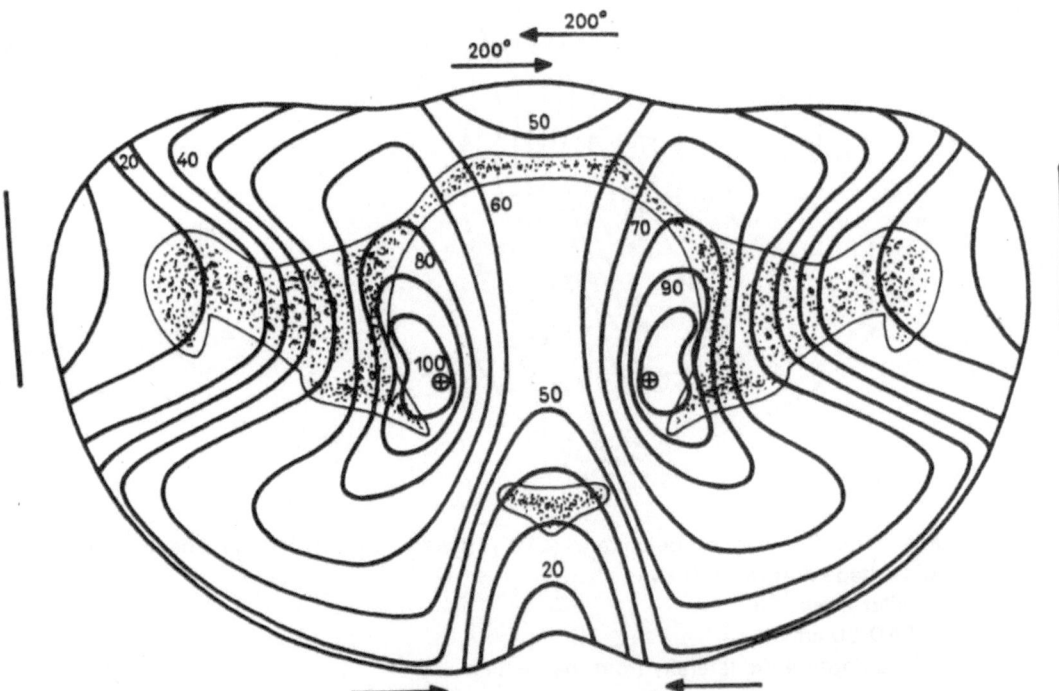

Fig. 197. Two-arc therapy of the parametrium with kilovoltage X-rays (200 kV). Neck of the femur shielded with lead blocks
  HVT 0.7 mm Cu, filter 0.2 mm Cu
  FAD 50 cm
  axis depth 11.5 cm
  two 200° arcs
  angle of convergence 60°
  field size 2.5 × 7 cm
  Plexiglas–water–bone phantom
  (Spechter 1957)

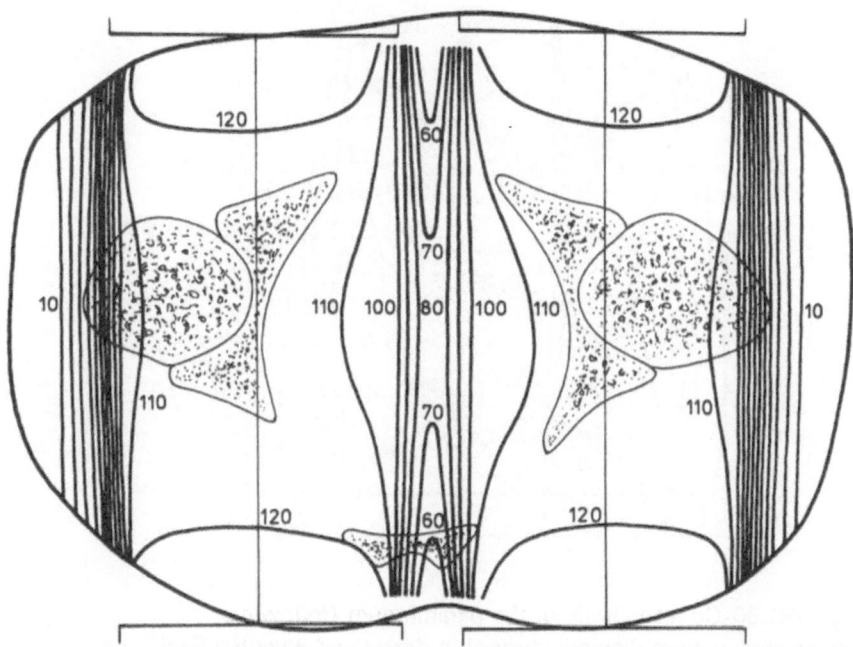

Fig. 198. 60-Co teletherapy of the parametrium through two dorsal and two ventral fields
   SSD 80 cm
   field size 10 × 15 cm
   Calculated isodoses
   (Nowakowski 1968)

Fig. 199. 60-Co teletherapy of the parametrium through two ventral and two dorsal fields
   SSD 50 cm
   field size
      6 × 14 cm each
   tilt of central
      beam 5° laterally
      for each
   Paraffin phantom
   (Frischkorn 1962)

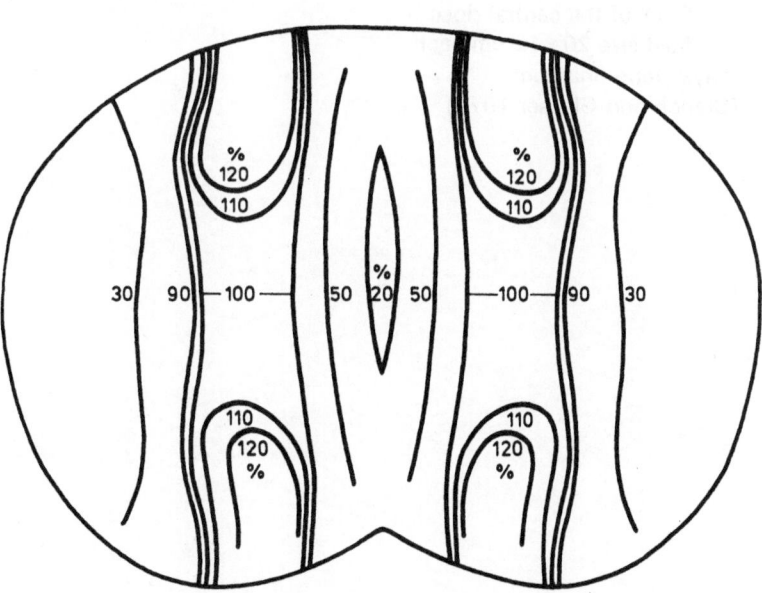

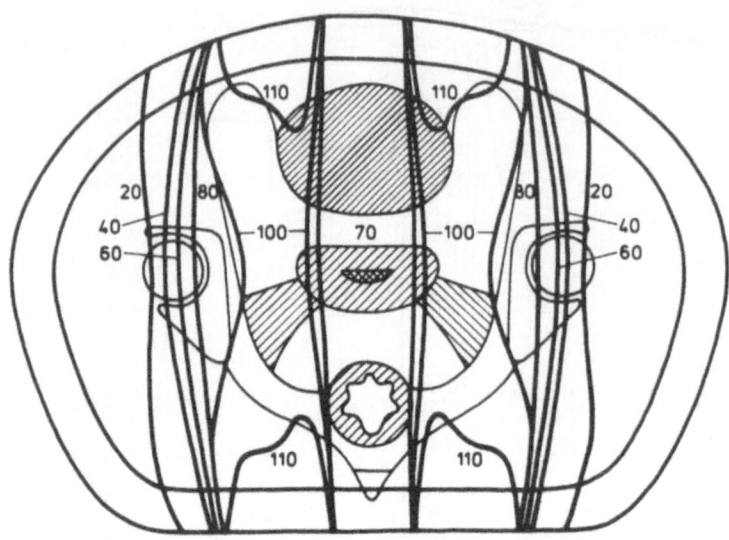

Fig. 200. 60-Co teletherapy of the parametrium (following intracavitary radium therapy) through a dorsal and a ventral field
SSD 60 cm

I. dorsal and ventral lower abdominal fields with 6/11 of the central dose
field size 20 × 12 cm each

II. dorsal and ventral lower abdominal fields, centre of the fields shielded with uranium blocks placed on a satellite platform close to the source (3 × 3 × 12.8 cm)
5/11 of the central dose
field size 20 × 12 cm each

Polystyrene phantom
(Stauch and Glaeser 1972)

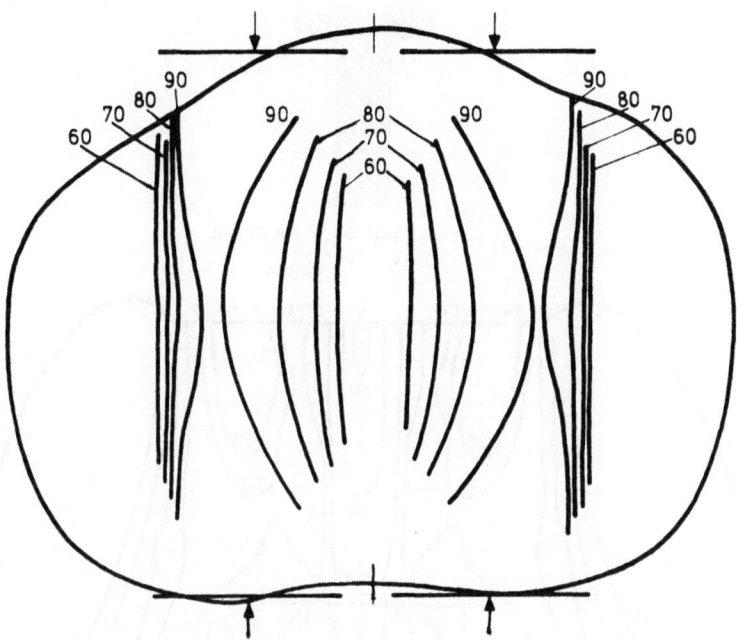

Fig. 201. 60-Co teletherapy of the parametrium through two ventral
and two dorsal wedge filtered fields
  SSD 50 cm
  field size 8 × 9 cm each
  wedges 5.5 cm wide, the thickest part measuring 1.5 cm
  Anatomical phantom
  (Kiviniitty and Unnérus 1968)

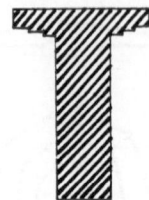

4 cm split at 10 cm depth

½ 45° wedges

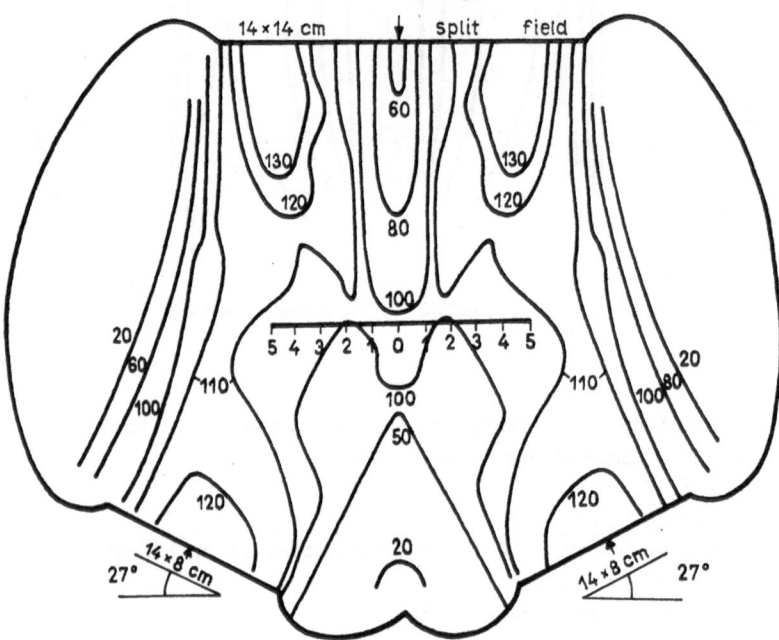

Fig. 202. 60-Co teletherapy of the parametrium for carcinoma of the uterine cervix, combined with intracavitary radium therapy. Split field technique with a ventral and two dorsal fields

SSD 60 cm

Ventral field: shielding of the centre with lead
field size 14 × 14 cm (split field)
central beam tilted 10° downwards
45° half-wedges

Dorsal fields: field size 8 × 14 cm each

Water phantom

(Fletcher 1962)

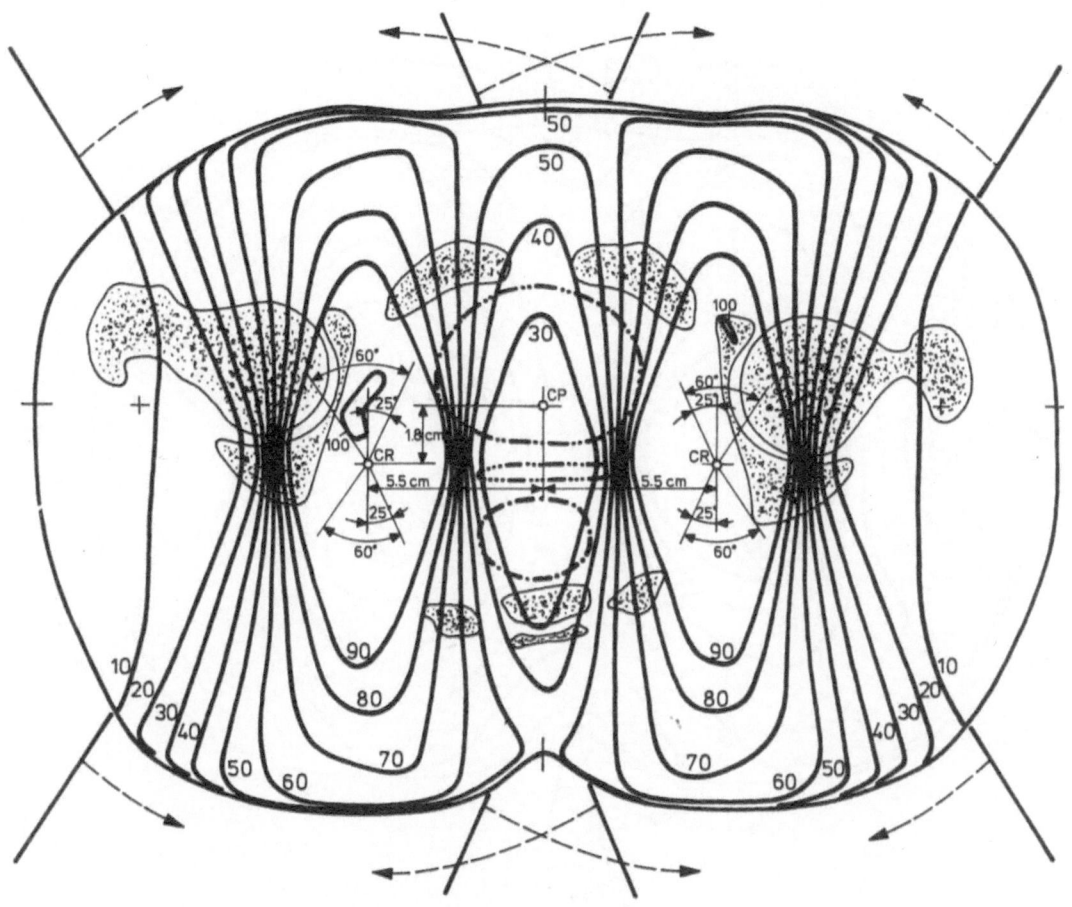

Fig. 203. Two-centre four-arc 60-Co therapy of the parametrium
  SAD 60 cm
  distance of axes 11 cm
  four 60° arcs
  field size 5 × 15 cm
  Alderson–Rando phantom
  (Brizel et al. 1963)

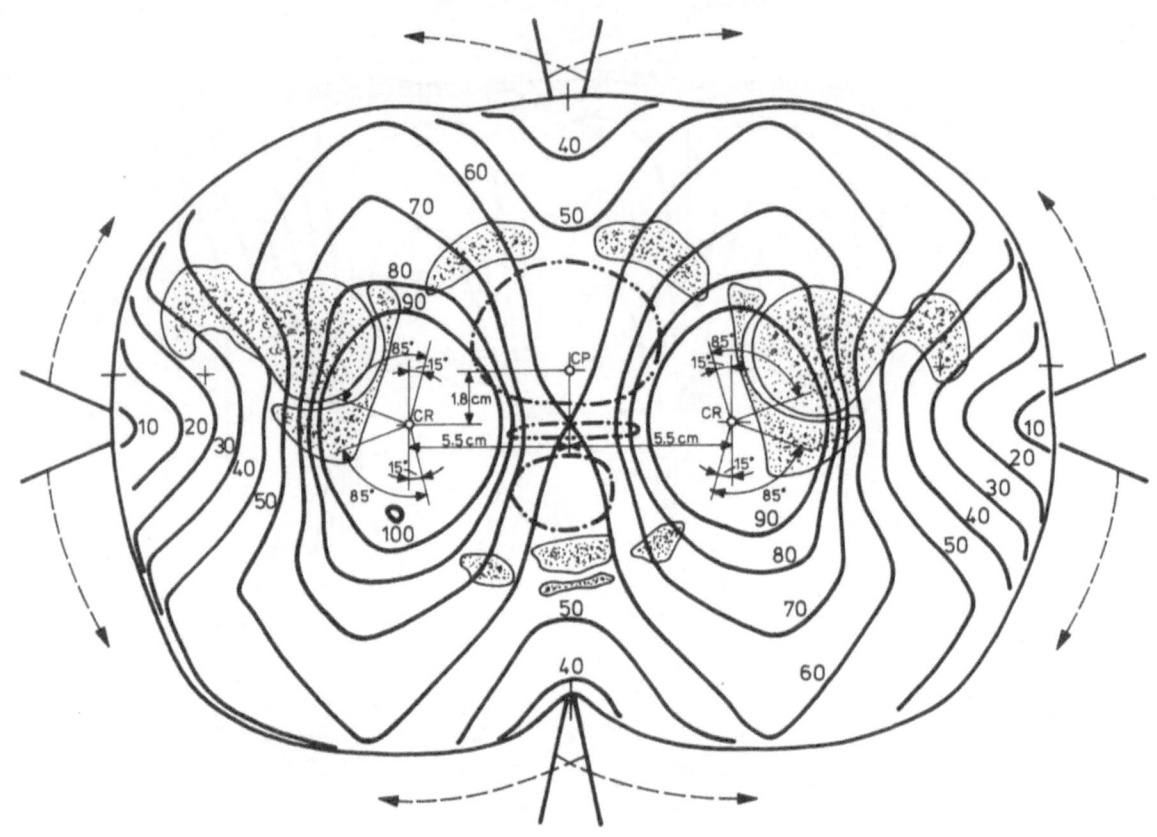

Fig. 204. Two-centre four-arc 60-Co therapy of the parametrium
   SAD 60 cm
   distance of axes 11 cm
   four 85° arcs
   field size 7 × 15 cm
   Alderson–Rando phantom
   (Brizel et al. 1963)

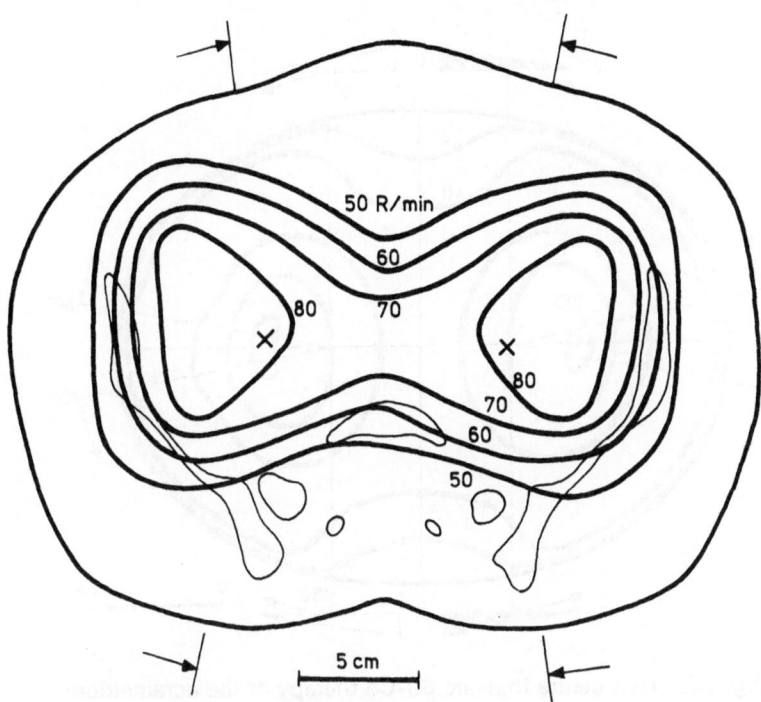

Fig. 205. Two-centre two-arc (160°) 60-Co therapy of the parametrium
SAD 65 cm
axes 5 cm on both
  sides of the midline
field size 6 × 10 cm on the surface
Anatomical phantom
(Kiviniitty and Unnérus 1968)

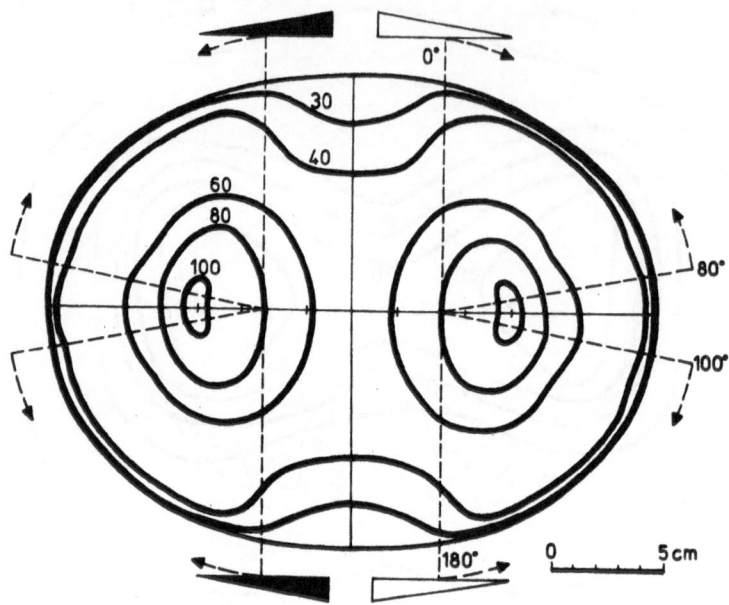

Fig. 206. Two-centre four-arc 60-Co therapy of the parametrium
SAD 60 cm
distance of axes 8 cm
four 80° arcs
field size 6 × 14 cm
17.5° lead wedges
Plexiglas phantom
(Kuttig et al. 1968)

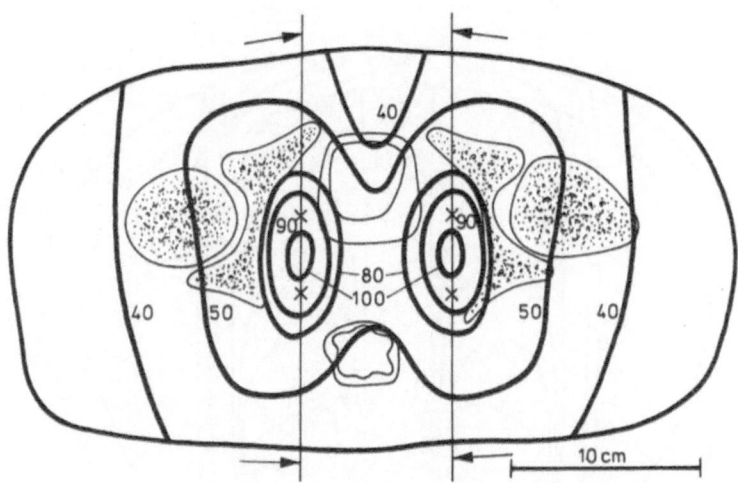

Fig. 207. Four-centre 60-Co teletherapy of the parametrium
  SAD 55 cm
  distance of axes
    8 cm horizontally
    4 cm vertically
  four 180° arcs
  field size 4 × 15 cm at axis
  (Welker and Eichhorn 1972*b*)

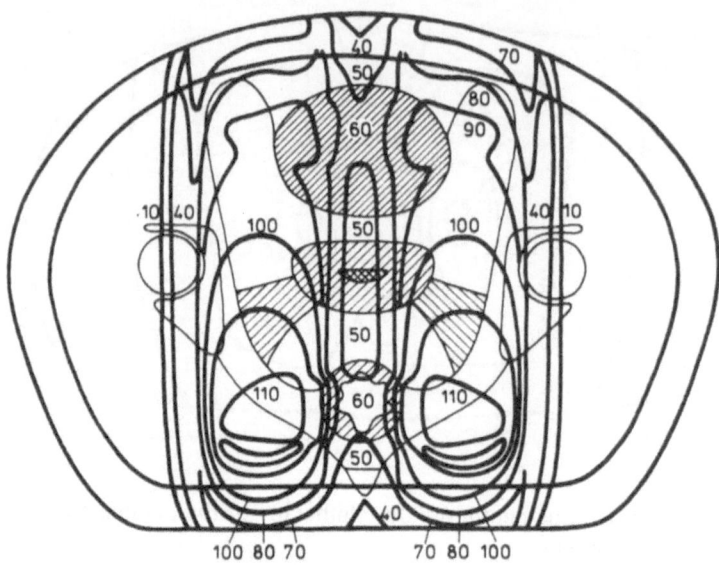

Fig. 208. High-energy X-ray (43 MV) therapy of the parametrium
through stationary fields (following intracavitary radium treatment)
  FSD 100 cm
  opposing ventral and dorsal lower abdominal fields
      with 50% of the focal dose
      field size 6 × 12 cm each
  dorsal parametrial fields with 50% of the focal dose
      field size 6 × 12 cm each
  Polystyrene phantom
  (Stauch and Glaeser 1972)

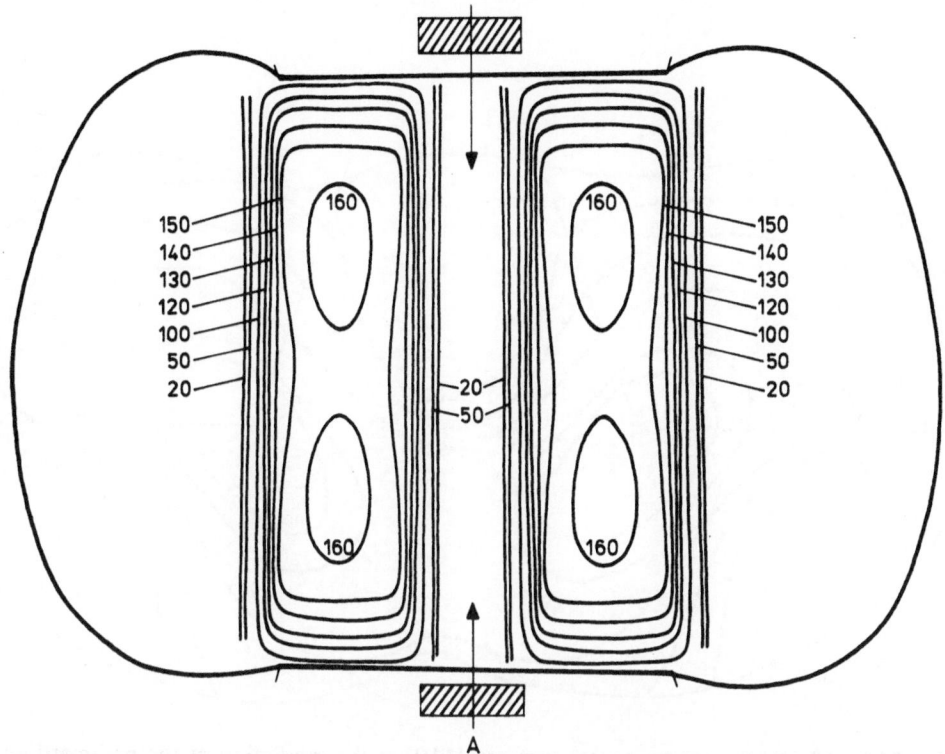

Fig. 209. Irradiation of the parametrium with 22 MV X-rays through opposing ventral and dorsal fields with central lead shielding
FSD 100 cm
field size 15 × 15 cm each (split field with 4 cm lead blocks)
Water phantom
(Fletcher 1962)

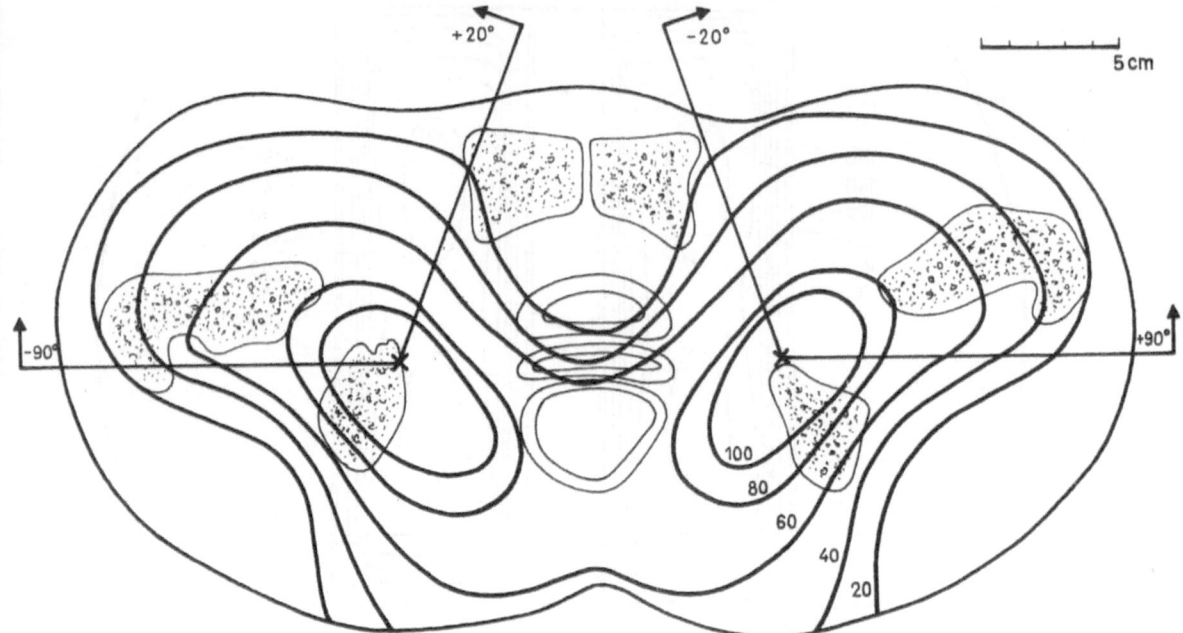

Fig. 210a. 42 MV X-ray two-centre two-arc (110° each) irradiation of the parametrium and pelvic lymph nodes. Axes cranially converging (cross-section at the level of the middle of the vagina)

    FAD 120 cm
    axis depth 9 cm from ventral
    distance of axes 13.2 cm
    field size 4 × 14 cm at axis
    Alderson–Rando phantom

Treatment planning: due to the 20° tilt of the central beam, the originally 10 cm distance
    of the axes becomes 13.2 cm at the caudal end and 5 cm at the cranial end. Axis depth
    9 cm from ventral corresponding to the parametrial level of the phantom
    (Németh et al. 1973*a*)

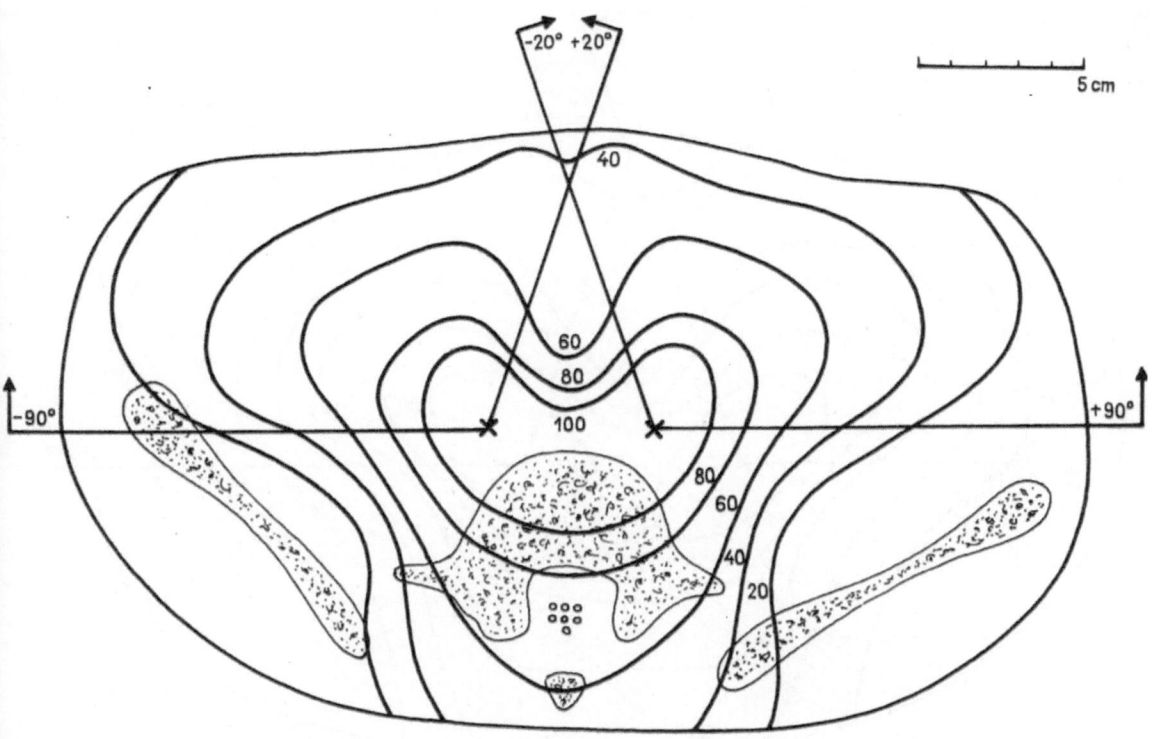

Fig. 210b. High-energy two-centre two-arc X-ray treatment of the parametrium and pelvic lymph nodes. Axes cranially converging (cross-section at the level of the middle of the uterus)
    axis depth 11 cm from ventral
    distance of axes 10 cm
    For treatment planning and other parameters see Fig. 210a
    (Németh et al. 1973a)

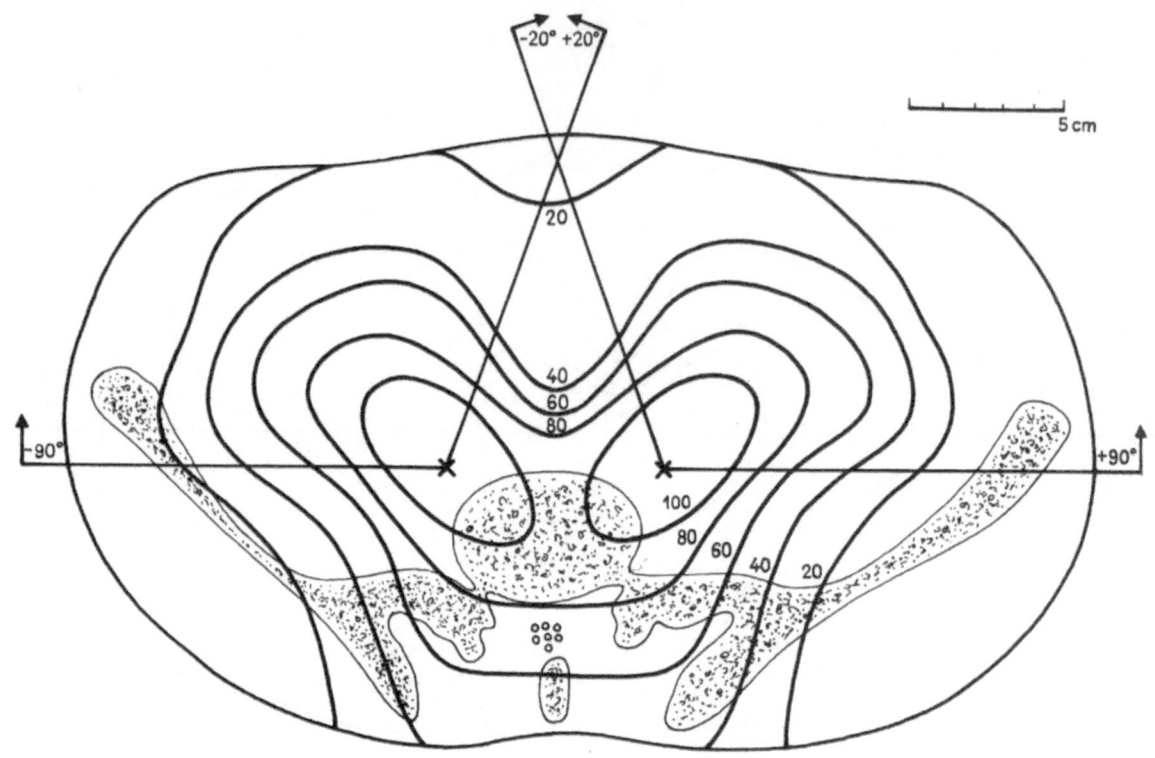

Fig. 210c. High-energy two-centre two-arc X-ray treatment of the parametrium and pelvic lymph nodes. Axes cranially converging (cross-section at the level of the upper end of the sacrum below the promontory)

    axis depth 10 cm from ventral

    distance of axes 7 cm

    For treatment planning and other parameters see Fig. 210a

    (Németh et al. 1973*a*)

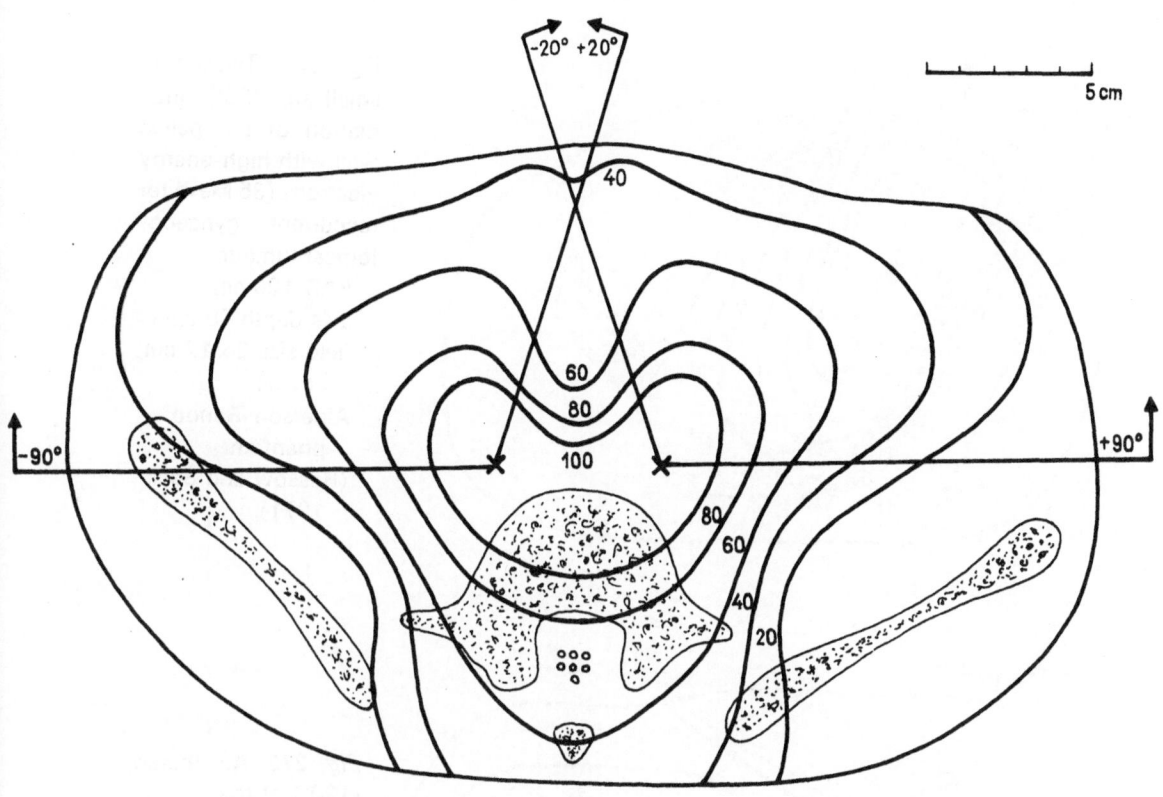

Fig. 210d. High-energy two-centre two-arc X-ray treatment of the parametrium and pelvic
lymph nodes. Cranially convergent axes (cross-section at the level of aortic bifurcation)
    axis depth 9 cm from ventral
    distance of axes 5 cm
    For treatment planning and other parameters see Fig. 210a
    (Németh et al. 1973*a*)

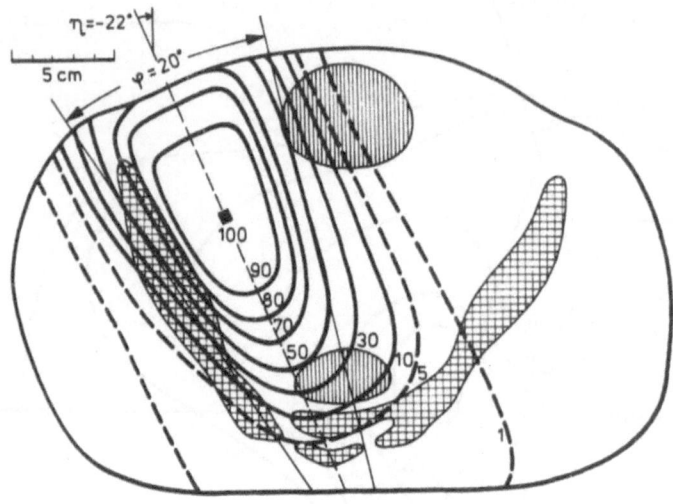

Fig. 211. Telecentric small-arc (20°) irradiation of the pelvic wall with high-energy electrons (35 MeV) for reccurrent gynaecological tumour
    FAD 120 cm
    axis depth 30 cm
    field size 3 × 12 cm
      at axis
    Alderson–Rando
      phantom
(Rassow and Sack 1971)

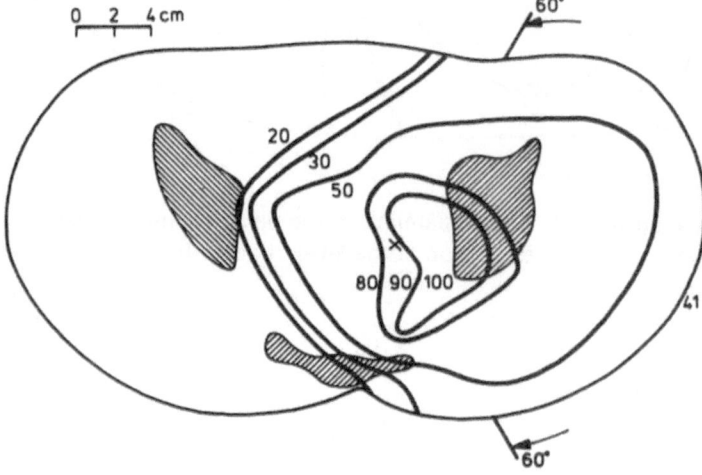

Fig. 212. Arc therapy (120°) of the parametrium with 42 MeV electrons
    FAD 120 cm
    axis depth 16 cm
    field size 8 × 14 cm
      at axis
    Alderson–Rando
      phantom
(Fehrentz et al. 1969)

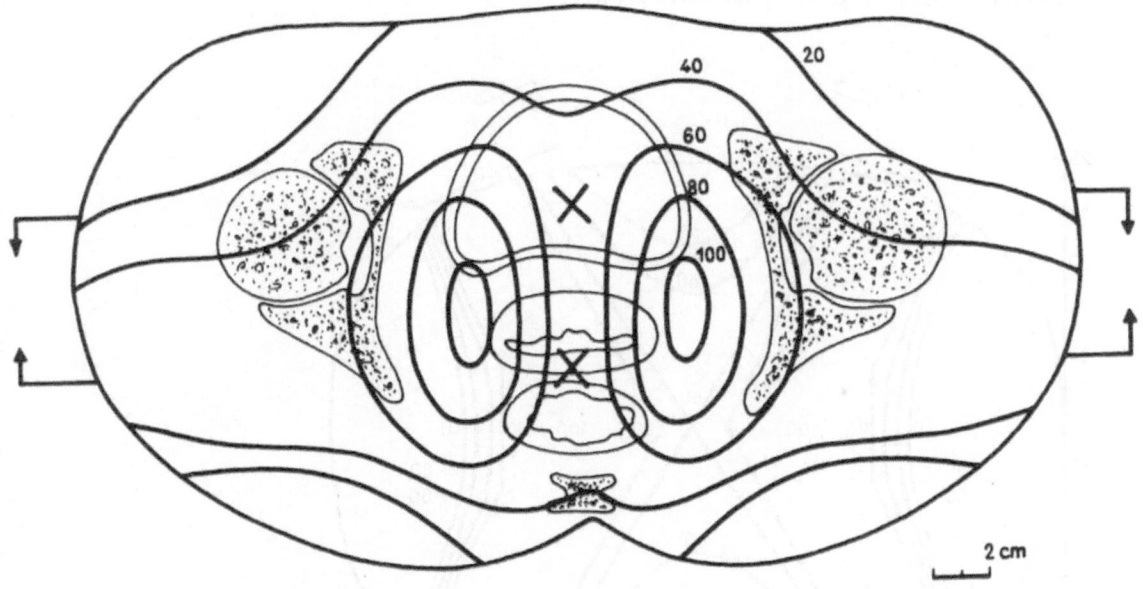

Fig. 213. Two-centre two-arc irradiation of the parametrium with 42 MeV electrons using a shutter tube (see Fig. 106b)

  FAD 120 cm
  distance of axes 6 cm
  two 180° arcs
  field size 7.5 × 16 cm
  Alderson–Rando phantom
  (Németh et al. 1973*b*)

Uterine cervix and parametrium

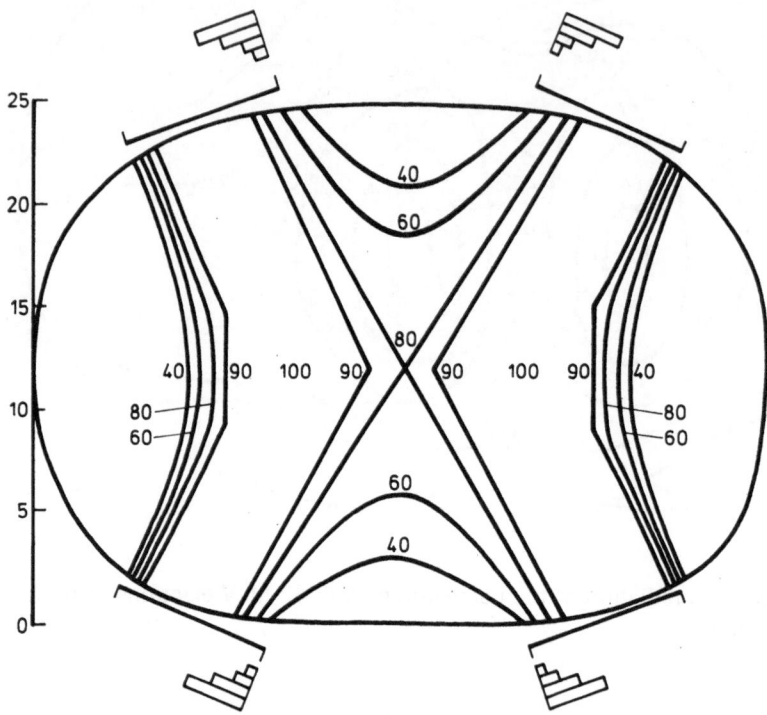

Fig. 214. 60-Co teletherapy of carcinoma of the uterine cervix through four oblique stationary fields (pre- and postoperative irradiation)

    SSD 50 cm

    field size 8 × 14 cm

    compensating filter consisting of four lead blocks each measuring
      5 mm in thickness

    angle of incidence of central beams 20°

    Paraffin–bone phantom

    (Frischbier and Kuttig 1964)

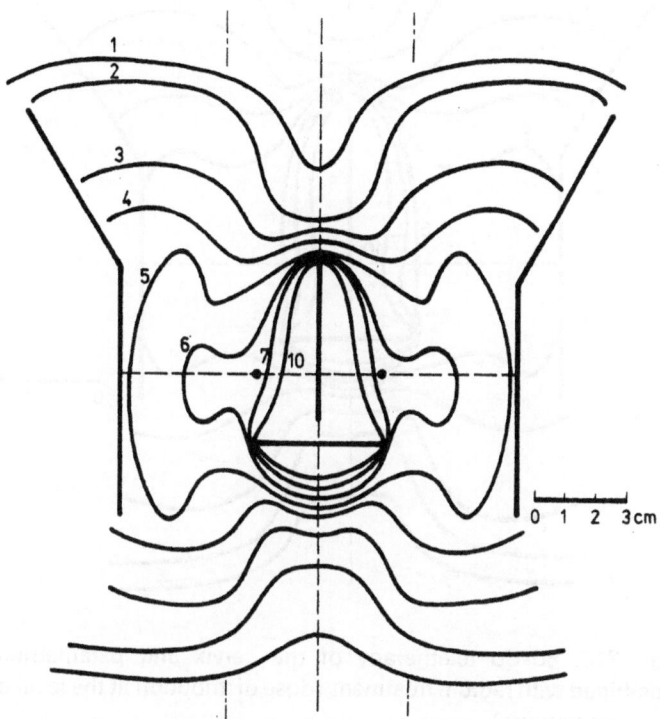

Fig. 215. 60-Co teletherapy of the cervix and parametrium combined with radium treatment (dose distribution at the level of the parametrium)

60-Co: SSD 50 cm

depth of focus 10 cm

field size 6 × 15 cm each (two ventral and two dorsal stationary fields)

distance of fields 6 cm on the surface

3.5° tilt of the central beam laterally (beam is perpendicular at the medial edge of the field)

4000 R per parametrium

Radium: 5000 mg-hrs (90 mg intrauterine tube and 130 mg intravaginal plate)

Plexiglas–water phantom

(Frischbier and Seifert 1965)

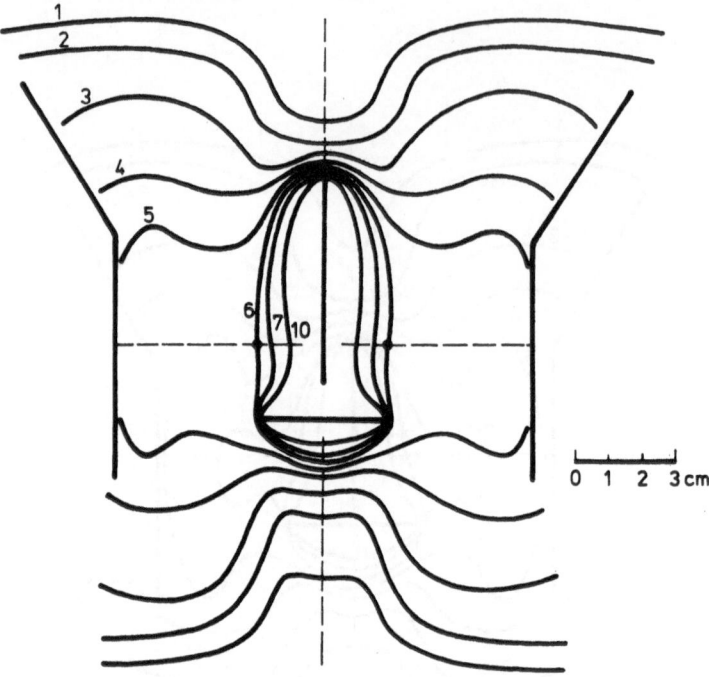

Fig. 216. 60-Co teletherapy of the cervix and parametrium combined with radium treatment (dose distribution at the level of the parametrium)

  60-Co: SSD 50 cm
        depth of focus 10 cm
        field size 8 × 15 cm (two ventral and two dorsal
           stationary fields. Beam is perpendicular at the medial
           edge of the field
        4000 R per parametrium
  Radium: 5000 mg-hrs (120 mg intrauterine tube, 90 mg
           intravaginal plate)
Plexiglas–water phantom
(Frischbier and Seifert 1965)

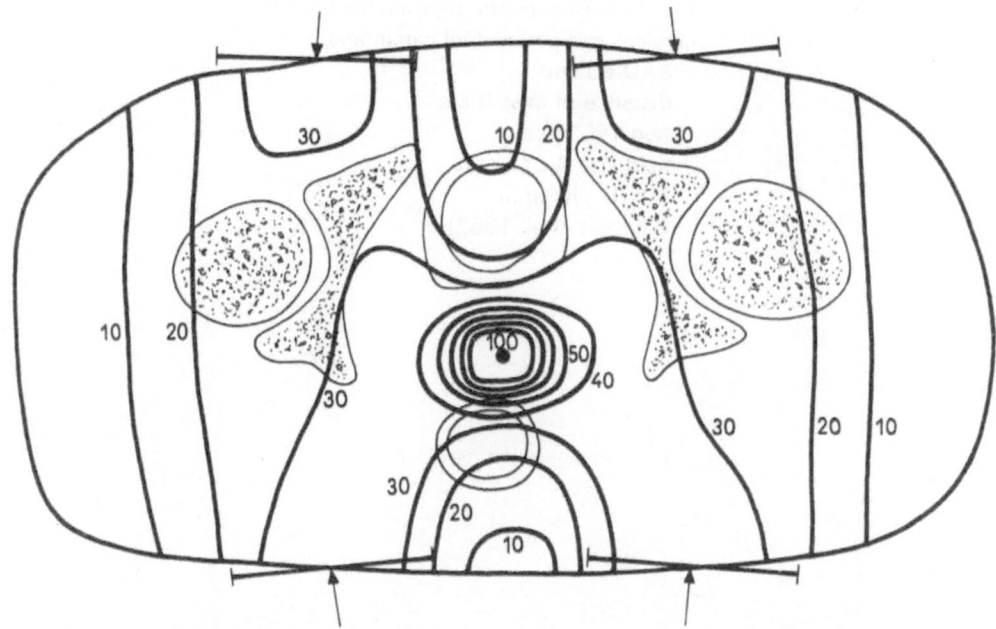

Fig. 217. 60-Co teletherapy of the cervix and parametrium combined with radium treatment
60-Co: SSD 55 cm
field size 8 × 15 cm each (two ventral and two dorsal stationary fields)
central beams tilted 4° laterally
Radium:140 mg-hrs (90 mg intrauterine tube, 50 mg intravaginal plate)
42.8 h insertion
(Welker and Eichhorn 1972*b*)

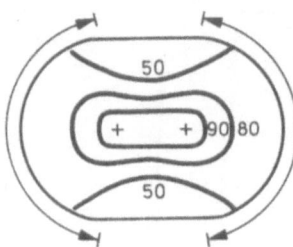

Fig. 218. Two-centre two-arc 60-Co therapy of cervical and parametrial carcinoma
    SAD 60 cm
    distance of axes 8 cm
    two 160° arcs
    field size 8 × 12 cm
    Mix-D phantom
    (Gietzelt et al. 1962)

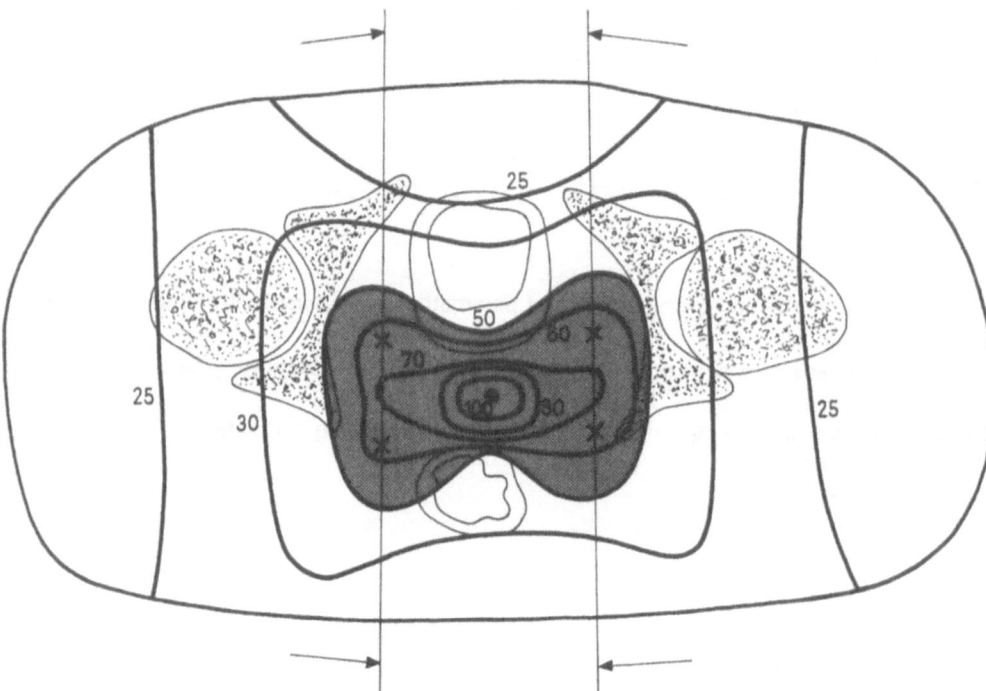

Fig. 219. Combined four-centre 60-Co arc (4 × 180°) therapy and radium treatment of carcinoma of the cervix and parametrium
    SAD 55 cm
    distance of axes 8 cm horizontal
                4 cm vertical
    field size 4 × 15 cm at axis
    Calculated isodoses
    (Welker and Eichhorn 1972*b*)

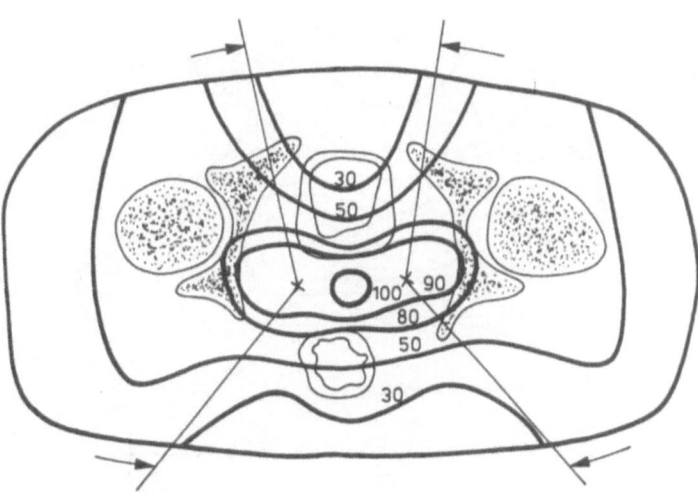

Fig. 220. Two-centre two-arc (130° both) 60-Co irradiation of the cervix and parametrium
    SAD 55 cm
       distance of axes 6 cm
       field size 6 × 15 cm at axis
    Calculated isodoses
    (Welker and Eichhorn 1972*b*)

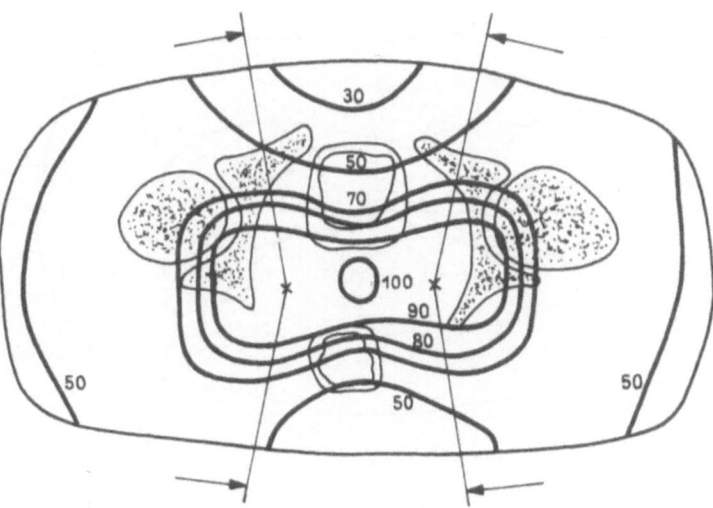

Fig. 221. Two-centre two-arc (160° each) 60-Co teletherapy of the cervix and parametrium
    SAD 55 cm
       distance of axes 8 cm
       field size 8 × 15 cm at axis
    Calculated isodoses
    (Welker and Eichhorn 1972*b*)

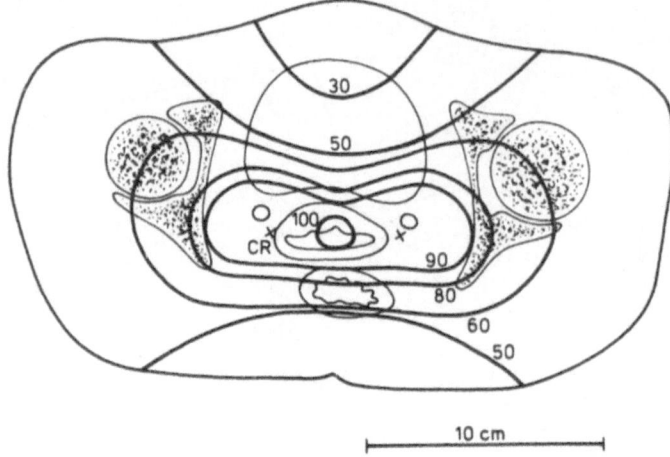

Fig. 222. Two-centre
two-arc (130° each)
60-Co teletherapy of a
carcinoma of the cervix
and parametrium
  SAD 55 cm
  distance of axes 7 cm
  field size 7 × 10 cm
    at axis
  (Richter and
    Schirrmeister 1965)

10 cm

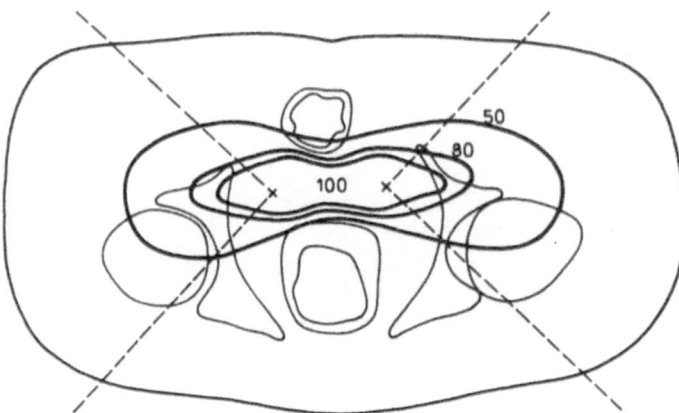

Fig. 223. Two-centre
two-arc (90° each)
60-Co irradiation of a
carcinoma of the cervix
and parametrium
  SAD 55 cm
  distance of axes 6 cm
  field size 4 × 15 cm
    at axis
  (Matschke and Welker
    1963)

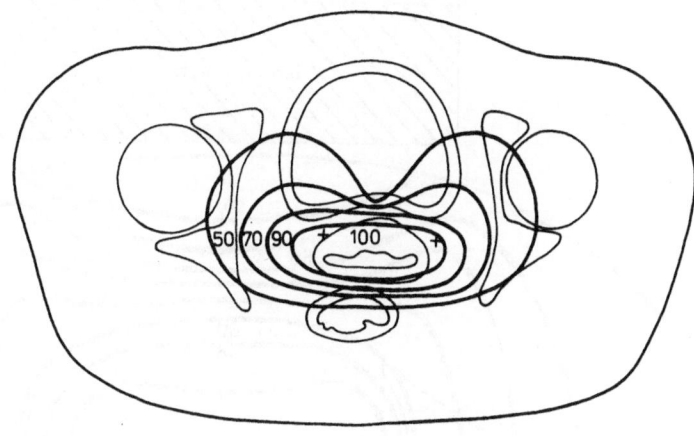

Fig. 224. Two-centre two-arc (125° each) 60-Co irradiation of a carcinoma of the cervix and parametrium
   SAD 55 cm
   distance of axes 5 cm
   field size 5 × 15 cm
   Calculated isodoses
   (Welker 1965)

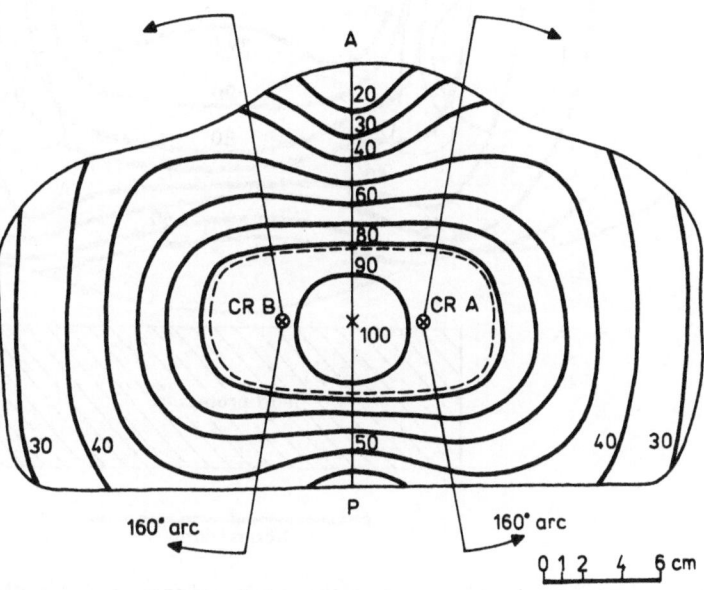

Fig. 225. Two-centre two-arc 60-Co irradiation of a cervical and parametrial carcinoma
   SAD 60 cm
   two 160° (10°/170°) arcs
   axis depth 11 cm from ventral
   distance of axes 8 cm
   field size 10 × 15 cm
   Calculated isodoses
   (Howarth and Wilson 1961)

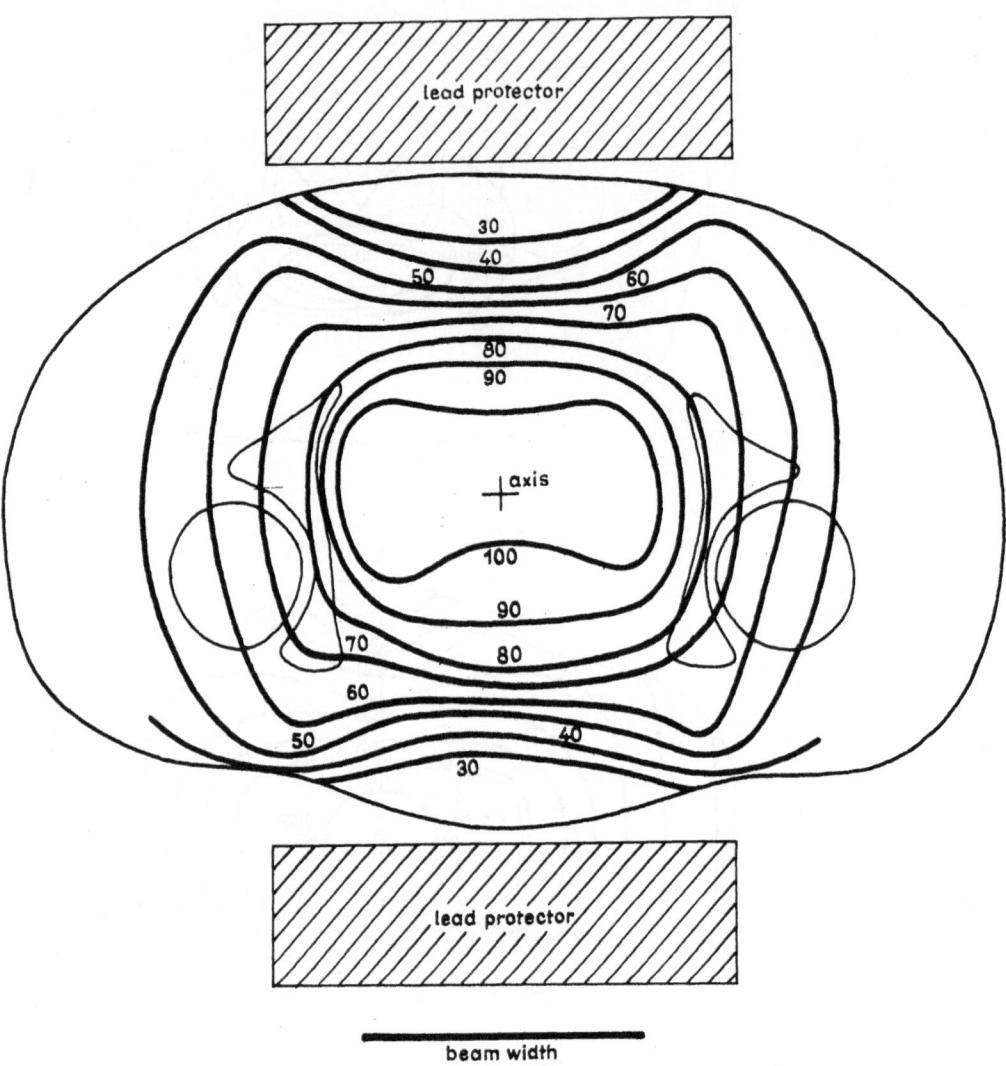

Fig. 226. Rotation (360°) therapy of the cervix and parametrium with 2 MV X-rays (bladder and rectum protected with lead blocks of 18 cm length anteriorly and posteriorly)

FAD 110 cm
axis depth 11.8 cm from ventral (in the midline)
field size 13.5 × 15 cm at 100 cm distance
Masonite phantom
(Trump et al. 1951)

Pelvis

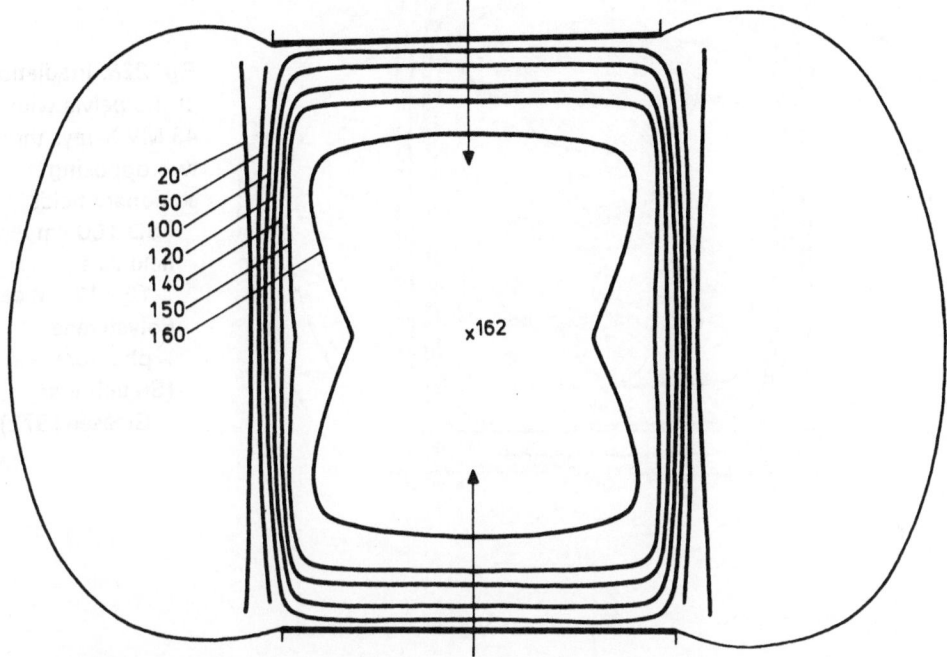

20
50
100
120
140
150
160

x162

Fig. 227. Irradiation of the pelvis with 22 MV X-rays through two opposing stationary fields
    FSD 100 cm
    field size 15 × 15 cm each
    Water phantom
    (Fletcher 1962)

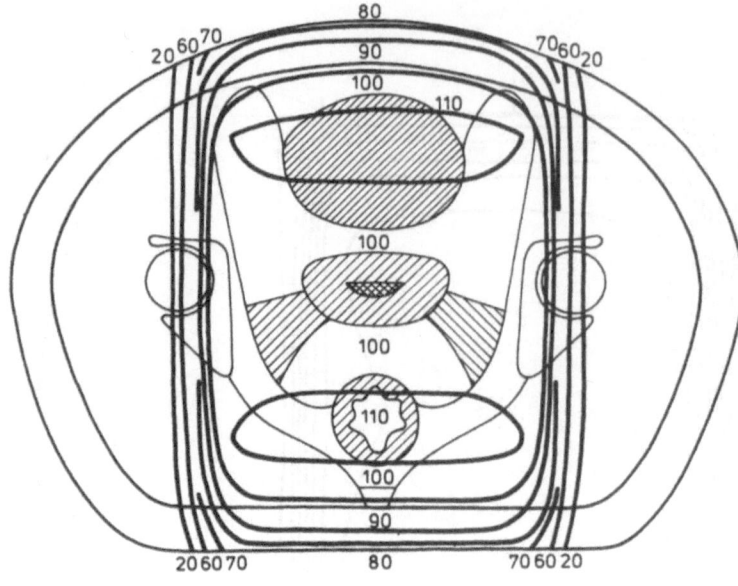

Fig. 228. Irradiation
of the pelvis with
43 MV X-rays through
two opposing
stationary fields
    FSD 100 cm
    field size
       16 × 12 cm each
    Polystyrene
      phantom
    (Stauch and
      Glaeser 1972)

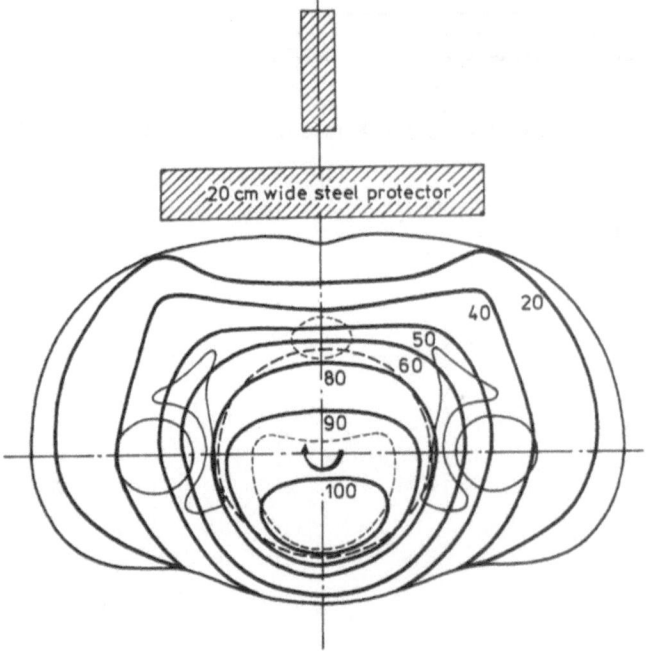

Fig. 229. Rotation
(360°) therapy of the
pelvis with 2 MV
X-rays (20 cm wide
lead protection
dorsally)
    FAD125 cm
    axis depth 9.5 cm
      from ventral
      in the midline
    field size 13 × 15 cm
      at axis
    Masonite phantom
    (Trump et al.
      1954)

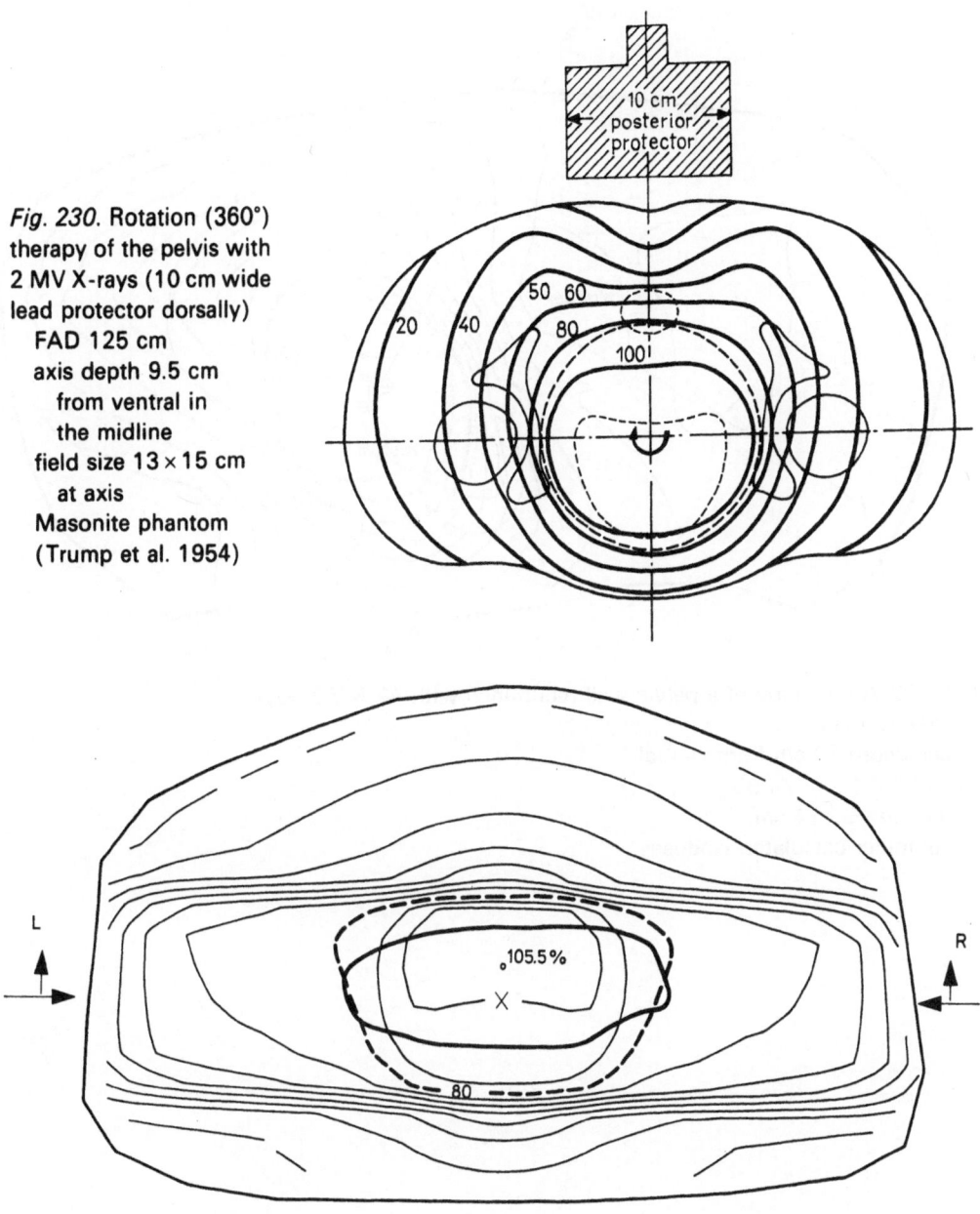

Fig. 230. Rotation (360°) therapy of the pelvis with 2 MV X-rays (10 cm wide lead protector dorsally)
 FAD 125 cm
 axis depth 9.5 cm
  from ventral in
  the midline
 field size 13 × 15 cm
  at axis
 Masonite phantom
 (Trump et al. 1954)

Fig. 231. Irradiation of the pelvis with 42 MV X-rays. Combination of arc therapy with two lateral isocentric stationary fields)
 FAD and focus-isocentre distance 120 cm
 axis depth 10 cm from ventral in the midline
 arc 180° (90°/90°)
 loading 2 :1 :1
 field size 8 × 14 cm each
 Computer calculated isodoses

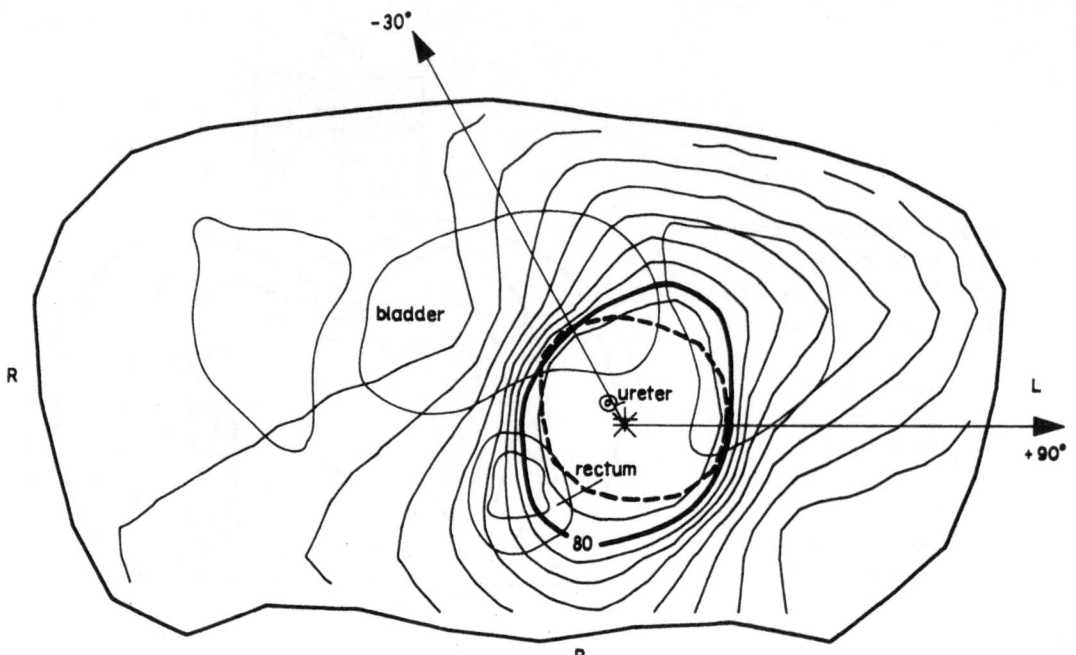

Fig. 232. Arc therapy of a pelvic wall recurrence with 42 MV X-rays
FAD 120 cm
axis depth 10 cm from ventral
arc 120° (−30°/+90°)
field size 6 × 14 cm
Computer calculated isodoses

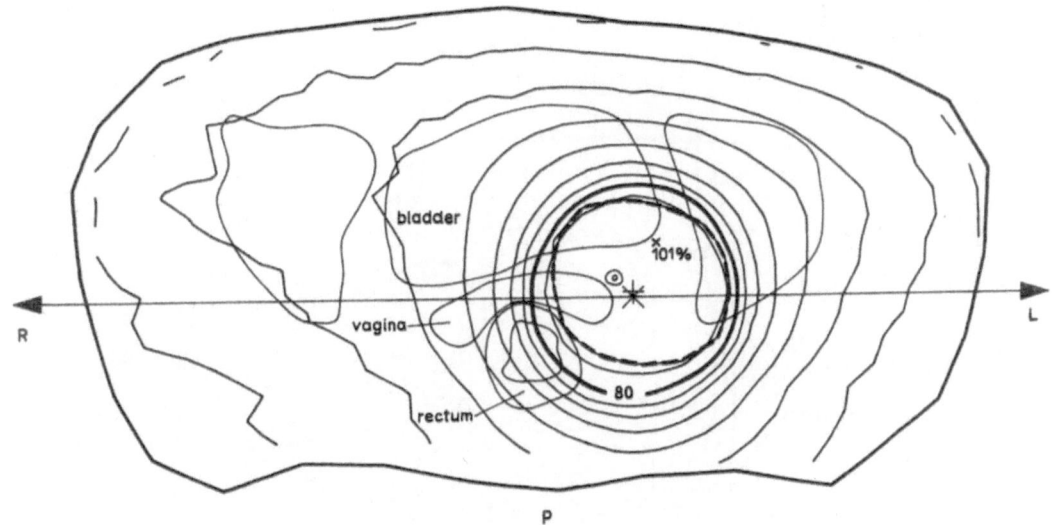

Fig. 233. Arc therapy of a pelvic wall recurrence with 42 MV X-rays
FAD 120 cm
axis depth 10 cm from ventral
arc 180° (90°/90°)
field size 6 × 14 cm
Computer calculated isodoses

Fig. 234. Two-centre
two-arc (120° each)
therapy of the pelvis
using 42 MeV
electrons
FAD 120 cm
axis depth 16 cm
in the midline
field size 8 × 14 cm
Alderson–Rando
phantom
(Fehrentz et al.
1969)

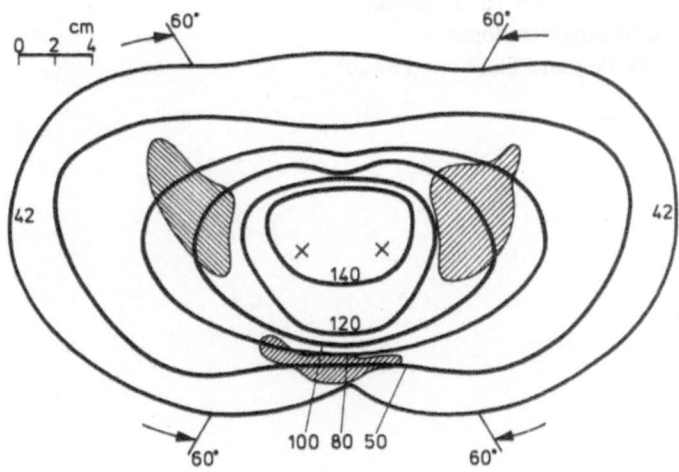

Ovary

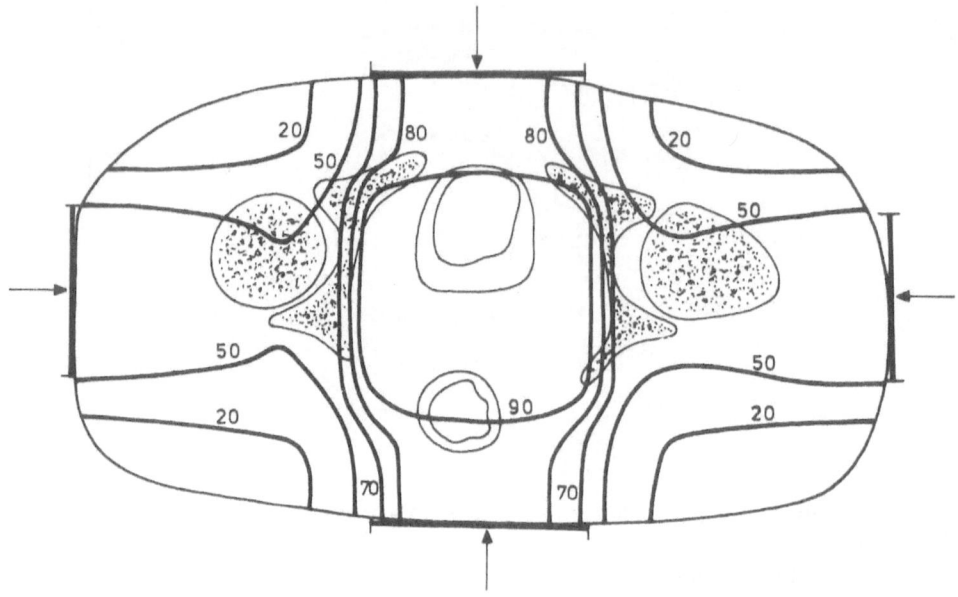

Fig. 235. 60-Co teletherapy of the ovary through four stationary fields
SSD 55 cm
field size 10 × 15 cm ventral and dorsal
        8 × 15 cm lateral
Calculated isodoses
(Welker and Eichhorn 1972*b*)

Fig. 236. 60-Co moving strip irradiation of abdominal metastases of ovarian tumour. *a* Strip fields. *b* Isodoses

SSD 60 cm
width of strips 2.5 cm
Calculated isodoses

Planning of treatment: 1st day — irradiation of first strip through both ventral and dorsal portals. 2nd day — irradiation of strips 1 and 2 through ventral and dorsal portals until strip 1 has received 3000 rads. Strip 1 is then omitted and strip 3 irradiated, etc. Renal shielding at 1500 rads when the height of the kidneys is reached
(Friedman et al. 1970)

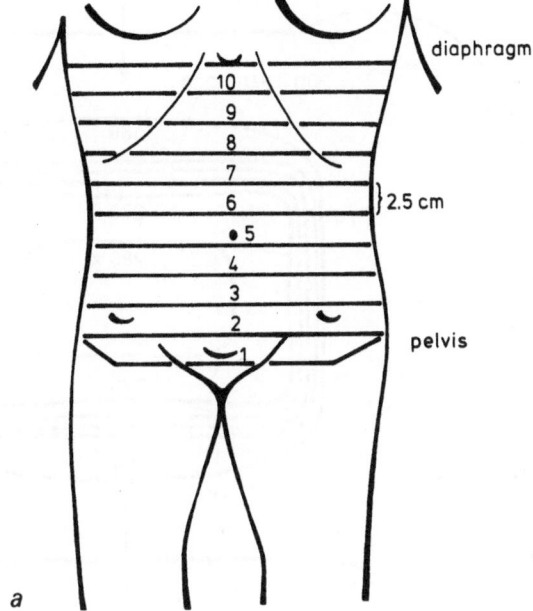

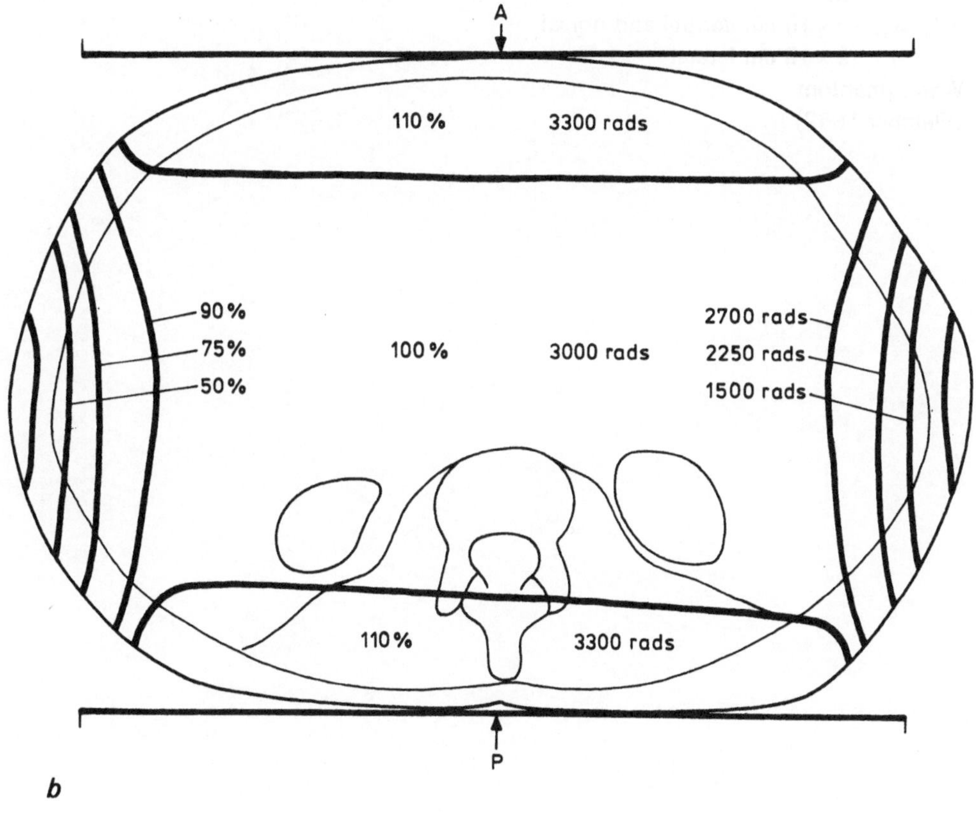

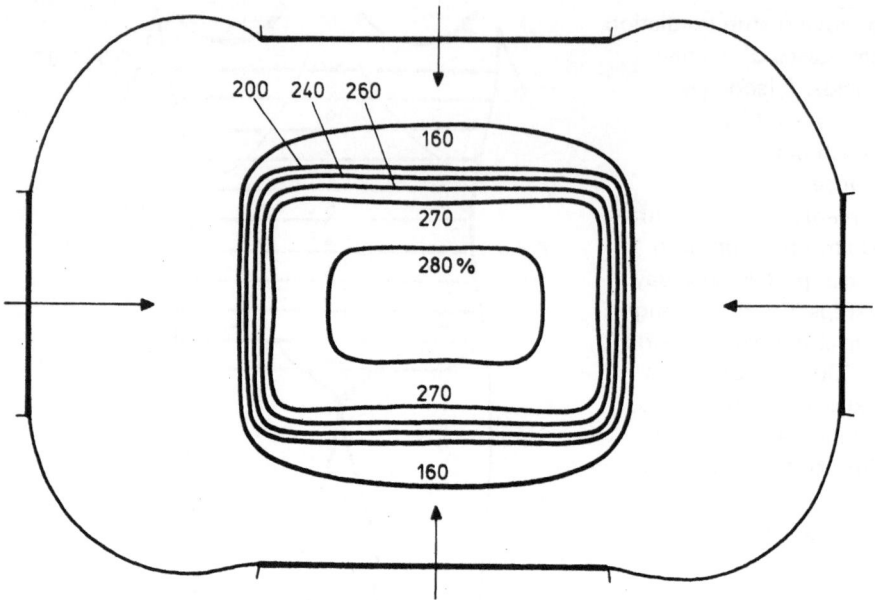

Fig. 237. Irradiation of the ovaries with high-energy X-rays (22 MV) through four stationary fields
   FSD 100 cm
   field size 15 × 15 cm ventral and dorsal
             9 × 15 cm lateral
   Water phantom
   (Fletcher 1962)

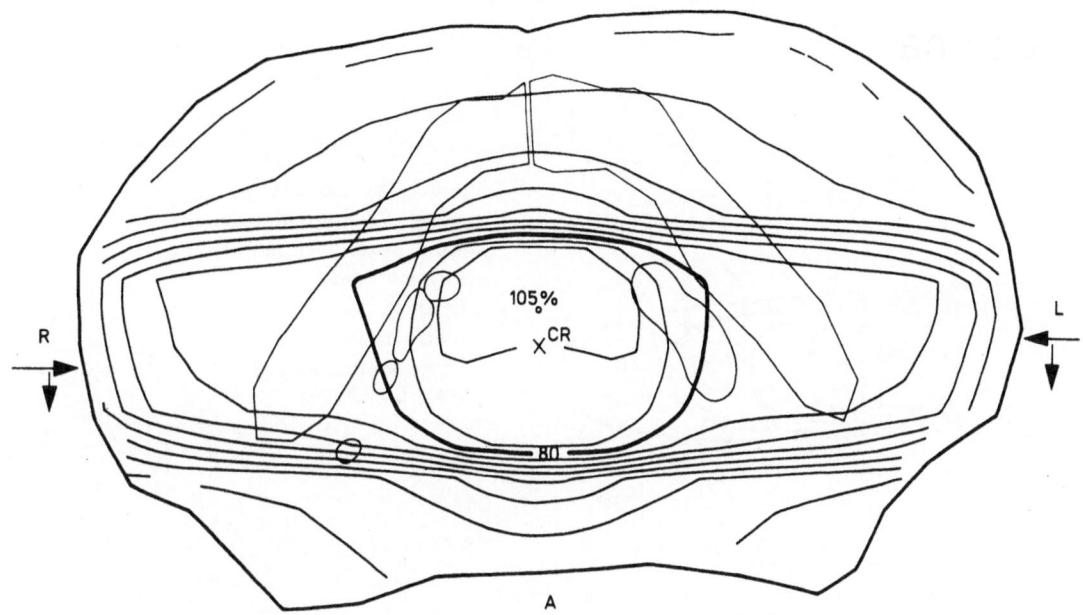

Fig. 238. High-energy X-ray (42 MV) whole pelvis irradiation for inoperable ovarian tumour. Combination of arc therapy and two lateral isocentric stationary fields
  FAD and axis-isocentre distance 120 cm
  arc 180° (90°/90°)
  field size 8 × 14 cm each
  loading 2:1:1

Vagina

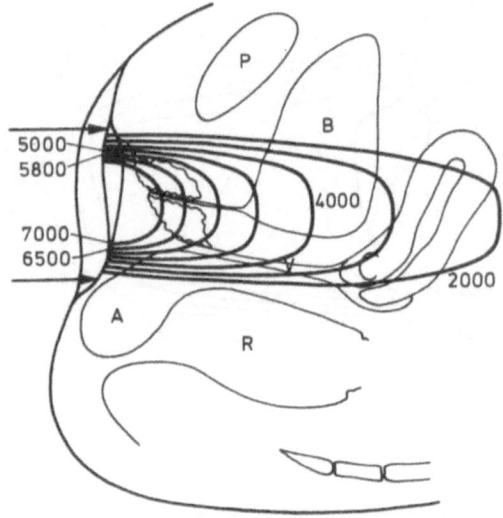

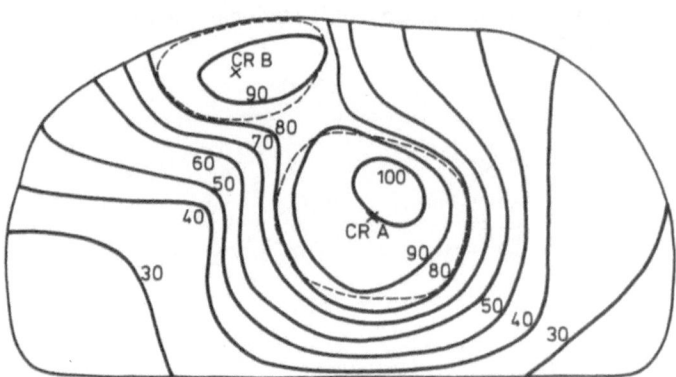

Fig. 239. 60-Co tele-
therapy of a vaginal-vulvar
tumour through a perineal
stationary field
    SSD 80 cm
    field size 6 × 8 cm
    Calculated isodoses
    (Nobler 1972)

Fig. 240. Two-centre four-arc 60-Co irradiation of inguinal
metastases of a vaginal tumour
    SAD 75 cm
    Vagina:
        axis depth 11 cm in the midline
        arcs: right 140° (+30°/+170°)
              left 180° (+10°/−170°)
        field size 10 × 15 cm each
    Metastasis:
        axis depth 2.5 cm under the skin
        arcs: right 60° (+30°/+90°)
              left 60° (−70°/−130°)
        field size 6 × 15 cm
    (Gough 1962)

Vulva

Fig. 241. 60-Co and 137-Cs therapy of the vulva through two stationary fields. 40% of the total dose to the Co field, and 60% to the Cs field
    Vulva:
        137-Cs
        SSD 40 cm
        field size 6 × 8 cm
    Suprasymphyseal field:
        60-Co
        SSD 60 cm
        field size 6 × 6 cm
    Polystyrene phantom
    (Halama and Rassow 1969)

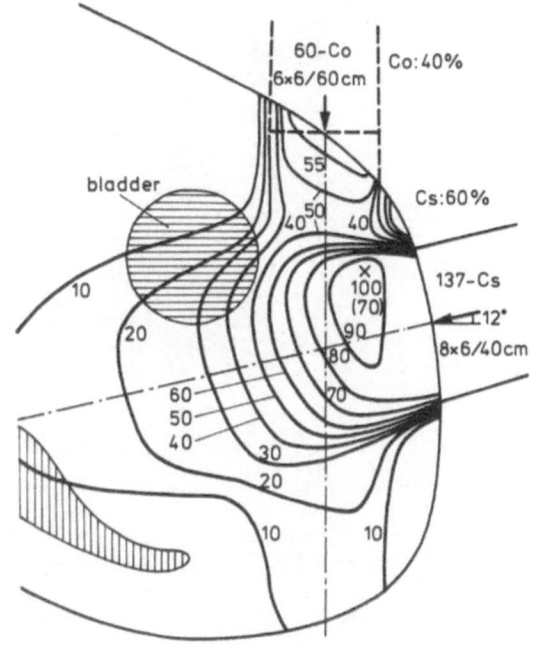

Fig. 242. 60-Co teletherapy of the vulva through two wedge fields
    SSD 60 cm
    field size 6 × 8 (vulva)
             6 × 6 (suprasymphyseal
                   field)
    15° wedges
    Polystyrene phantom
    (Halama and Rassow 1969)

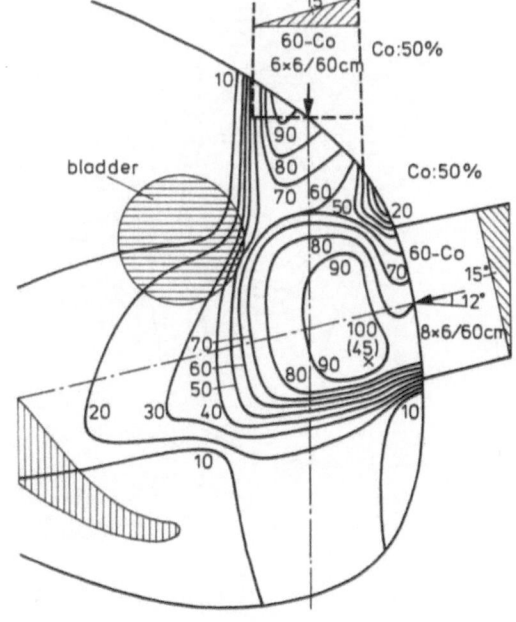

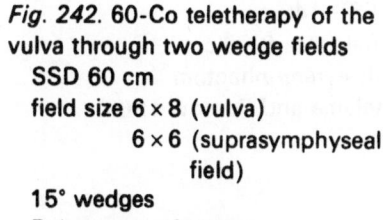

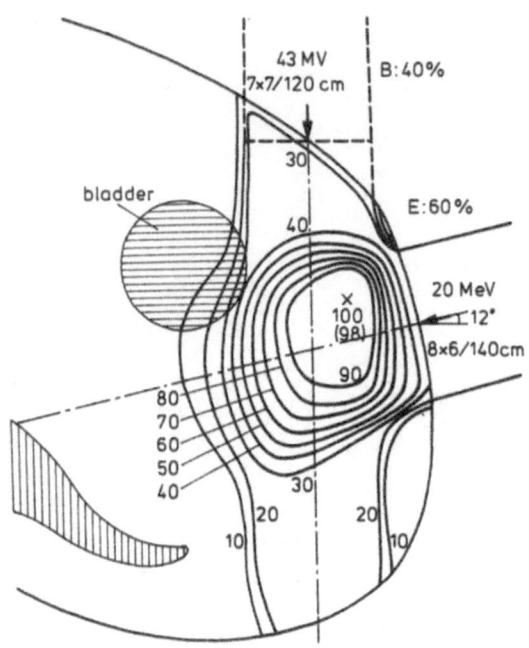

Fig. 243. Combined electron beam and high-energy X-ray therapy of the vulva through two stationary fields. 40% of the total dose to the X-ray field and 60% to the electron field
  X-rays:
    43 MV
    FSD 120 cm
    field size 7 × 7 cm
  Electrons:
    20 MeV
    FSD 140 cm
    field size 6 × 8 cm
  Polystyrene phantom
  (Halama and Rassow 1969)

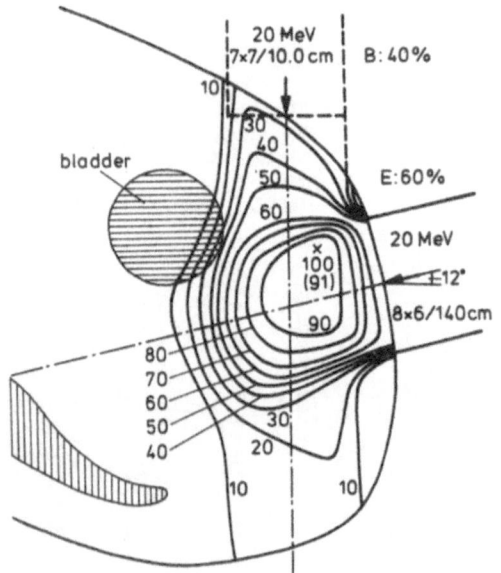

Fig. 244. Combined electron beam and high-energy X-ray therapy of the vulva through two stationary fields. 60% of the total dose to the electron field and 40% to the X-ray field
  X-ray:
    20 MV
    FSD 100 cm
    field size 7 × 7 cm
  Electrons:
    20 MeV
    FSD 140 cm
    field size 8 × 6 cm
  Polystyrene phantom
  (Halama and Rassow 1969)

174 | Vulva

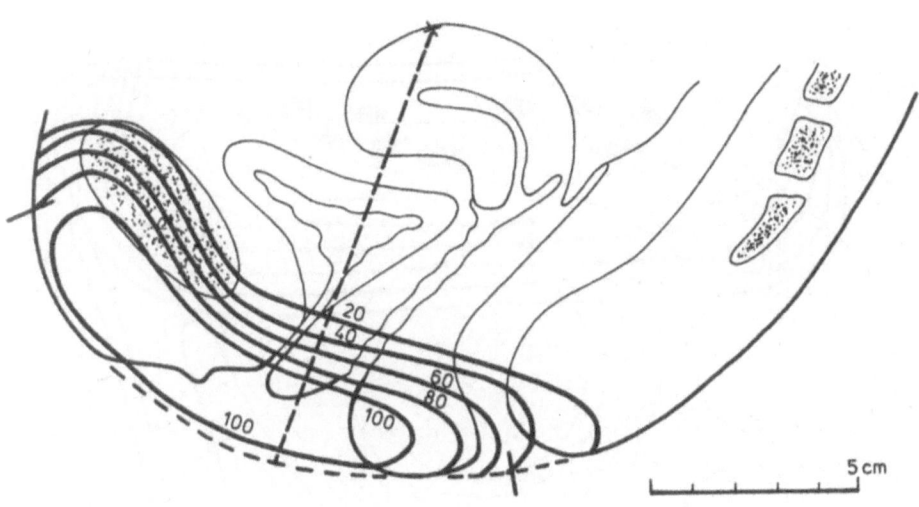

Fig. 245. Arc (70°) therapy of the vulva with 7.5 MeV electrons
   FAD 120 cm
   axis depth 11 cm
   3° caudal tilt of the central beam
   field size 3 × 12 cm at axis
   Paraffin phantom

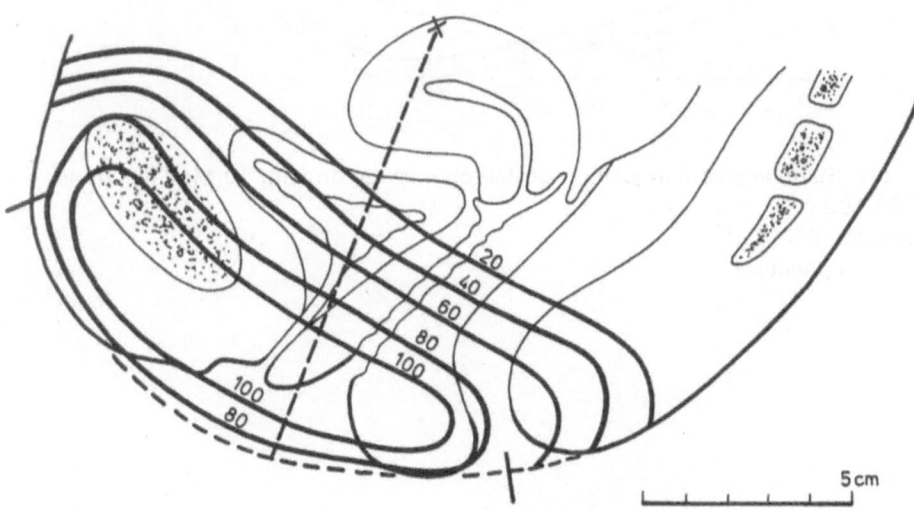

Fig. 246. Arc (70°) therapy of the vulva with 15 MeV electrons
   SAD 120 cm
   axis depth 11 cm
   3° caudal tilt of the central beam
   field size 3 × 12 cm at axis
   Paraffin phantom

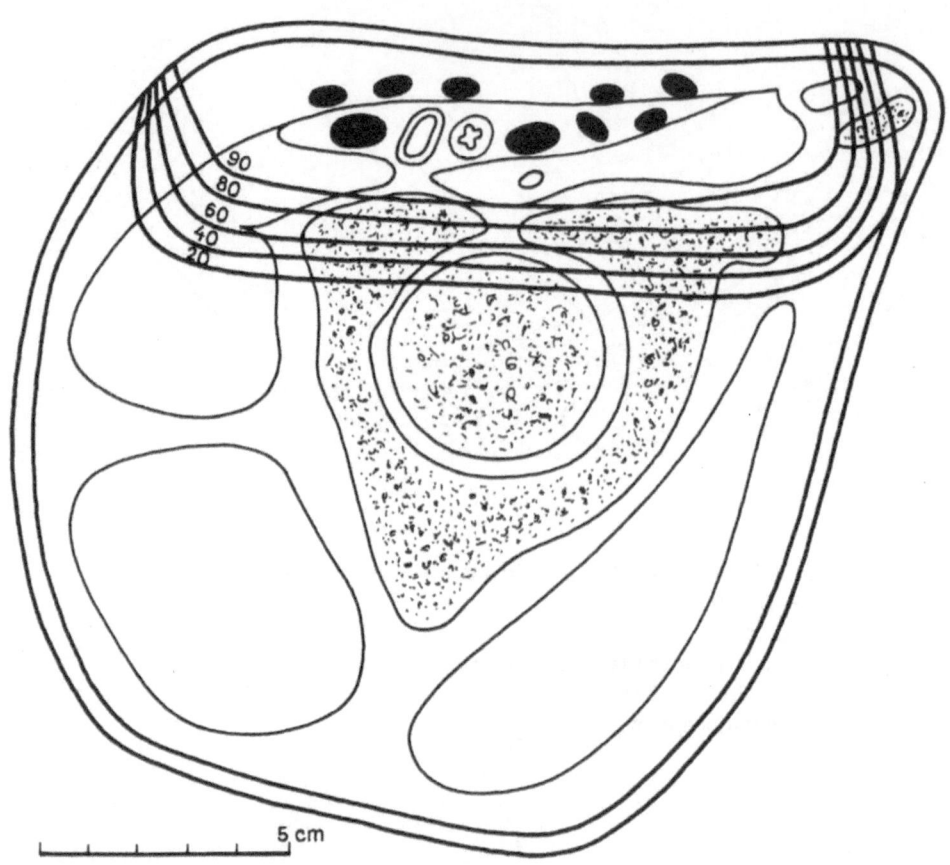

Fig. 247. Stationary field irradiation of the inguinal region with 10 MeV electrons
FSD 100 cm
field size 8 × 12 cm
Paraffin phantom

Male genital organs

Prostate

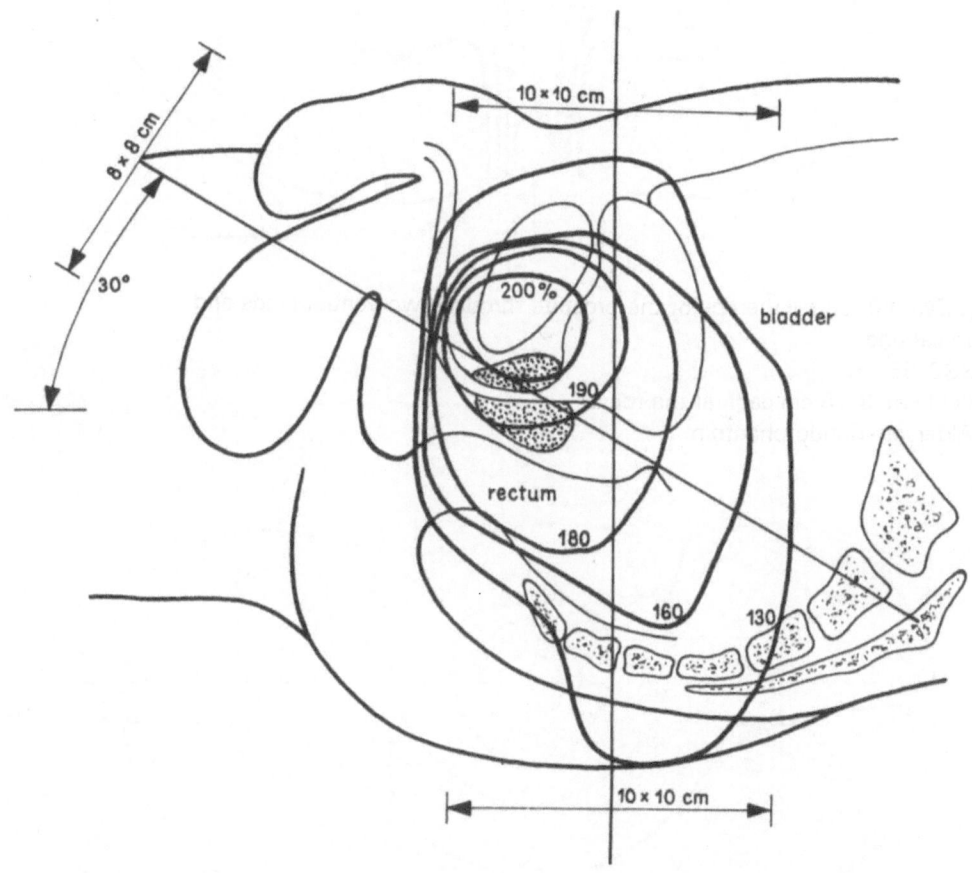

Fig. 248. 60-Co teletherapy of the prostate through three stationary fields
SSD 80 cm
field size   8 × 8 cm (perineal field)
        10 × 10 cm (ventral and dorsal fields)
(Rodriguez-Antunez et al. 1973)

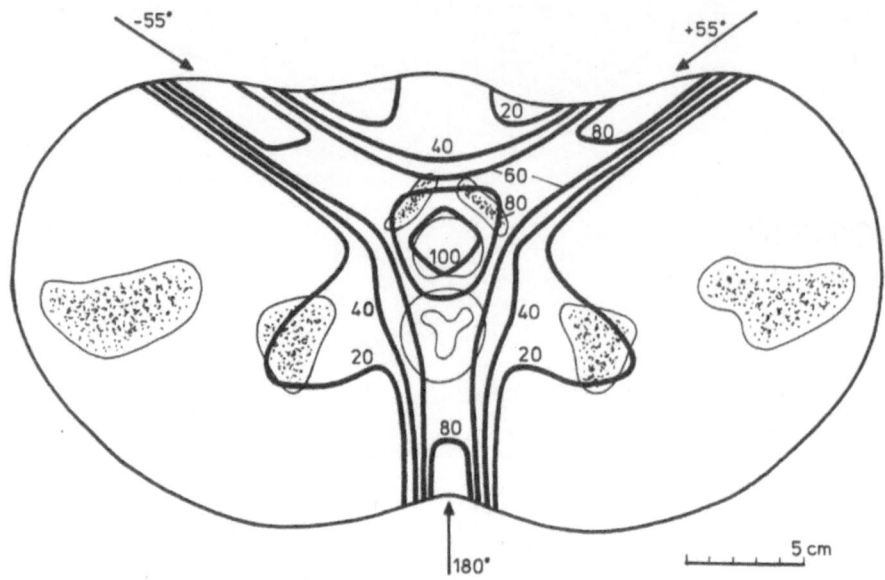

Fig. 249. 60-Co teletherapy of the prostate through two ventral fields and
a dorsal one
   SSD 55 cm
   field size 3 × 8 cm each at the focus
   Alderson–Rando phantom

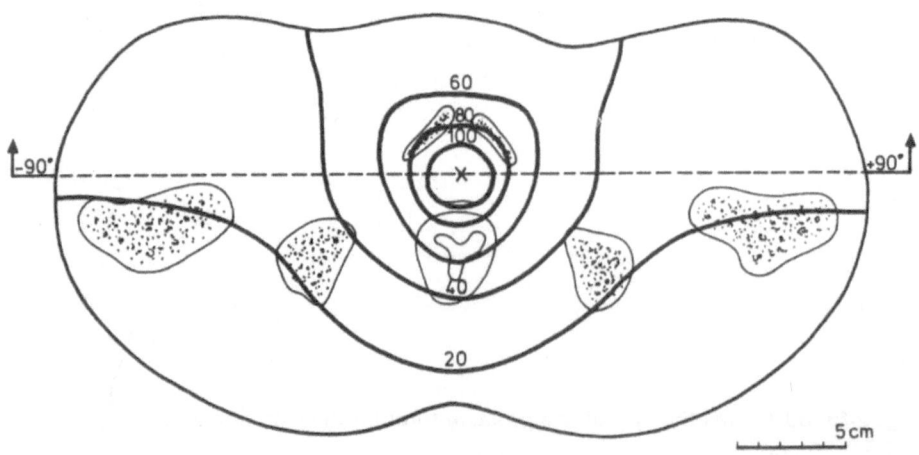

Fig. 250. 60-Co arc (180°) therapy of the prostate
   SAD 60 cm
   axis depth 7 cm in the midline
   field size 3 × 8 cm
   Alderson–Rando phantom

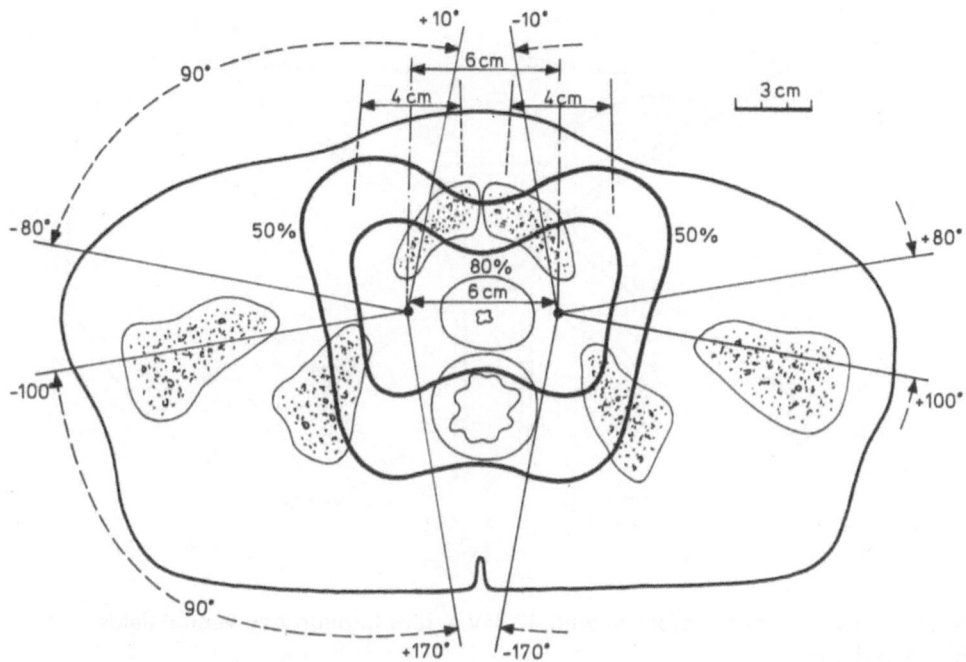

Fig. 251. Two-centre four-arc 60-Co therapy of the prostate
  SAD 65 cm
  axis depth 8 cm in the midline
  distance of axes 6 cm (3 cm left and right from the midline)
  four 90° arcs
  field size 4 × 5 cm on the skin at 0°
  Alderson–Rando phantom
  (Kling et al. 1971)

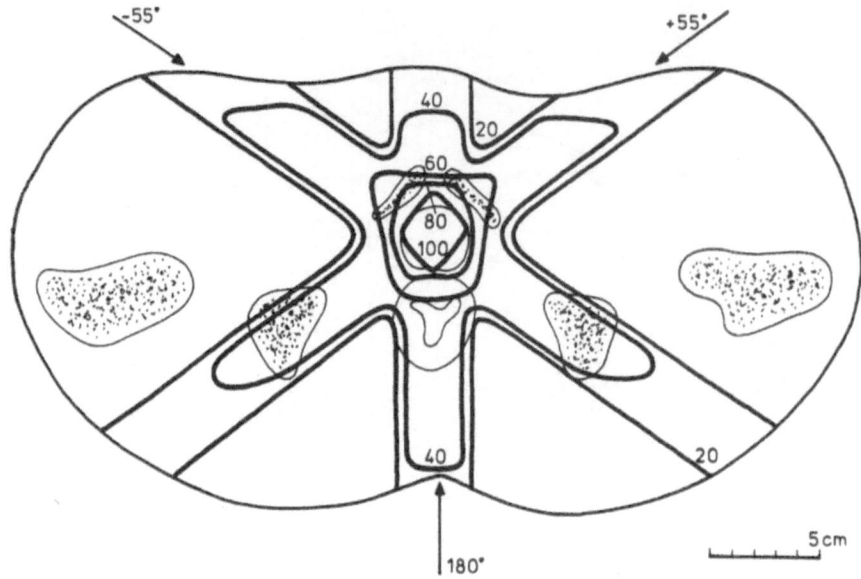

Fig. 252. Irradiation of the prostate with 42 MV X-rays through two ventral fields and a dorsal one
FSD 100 cm
field size 3×8 cm on the surface
Alderson–Rando phantom

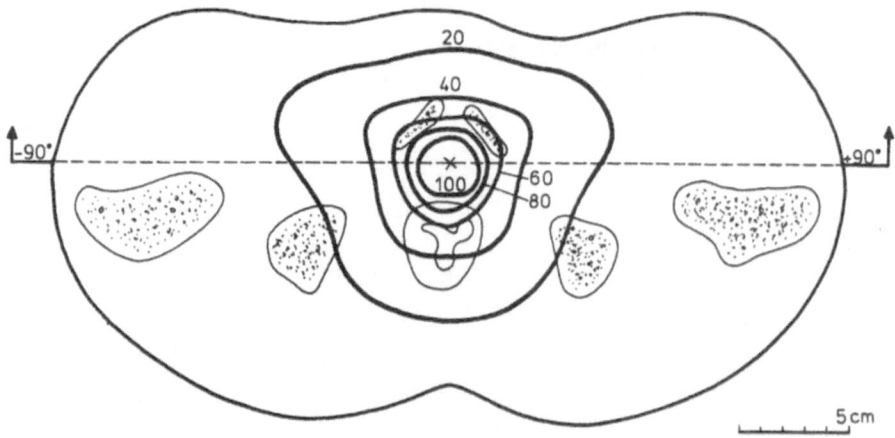

Fig. 253. Arc therapy (180°) of the prostate with high-energy X-rays (42 MV)
FAD 120 cm
axis depth 7 cm in the midline
field size 3×8 cm at axis
Alderson–Rando phantom

Urinary tract

Kidney

Fig. 254. 60-Co
teletherapy of the
kidney through a
ventral and a dorsal
field
  SSD 50 cm
  field size 10 × 14 cm
  central beam
    vertical for the
    ventral field
  angle of incidence
    20° for the dorsal
    field
  Alderson–Rando
    phantom
  (Kuttig 1968)

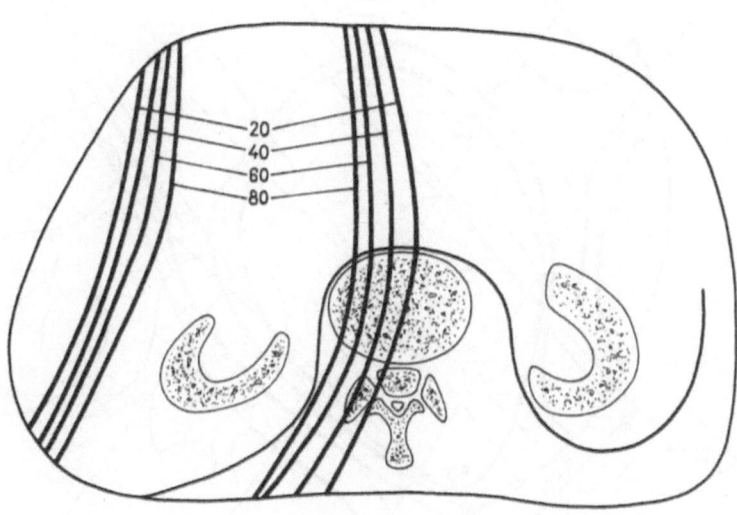

Fig. 255. 60-Co arc
(210°) therapy of the
kidney
  SAD 60 cm
  axis depth 8 cm
  field size 8 × 14 cm
  Alderson–Rando
    phantom
  (Kuttig 1968)

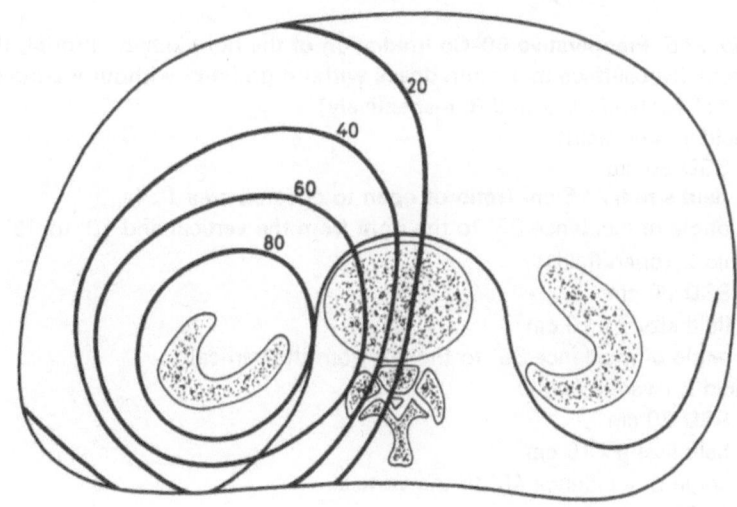

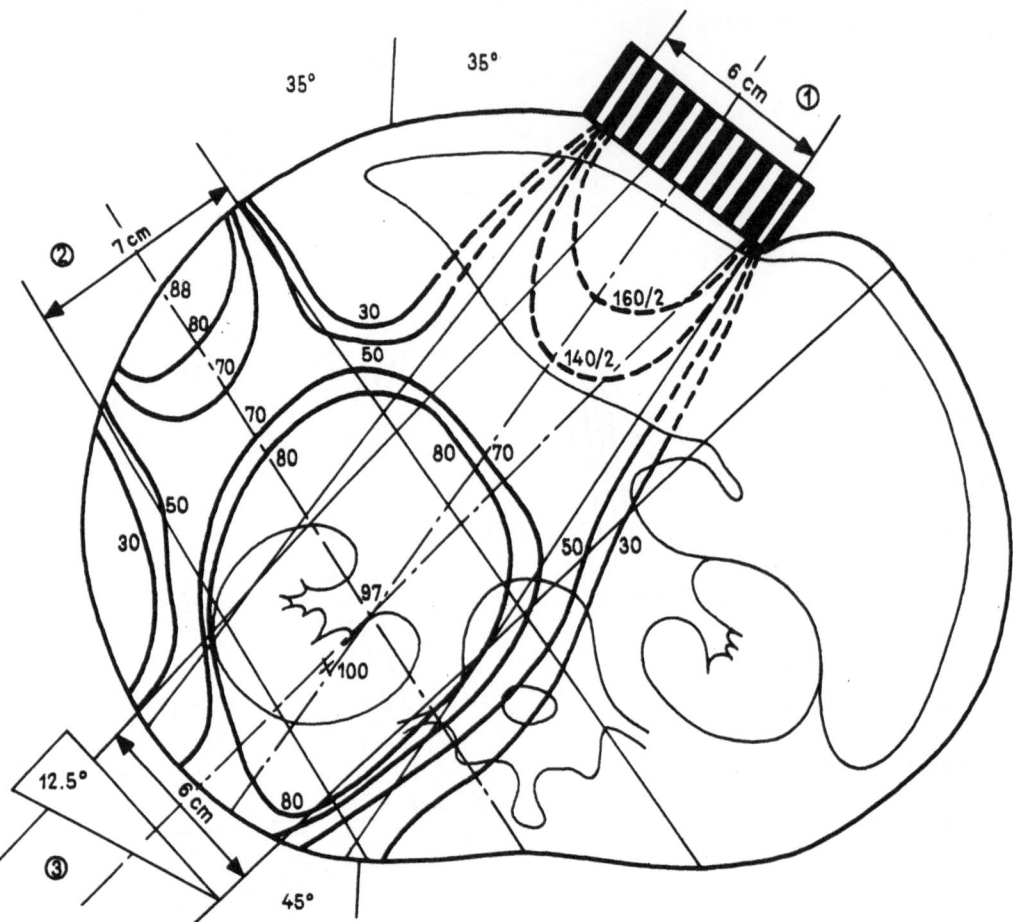

Fig. 256. Preoperative 60-Co irradiation of the right kidney through three stationary fields (Subsurface maximum doses without grid and without wedge should be 2:1:1 for fields 1, 2 and 3, respectively)

Field 1 (grid field):
  SSD 50 cm
  field size 6 × 16 cm (ratio of open to covered area 1 : 1)
  angle of incidence 35° to the right from the vertical and 10° to 15° craniad

Field 2 (open field):
  SSD 60 cm
  field size 7 × 16 cm
  angle of incidence 35° to the left from the vertical

Field 3 (wedge field):
  SSD 60 cm
  field size 6 × 16 cm
  angle of incidence 45° to the vertical
  12.5° wedge

Alderson–Rando phantom
(Rödel and Ringleb 1970)

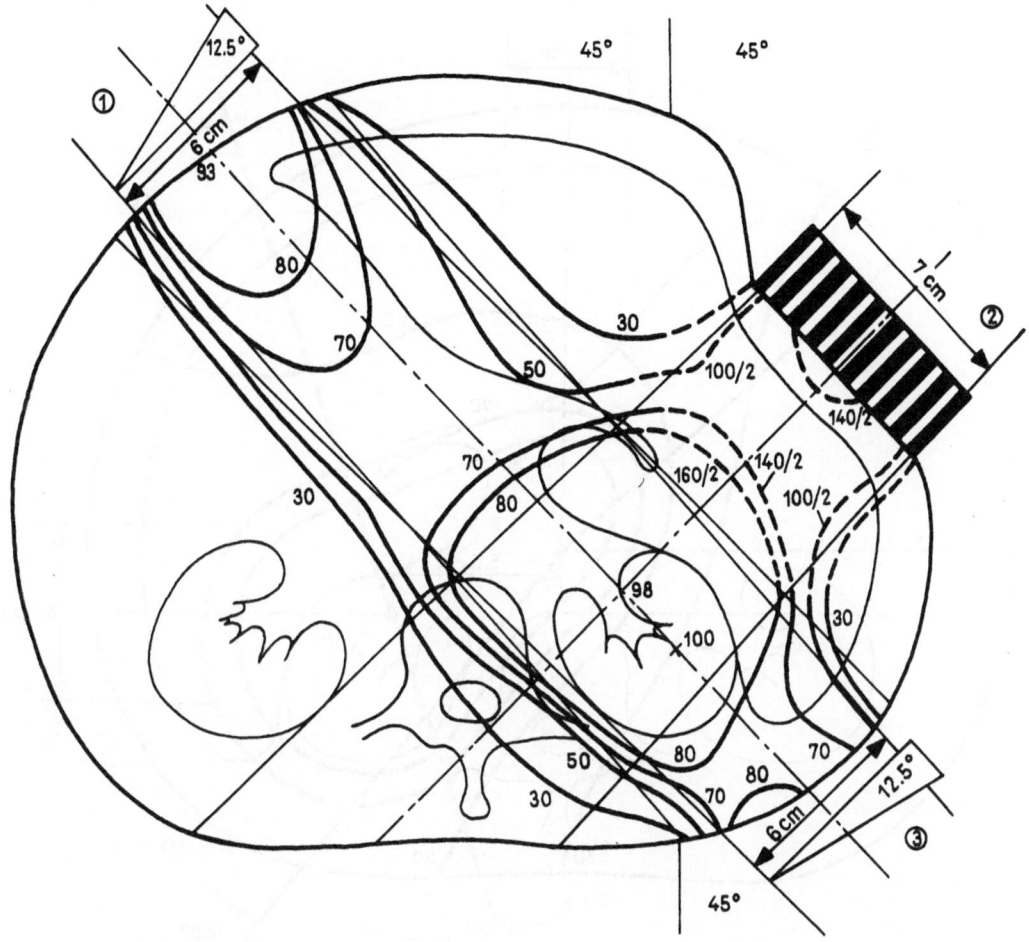

Fig. 257. Preoperative 60-Co irradiation of the left kidney through three stationary fields (irradiation time for right ventrolateral grid field is twice as long as that for the two wedge fields)

Field 1 (wedge field):
  SSD 60 cm
  field size 6 × 16 cm
  central beam angulates 45° to the left from the vertical
  12.5° wedge

Field 2 (grid field):
  SSD 50 cm
  field size 7 × 16 cm (ratio of open to covered area 1:1)
  central beam angulates 45° upwards from the horizontal and 10° to 15° craniad

Field 3 (wedge field):
  SSD 60 cm
  field size 6 × 16 cm
  central beam angulates 45° from the vertical
  12.5° wedge

Alderson–Rando phantom
(Rödel and Ringleb 1970)

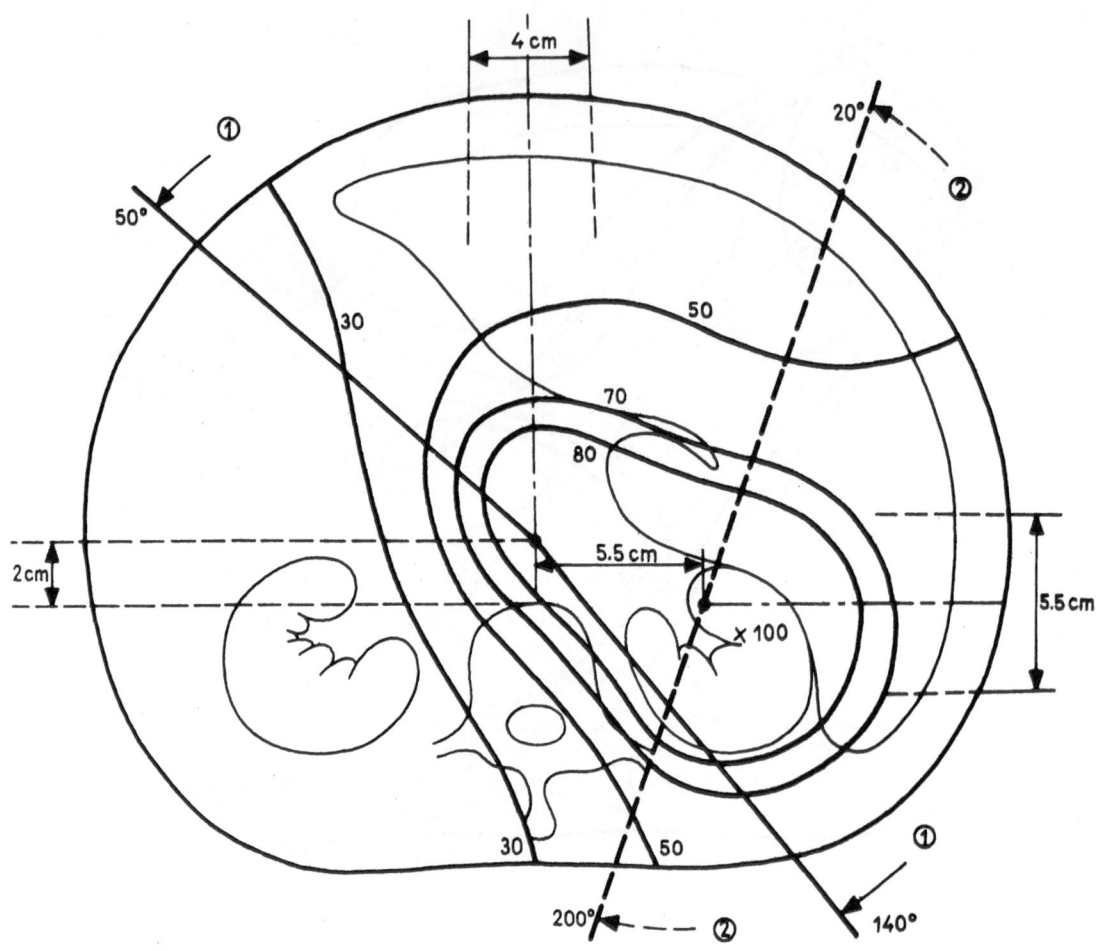

Fig. 258. Postoperative two-centre two-arc 60-Co irradiation of the kidney (loading
4 : 3 for the "central" and "kidney" arcing, respectively)
"Central" arcing:
  SAD 65 cm
  axis depth 2 cm from the edge of vertebral body in the midline
  arc 190°
  field size 4 × 16 cm
"Kidney" arcing:
  SAD 65 cm
  axis depth 5.5 cm from the midline on the involved side at the level of the anterior
    edge of the vertebral body
  arc 180°
  field size 5.5 × 16 cm
  Alderson–Rando phantom
  (Rödel and Ringleb 1970)

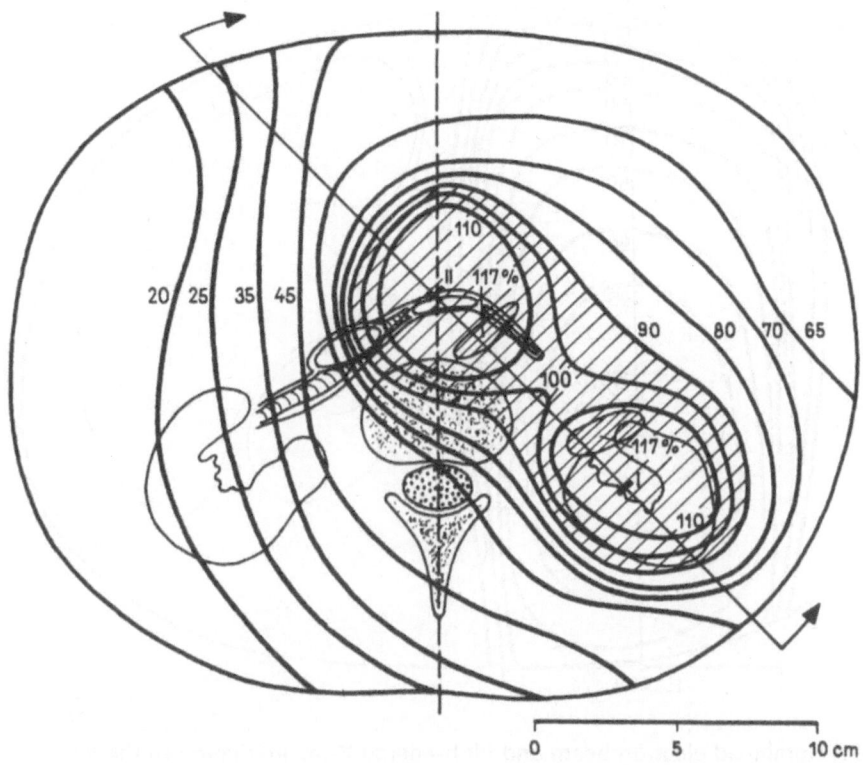

Fig. 259. Two-centre two-arc (180° each) 60-Co treatment of the left kidney and paraaortal lymph nodes
    SAD 60 cm
    axis depth: ventral axis 15 cm in the midline; the straight line connecting the
       axes angulates 45° from the midline
    distance of axes 10 cm
    field size 5 × 14 cm each
    (Gauwerky and Adam 1971)

Fig. 260. Eccentric high-energy
X-ray (42 MV) arcing of the kidney
    FAD 120 cm
    axis depth 7 cm, 1 cm
      contralaterally
    arc 90° (0°/–90°)
    central beam tilted to be shifted
      5 cm on the surface towards
      the target volume
    field size 4 × 14 cm
    Alderson–Rando phantom
    (Heuss and Hoeffken 1972)

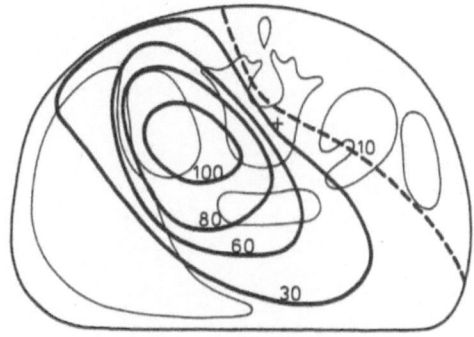

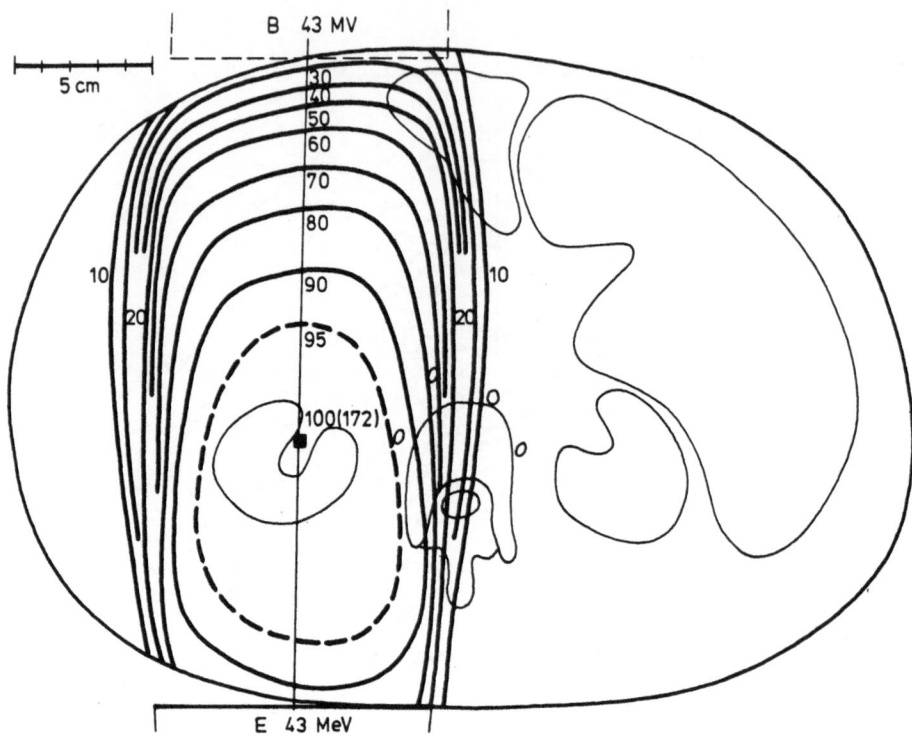

Fig. 261. Combined electron beam and high-energy X-ray irradiation of the left kidney through a ventral and a dorsal stationary field
Dorsal field: 43 MeV electrons
        FSD 120 cm
        field size 10 × 14 cm
Ventral field: 43 MV X-rays
        FSD 120 cm
        field size 10 × 14 cm
  Alderson–Rando phantom
  (Sack and Rassow 1972)

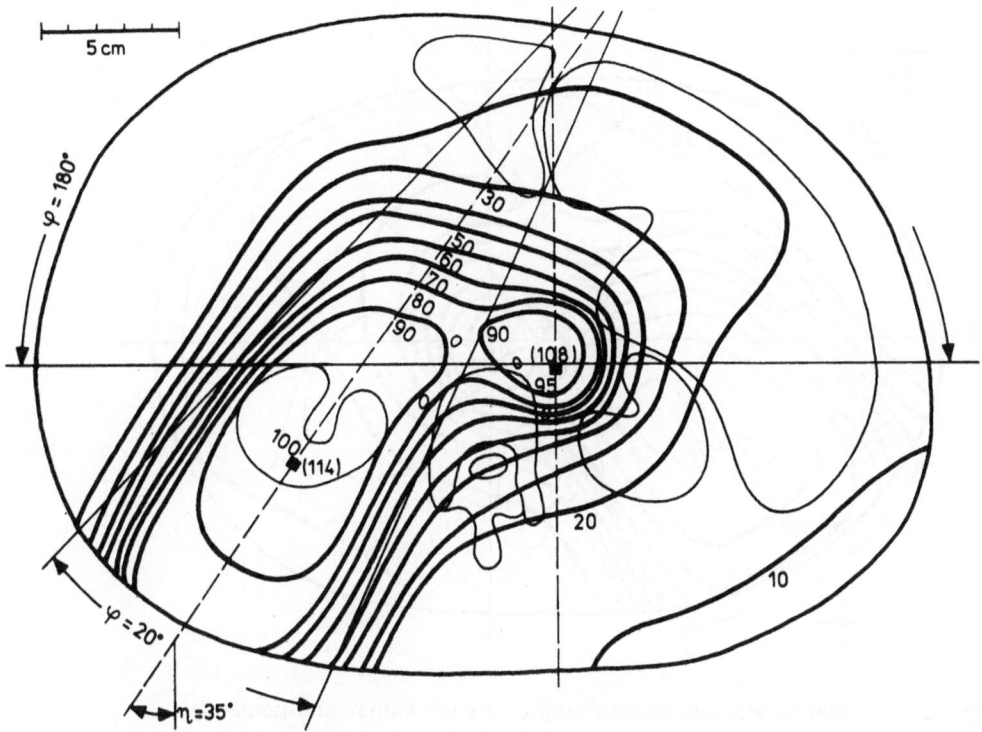

Fig. 262. Telecentric electron beam arcing of the left kidney and paraaortal lymph nodes combined with high-energy X-ray arcing

Electron beam: 35 MeV

             FAD 120 cm

             arc 20°

             axis depth 30 cm

             field size 3 × 12 cm at axis

X-ray: 43 MV

        FAD 120 cm

        axis depth 12 cm ventrally, 2 cm from the centre of the phantom laterally

        arc 180°

        field size 4 × 12 cm

Alderson–Rando phantom

(Sack and Rassow 1972)

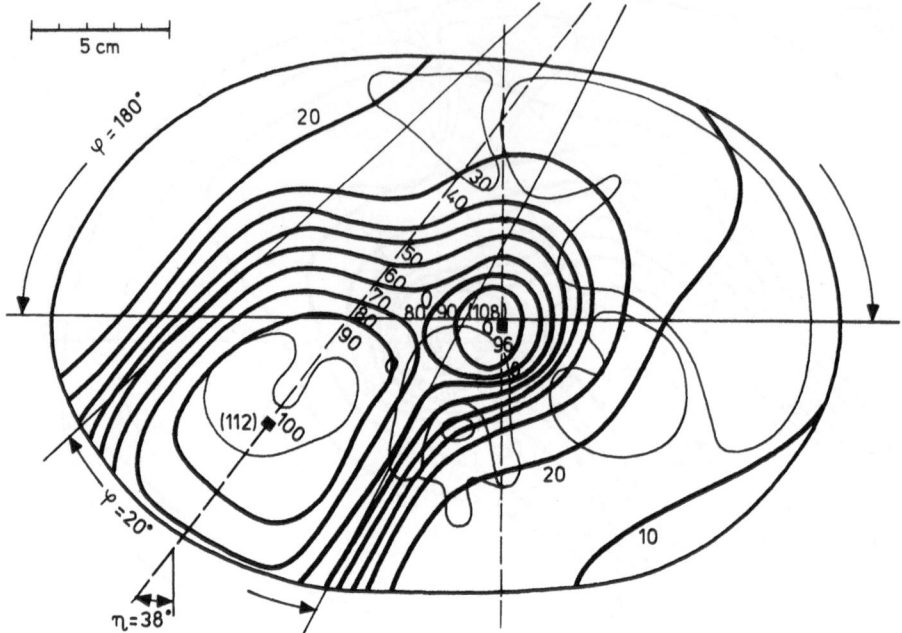

Fig. 263. Telecentric electron beam arcing of the left kidney and paraaortal lymph nodes combined with high-energy X-ray arcing

Electron beam: 25 MeV

                FAD 120 cm

                arc 20°

                axis depth 30 cm

                field size 3 × 12 cm at axis

X-ray: 43 MV

        FAD 120 cm

        axis depth 9 cm ventrally, 2 cm from the centre of the phantom
           laterally

        arc 180°

        field size 4 × 12 cm at axis

Alderson–Rando phantom

(Sack and Rassow 1972)

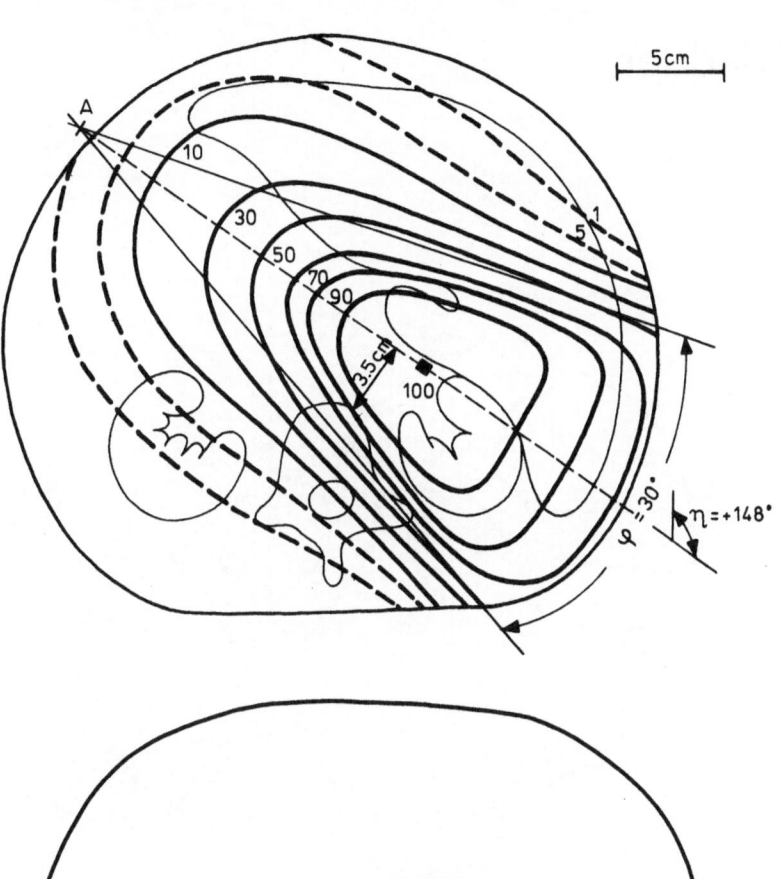

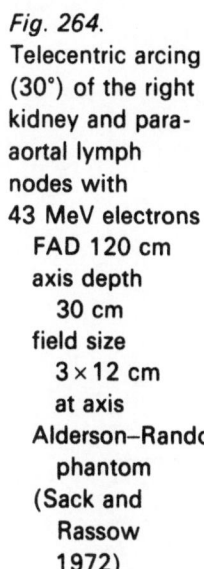

Fig. 264.
Telecentric arcing (30°) of the right kidney and para-aortal lymph nodes with 43 MeV electrons
FAD 120 cm
axis depth
30 cm
field size
3 × 12 cm
at axis
Alderson–Rando phantom
(Sack and Rassow 1972)

5 cm

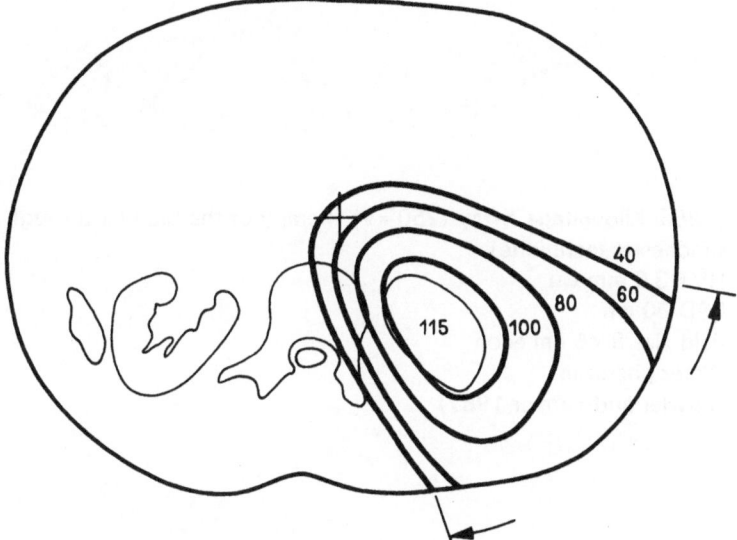

Fig. 265.
Postoperative electron beam (35 MeV) arcing (60°) of the kidney
FAD 120 cm
axis depth
11 cm
field size
4 × 14 cm
Alderson–Rando phantom
(Heuss and Hoeffken 1972)

Bladder

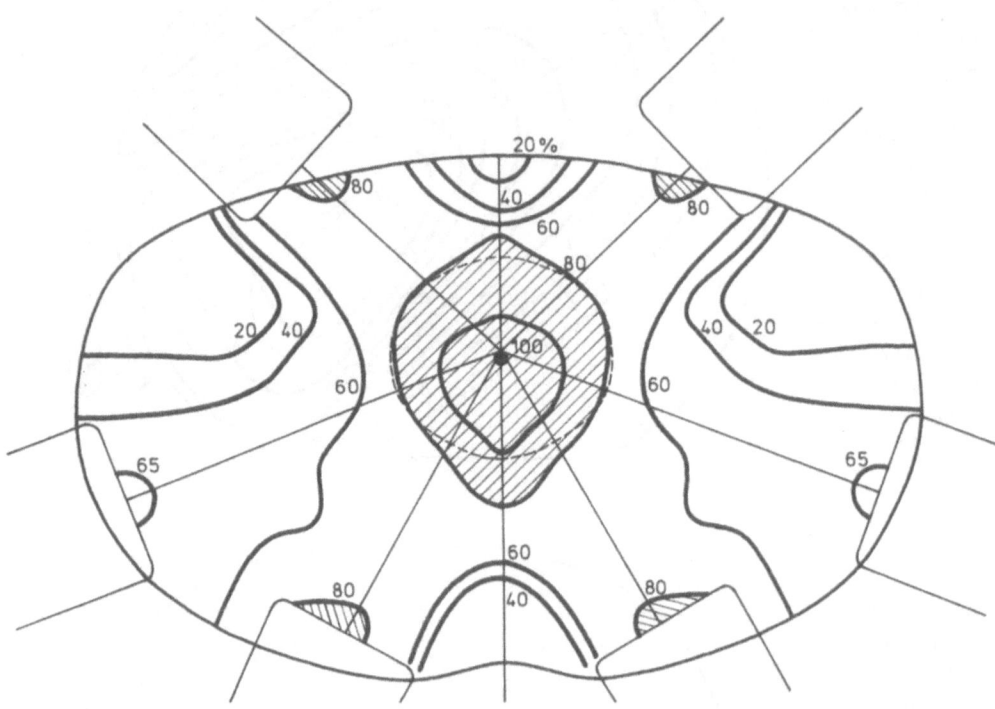

Fig. 266. Kilovoltage X-ray (250 kV) therapy of the bladder through six stationary fields
(Manchester technique)
   HVT 3.6 mm Cu
   FSD 50 cm
   field size 8 × 6 cm each
   Water phantom
   (Fowler and Farmer 1957)

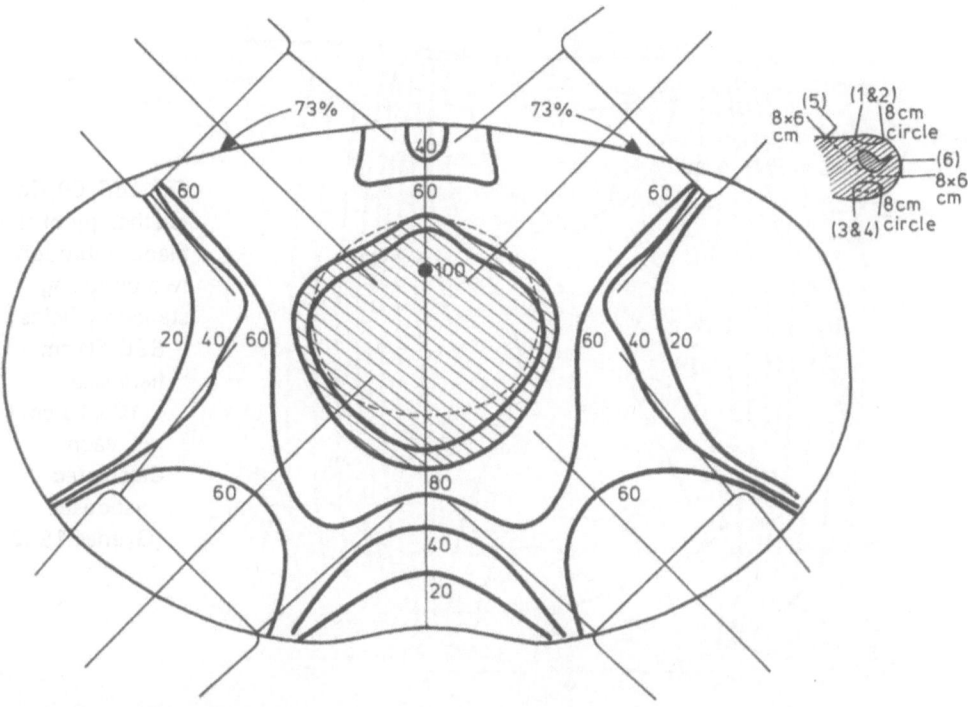

Fig. 267. Kilovoltage X-ray (250 kV) therapy of the bladder through six stationary fields (Newcastle technique)

    HVT 3.6 cm Cu

    FSD 50 cm

    field size 8 × 6 cm (perineal field and anterior oblique field)

           8 cm diam. circles (opposing fields)

    Water phantom

    (Fowler and Farmer 1957)

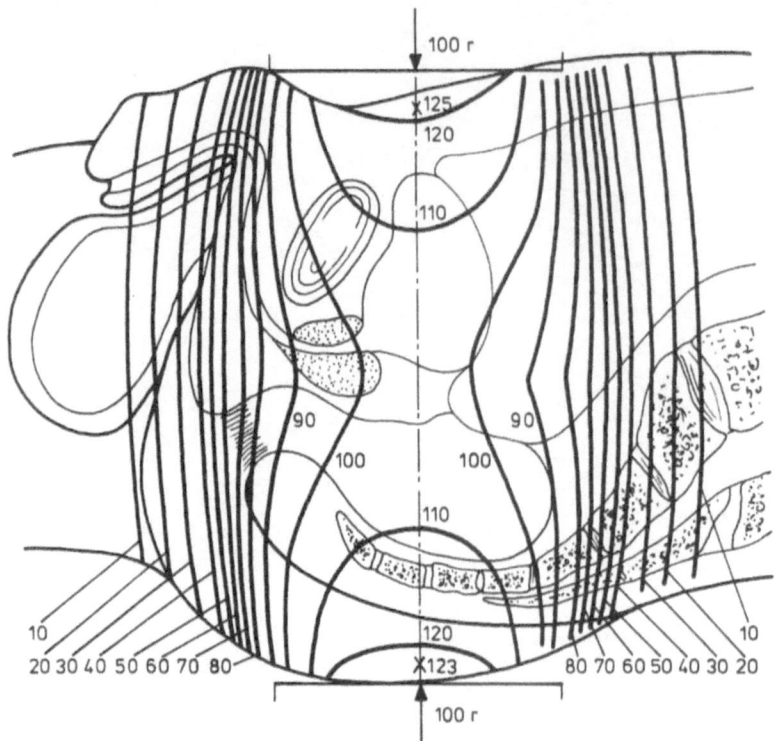

Fig. 268. 60-Co teletherapy of the bladder through two opposing stationary fields SSD 50 cm field size 10 × 15 cm each Calculated isodoses (Gyenes 1962)

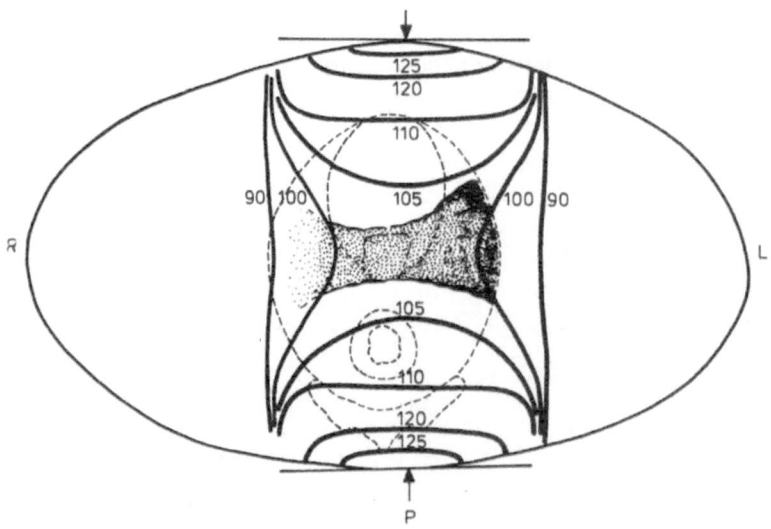

Fig. 269. 60-Co teletherapy of an extensive tumour of the posterior bladder wall in-filtrating the pros-tate, through two opposing stationary fields SSD 50 cm field size 12 × 12 cm Water phantom (Fletcher 1956a)

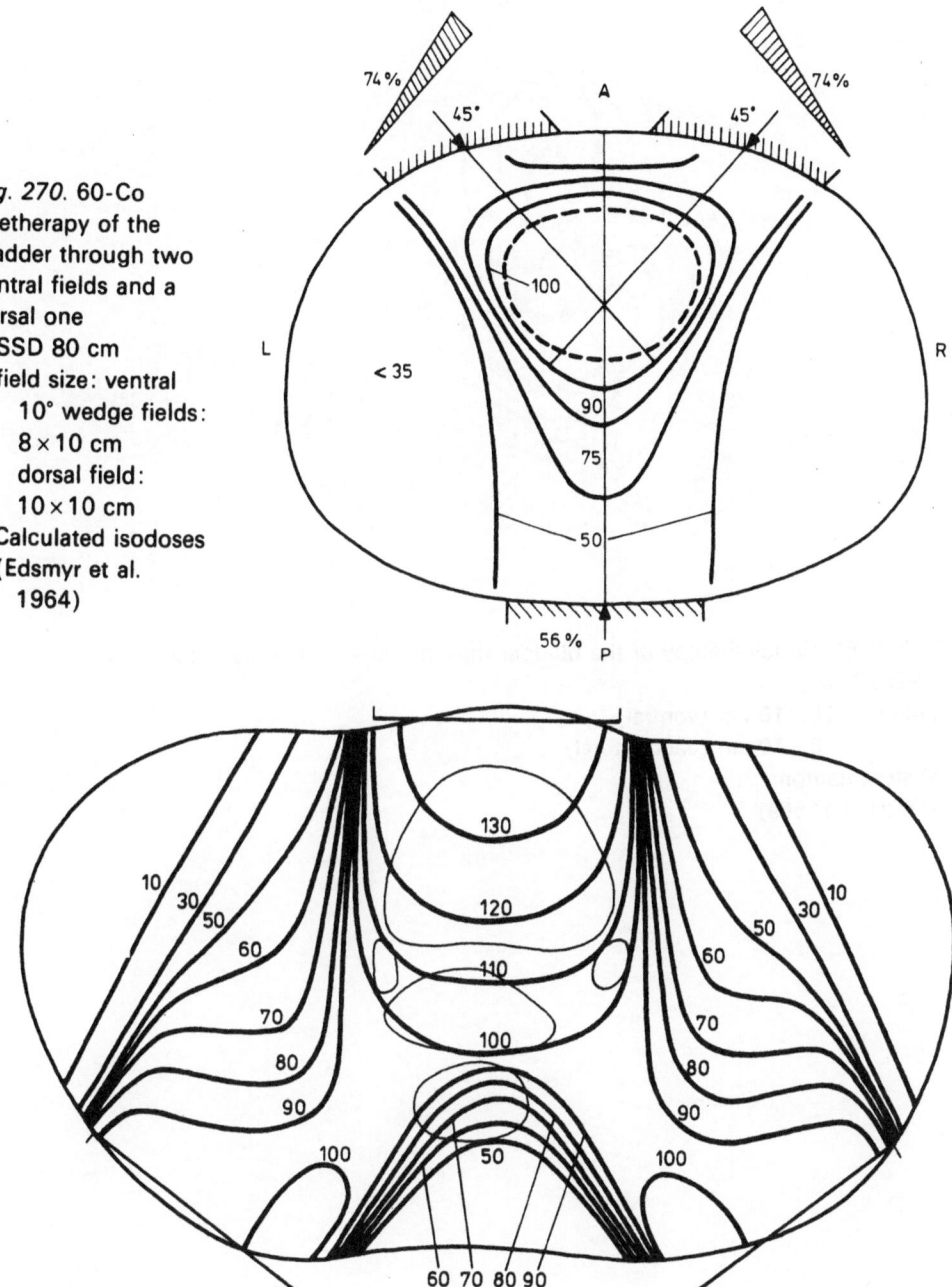

Fig. 270. 60-Co teletherapy of the bladder through two ventral fields and a dorsal one
  SSD 80 cm
  field size: ventral
    10° wedge fields:
    8 × 10 cm
    dorsal field:
    10 × 10 cm
  Calculated isodoses
  (Edsmyr et al. 1964)

Fig. 271. 60-Co teletherapy of the bladder through a ventral field and two stationary dorsal fields
  SSD 50 cm
  field size 10 × 8 cm each
  Calculated isodoses
  (Gyenes 1962)

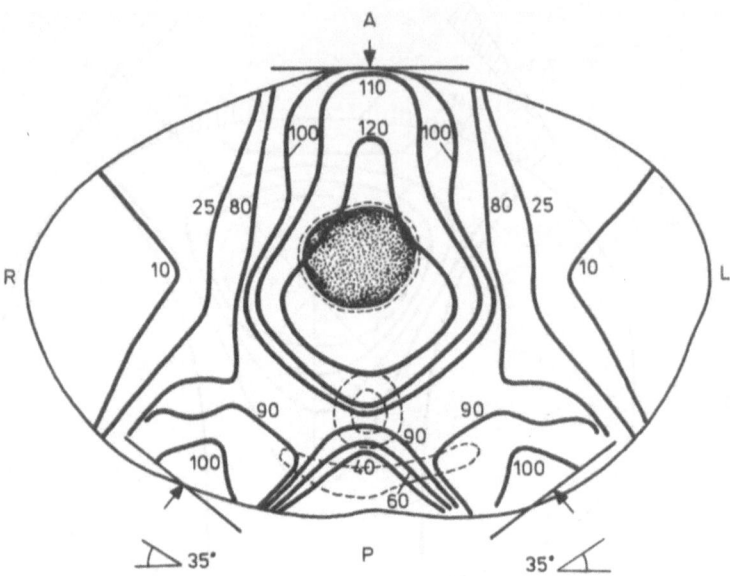

Fig. 272. 60-Co teletherapy of the bladder through three stationary fields
SSD 70 cm
field size 10 × 10 cm (ventral)
         8 × 10 cm (each lateral)
Water phantom
(Fletcher 1956*a*)

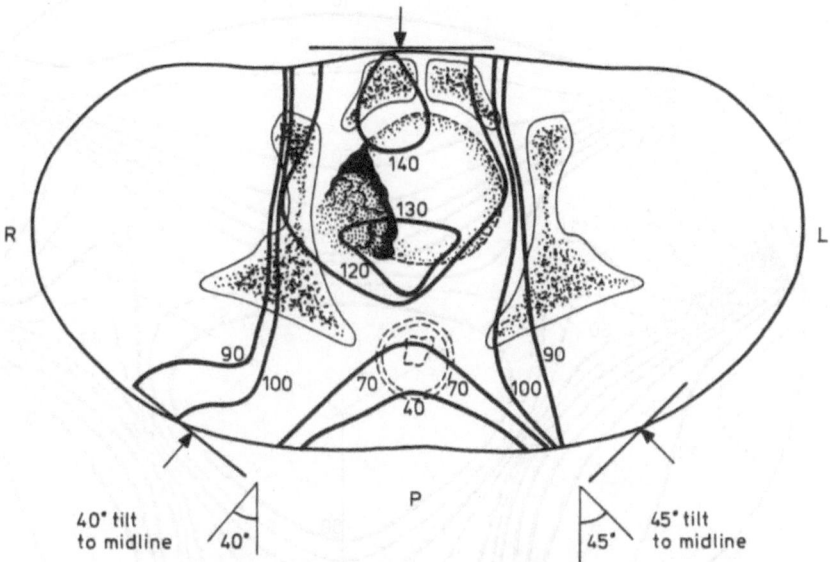

Fig. 273. 60-Co teletherapy of a tumour on the right side of the bladder through a ventral field and two stationary dorsal fields

Ventral field: SSD 70 cm

　　　　　　field size 8 × 8 cm

Dorsal fields: SSD 50 cm

　　　　　　field size 6 × 8 cm each

Water phantom

(Fletcher 1956*a*)

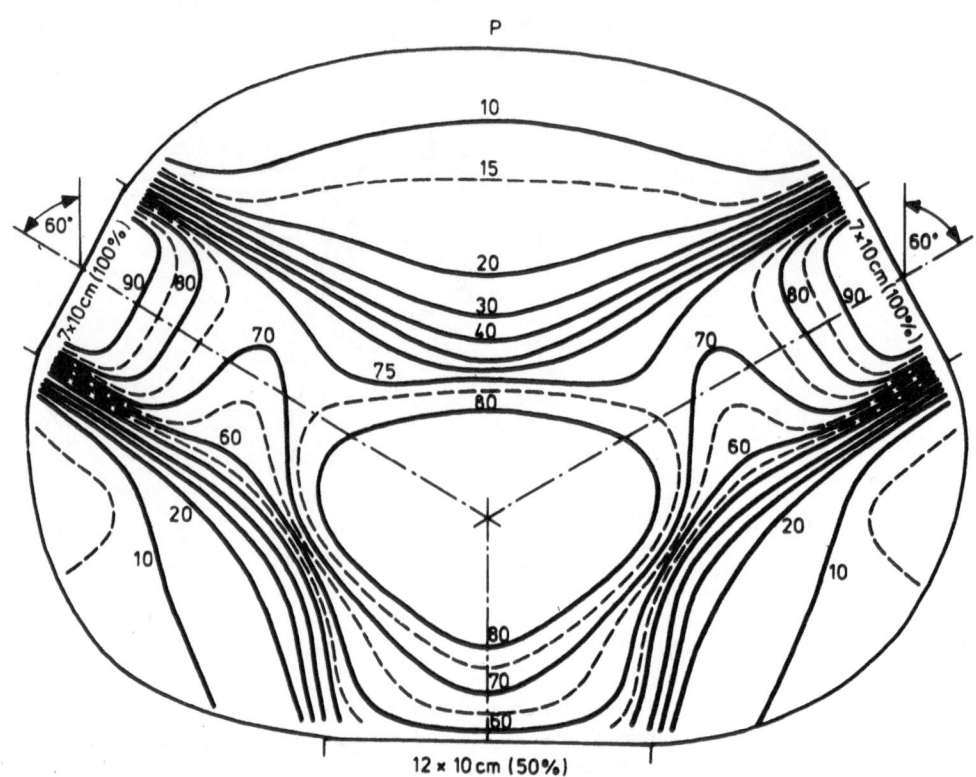

Fig. 274. 60-Co teletherapy of the bladder through three stationary fields (load to the ventral field 50% of that of the individual dorsal fields)
 SSD 50 cm
 field size 7 × 10 cm (each dorsolateral)
         12 × 10 cm (ventral)
 Water phantom
 (Birkner et al. 1964)

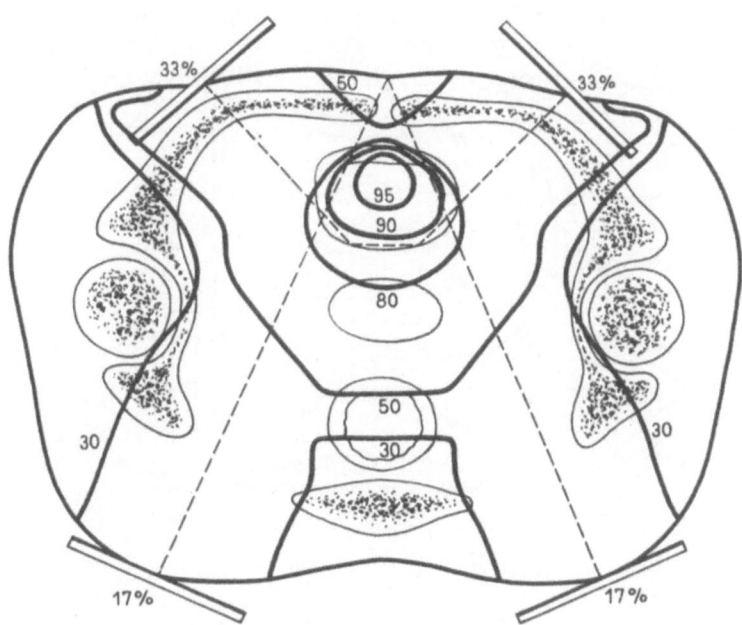

Fig. 275. 60-Co teletherapy of the bladder through four stationary fields (central beams of the ventral fields intercept 2 cm dorsally to the posterior bladder wall. Load 2:1 to the ventral and dorsal fields, respectively)
  SSD 60 cm
  field size 10 × 15 cm
  (Kriester et al. 1969)

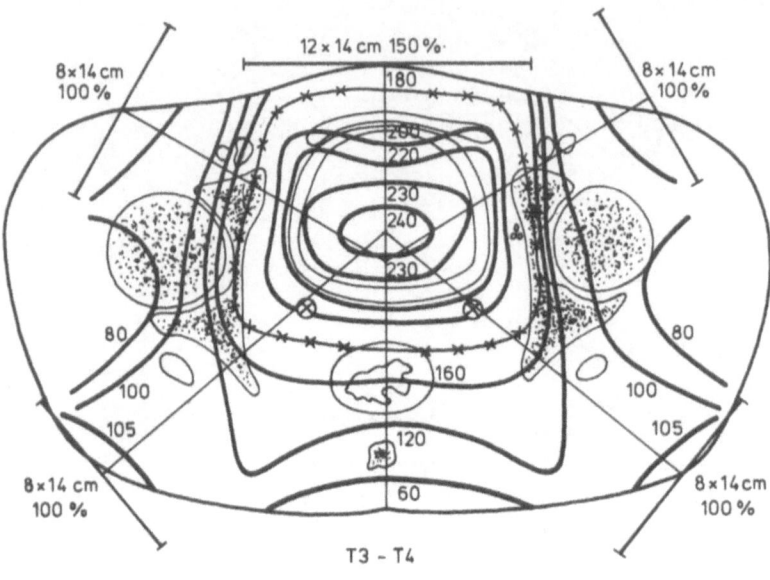

8×14 cm 100 %

12 × 14 cm 150 %·

180

8×14 cm 100 %

200

220

230

240

230

80

160

80

100

100

105

105

120

8×14 cm 100 %

60

8×14cm 100 %

T3 – T4

—✕—✕— Isodose + –minimum

Fig. 275. 60-Co teletherapy of the bladder through four stationary fields (central beams of the ventral fields intercept 2 cm dorsally to the posterior bladder wall. Load 2 : 1 to the ventral

SSD 80 cm

field size

    12 × 14 cm (ventral)

    8 × 14 cm (each lateral)

Calculated isodoses

(Wasilewski et al. 1968)

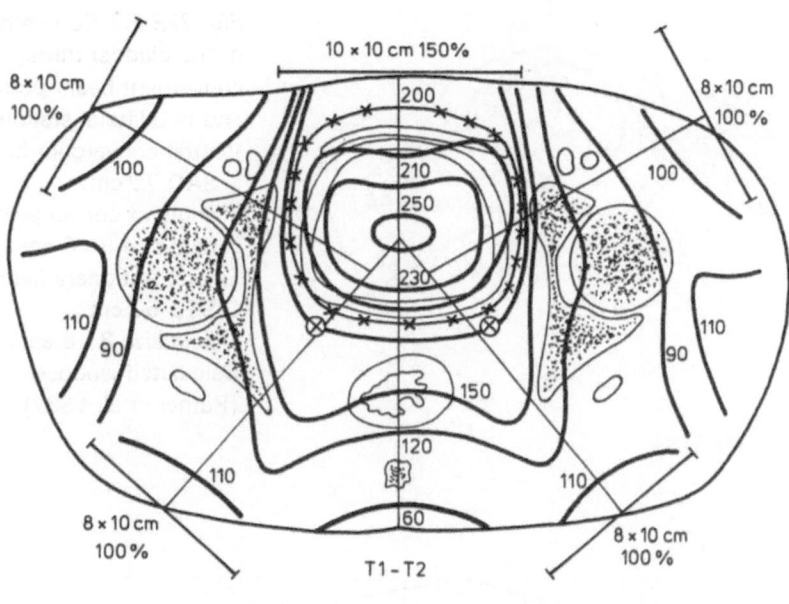

10 × 10 cm 150%

8 × 10 cm
100%

8 × 10 cm
100%

200

100

210

100

250

110

230

110

90

90

150

120

110

110

60

8 × 10 cm
100%

8 × 10 cm
100%

T1 – T2

⸻ ✳✳ Isodose + –minimum

Fig. 277. 60-Co teletherapy of a localized bladder tumour
through five stationary fields (load to ventral field 50% higher
than to the rest of the fields)
  SSD 80 cm
  field size
    10 × 10 cm (ventral)
     8 × 10 cm (each lateral)
  Calculated isodoses
  (Wasilewski et al. 1968)

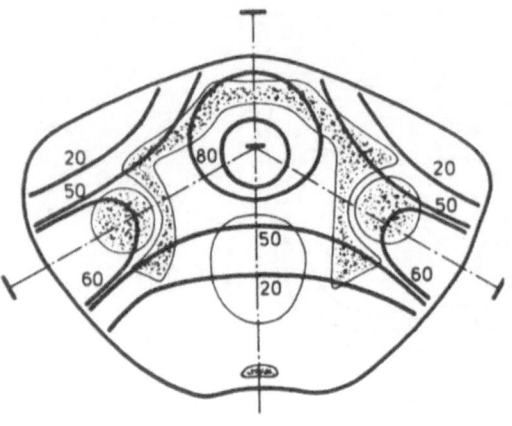

Fig. 278. 60-Co teletherapy
of the bladder through a ventral
convergent beam portal
and two lateral stationary fields
Ventral convergent beam field:
  SAD 75 cm
  angle of convergence 30°
  field size 8 × 8 cm at axis
Lateral stationary fields:
  SSD 50 cm
  field size 8 × 8 each
Calculated isodoses
(Ratner et al. 1967)

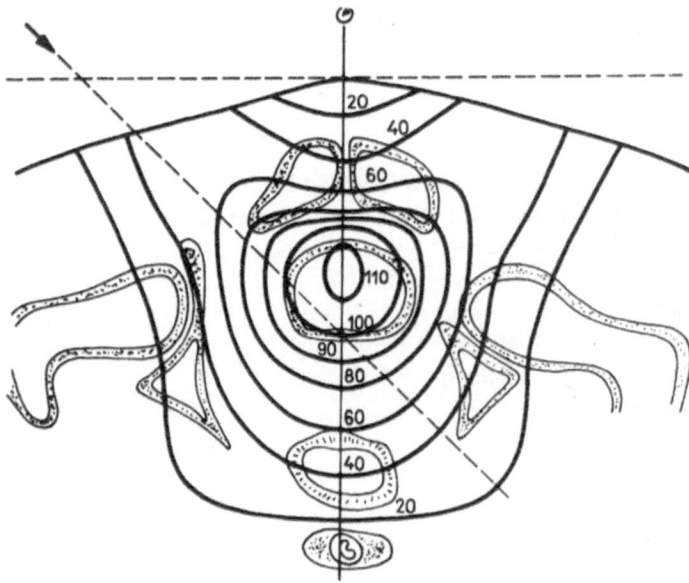

Fig. 279. 60-Co conical rotation treatment of the bladder
  SSD 70 cm
  axis depth 10 cm in the midline
  angle of incidence 45°
  field size 5 × 5 cm at the surface
  Pressdwood phantom
  (Castro and Whitcomb 1963)

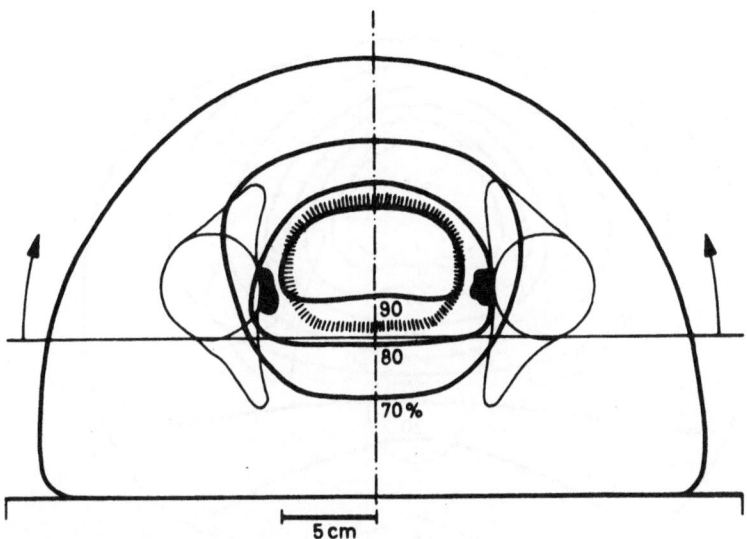

Fig. 280. 60-Co arc (180°) therapy of the bladder
SAD 60 cm
axis depth 14 cm
field size 12 × 14 cm at the focus
Calculated isodoses
(Mau and Fürst 1973)

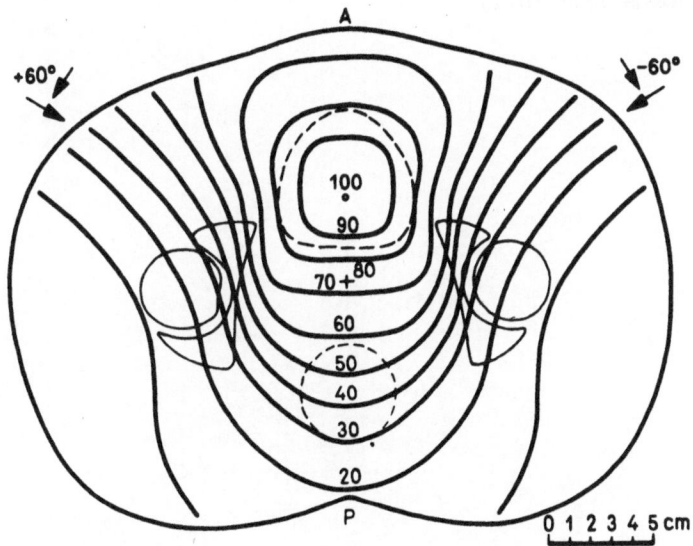

Fig. 281. 60-Co arc (120°) therapy of the bladder
SAD 60 cm
axis depth 11.5 cm
field size 8.4 × 12 cm at axis
Alderson–Rando phantom
(Frössler et al. 1972)

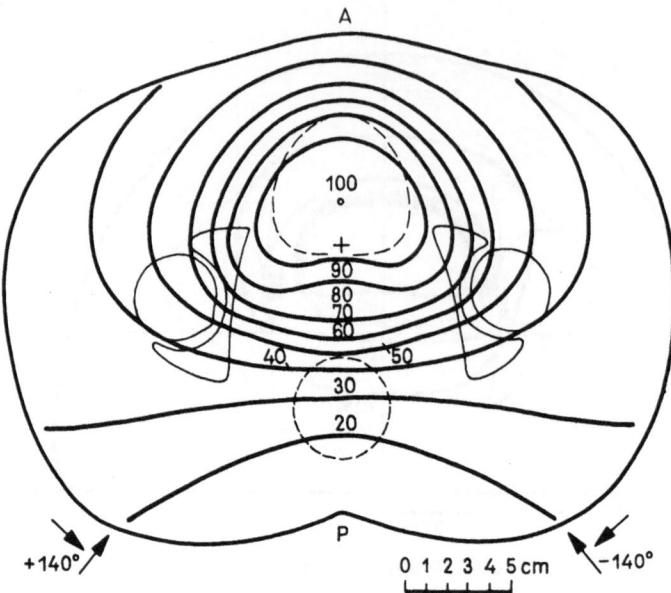

Fig. 282. 60-Co arc (280°) therapy of the bladder
SAD 60 cm
axis depth 9.5 cm
field size 8.4 × 12 cm at axis
Alderson–Rando phantom
(Frössler et al. 1972)

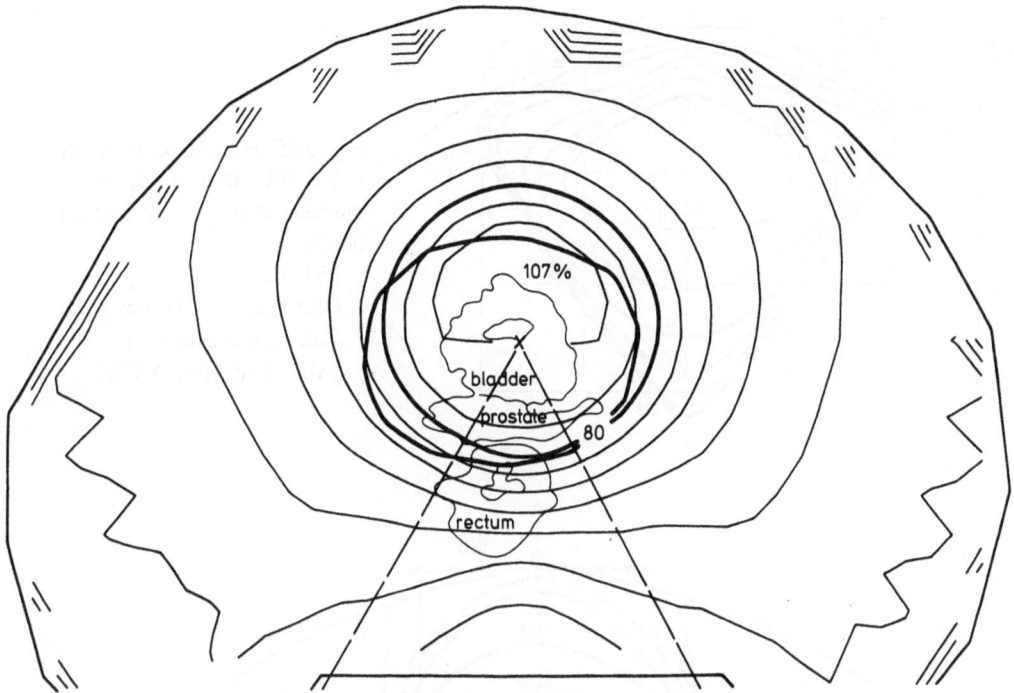

Fig. 283. 60-Co arc therapy of the bladder
   SAD 80 cm
   axis depth 12 cm
   arc 300° (150°/150°)
   field size 9 × 14 cm
   Computer calculated isodoses

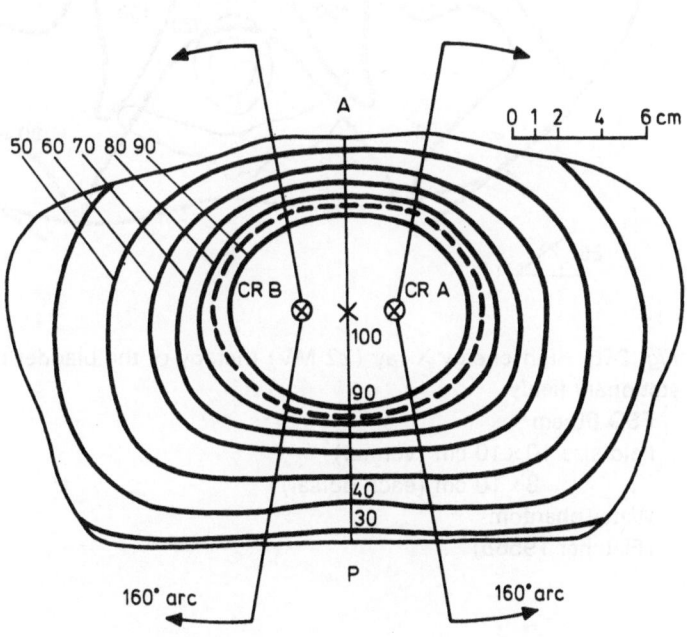

Fig. 284. Two-centre
two-arc (both 160°)
60-Co treatment of the
bladder
   SAD 60 cm
   axis depth 7.5 cm
      from ventral each
   distance of axes 4 cm
   field size 10 × 12 cm
   Calculated isodoses
   (Howath and Wilson
      1961)

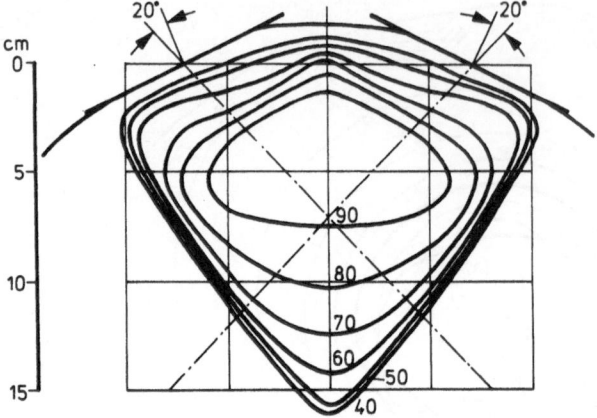

Fig. 285. High-energy X-ray (15.5 MV) therapy of the bladder through two stationary fields
    FSD 65 cm
    field size 10 × 10 cm each
    Calculated isodoses
    (Mau and Fürst 1973)

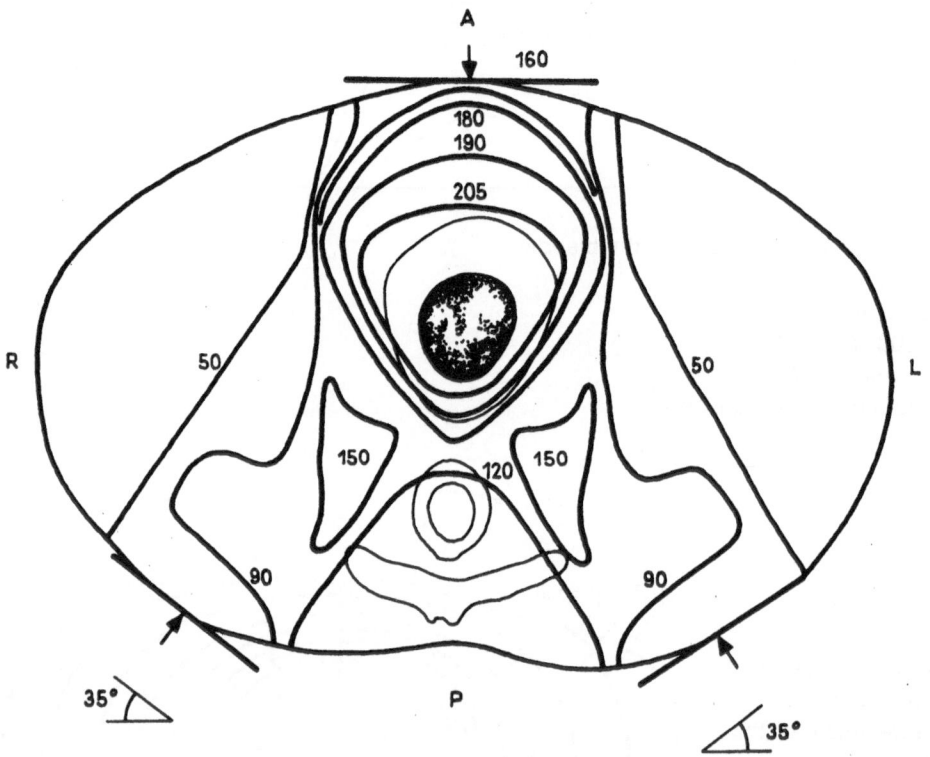

Fig. 286. High-energy X-ray (22 MV) therapy of the bladder through three stationary fields
    FSD 80 cm
    field size 10 × 10 cm (ventral)
                8 × 10 cm (each dorsal)
    Water phantom
    (Fletcher 1956*b*)

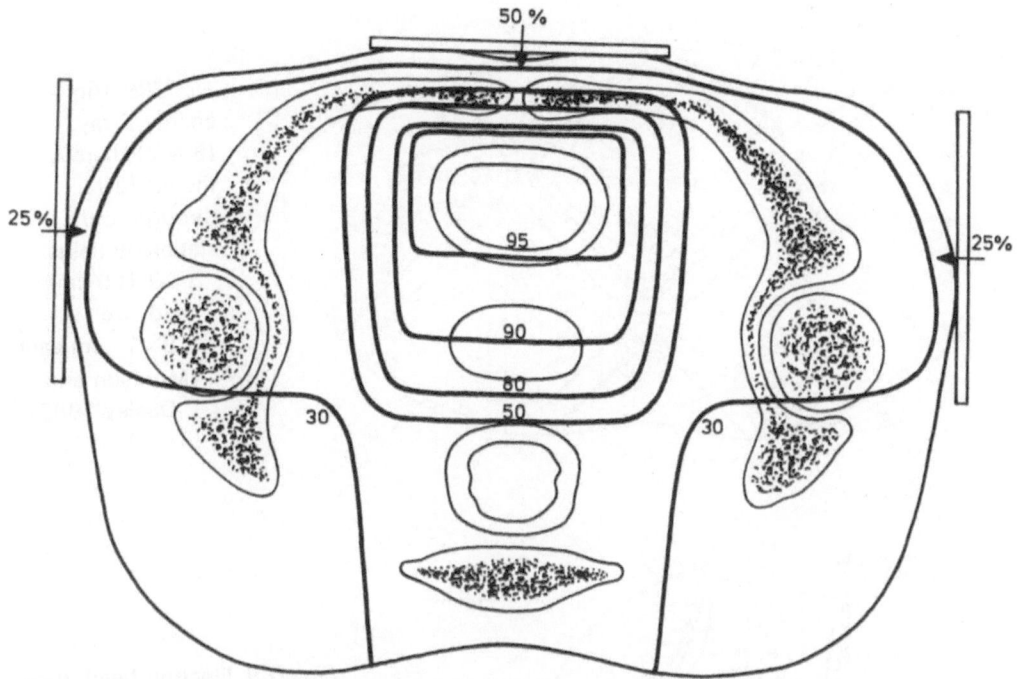

Fig. 287. High-energy X-ray (27.5 MV) therapy of the bladder through three stationary fields (1 : 2 load to the lateral and ventral fields, respectively)
FSD 120 cm
field size 10 × 15 cm
(Kriester et al. 1969)

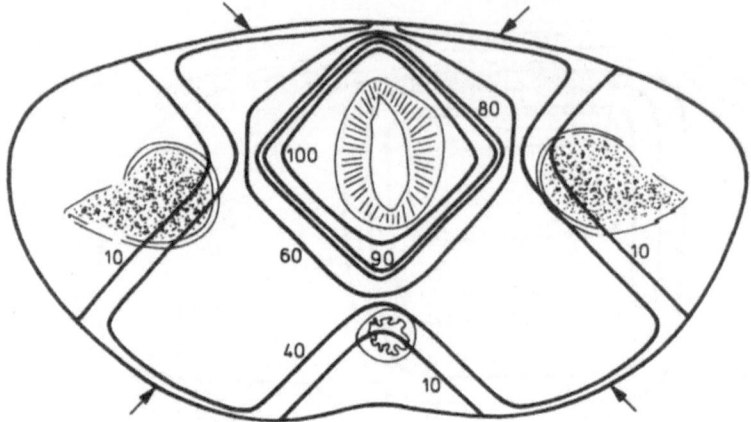

Fig. 288. High-energy X-ray (8 MV) therapy of the bladder through four stationary fields
    FSD 100 cm
    field size
        8 × 10 cm each
(Morrison and Deeley 1965)

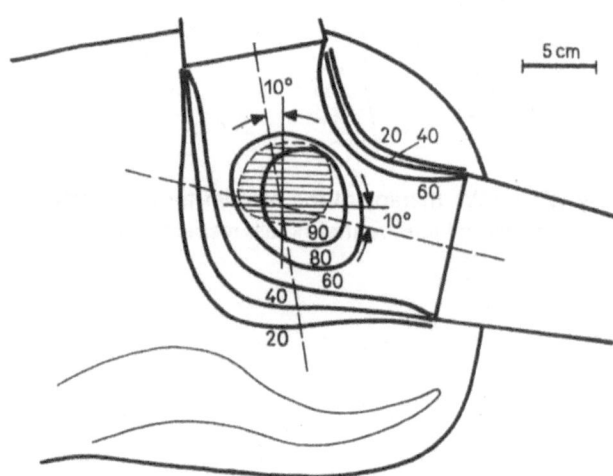

Fig. 289. Electron beam therapy (43 MeV) of the bladder through two stationary fields
    FSD 120 cm
    field size 10 × 14 cm
    Polystyrene phantom
    (Scherer et al. 1972)

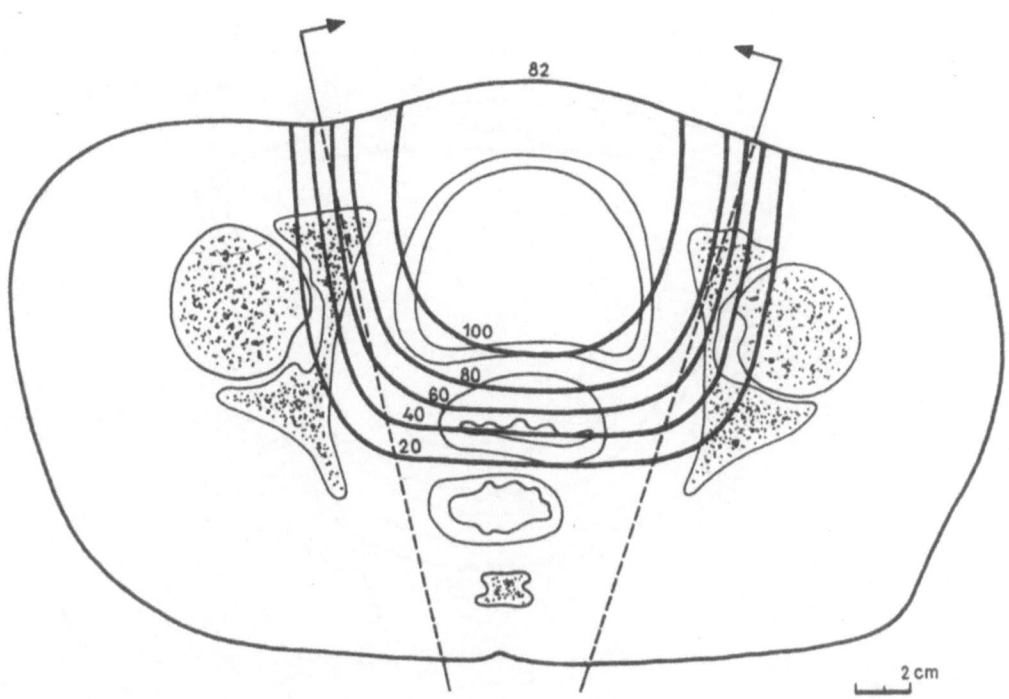

Fig. 290. Telecentric small-arc (30°) irradiation of the bladder with high-energy electrons (25 MeV)

FAD 120 cm
axis depth 30 cm
field size 3 × 14 cm
supposed depth of focus 9 cm
Alderson–Rando phantom
(Poser et al. 1973*b*)

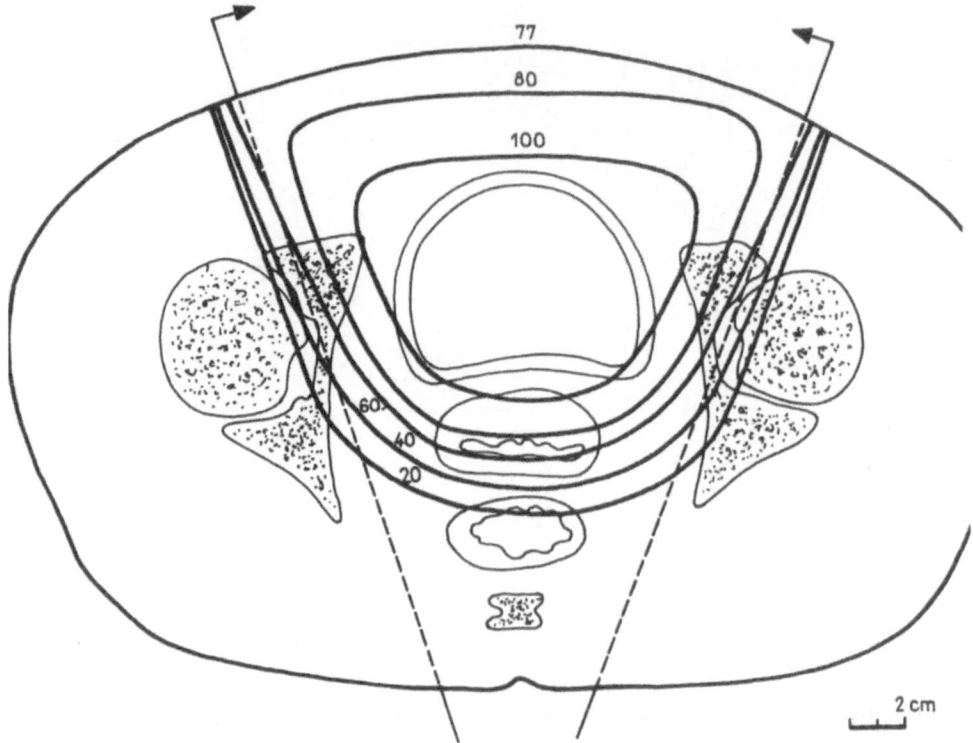

Fig. 291. Telecentric small-arc (40°) therapy of the bladder with high-energy electrons (30 MeV) (a-p diam of phantom 22 cm)

FAD 120 cm
axis depth 30 cm
field size 3 × 14 cm
supposed depth of focus 11 cm
Alderson–Rando phantom
(Poser et al. 1973*b*)

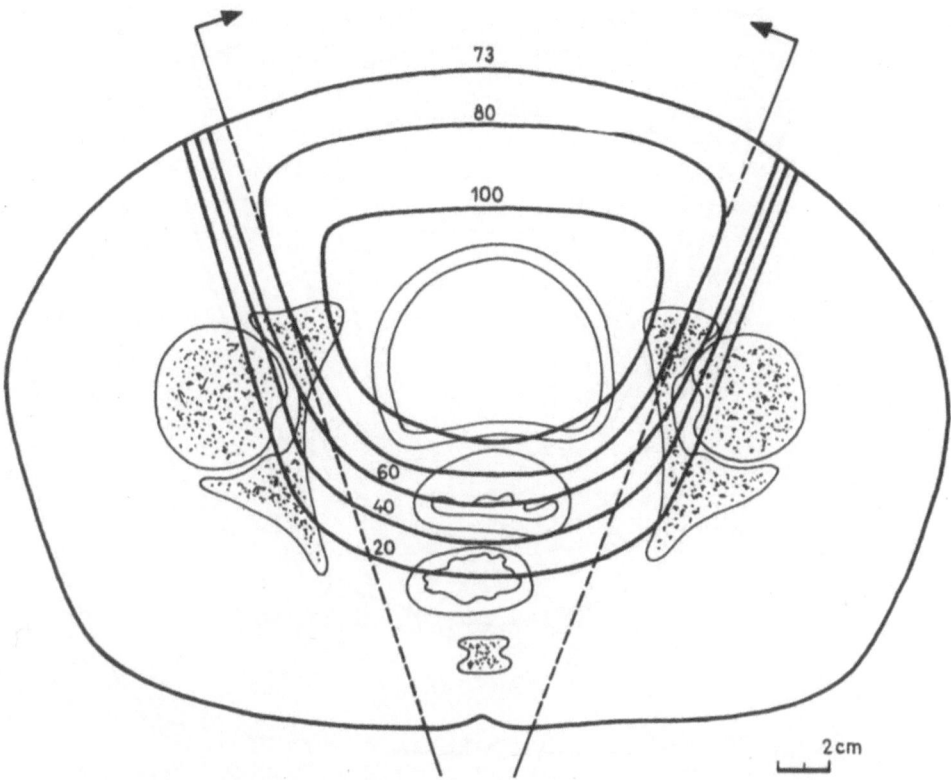

Fig. 292. Telecentric small-arc (40°) irradiation of the bladder with high-energy electrons (35 MeV) (a-p diam of phantom 24 cm)
  FAD 120 cm
  axis depth 30 cm
  field size 3 × 14 cm
  supposed depth of focus 13 cm
  Alderson–Rando phantom
  (Poser et al. 1973*b*)

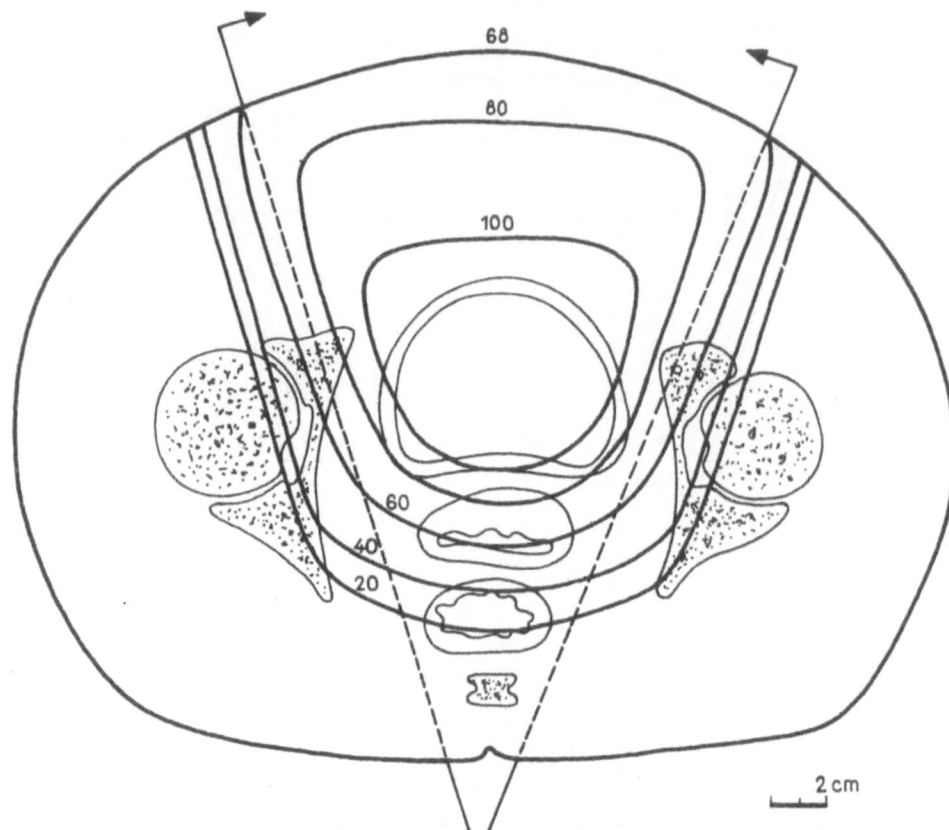

Fig. 293. Telecentric small-arc (40°) irradiation of the bladder with high-energy electrons (42 MeV) (a-p diam of phantom 26 cm)

    FAD 120 cm
    axis depth 30 cm
    field size 3 × 14 cm
    supposed depth of focus 15 cm
    Alderson–Rando phantom
    (Poser et al. 1973*b*)

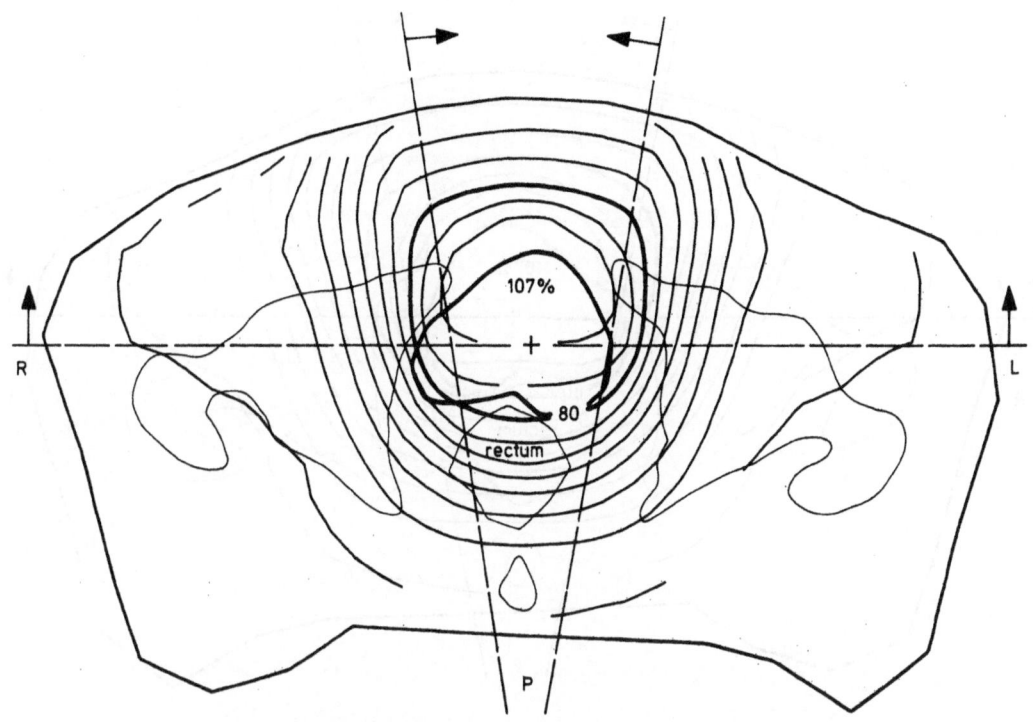

Fig. 294. Combined electron beam and high-energy X-ray therapy of the bladder
Electron beam: 30 MeV
                FAD 120 cm
                axis depth 30 cm from ventral in the midline
                arc 30° (15°/15°) telecentric
                field size 3 × 10 cm
X-ray: 42 MV
        FAD 120 cm
        axis depth 12 cm
        arc 180° (90°/90°)
        field size 8 × 10 cm
Computer calculated isodoses

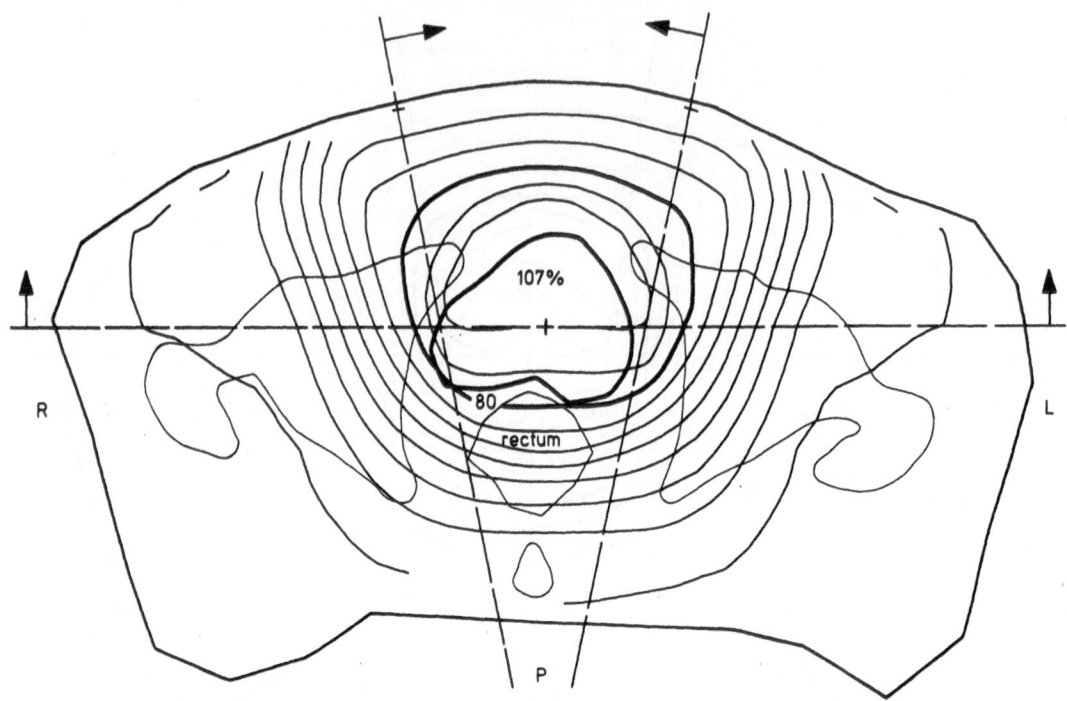

Fig. 295. Combined electron beam and high-energy X-ray therapy of the bladder
Electron beam: 30 MeV
                FAD 120 cm
                axis depth 30 cm from ventral in the midline
                arc 40° (20°/°20°) telecentric
                field size 3 × 10 cm
X-ray: 42 MV
       FAD 120 cm
       axis depth 12 cm
       arc 180° (90°/90°)
       field size 8 × 10 cm
Computer calculated isodoses

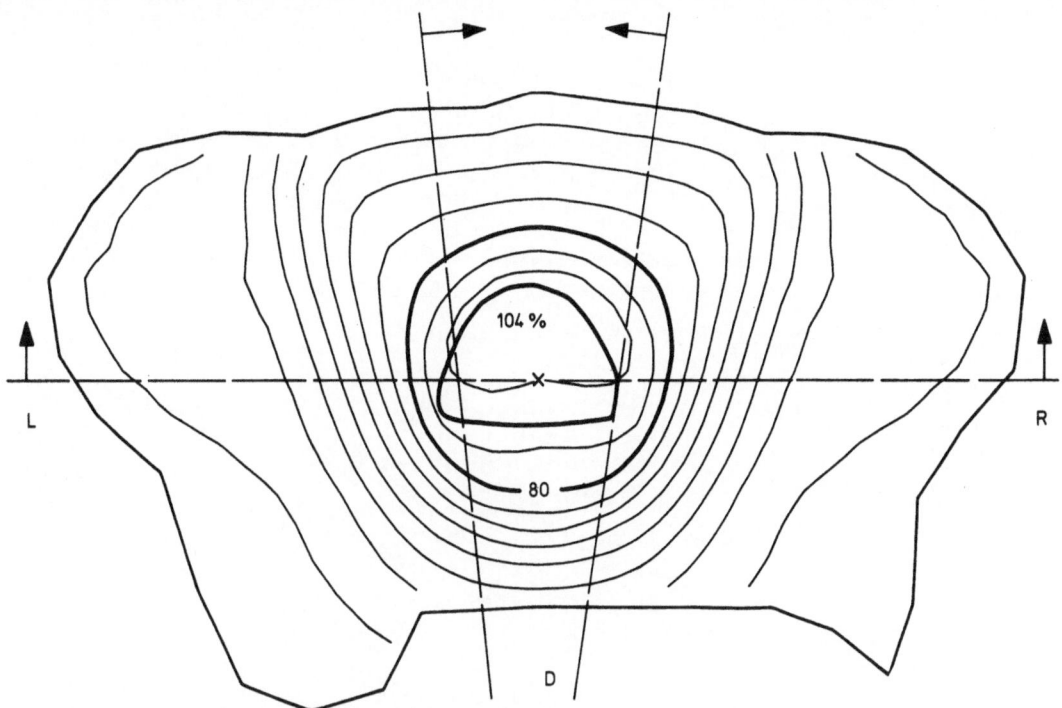

Fig. 296. Combined electron beam and high-energy X-ray irradiation of the bladder
Electron beam: 35 MeV
                FAD 120 cm
                axis depth 30 cm from ventral in the midline
                arc 40° (20°/20°) telecentric
                field size 3 × 10 cm
X-ray: 42 MV
        FAD 120 cm
        axis depth 12 cm
        arc 180° (90°/90°)
        field size 3 × 10 cm
Computer calculated isodoses

Paraaortic lymph nodes

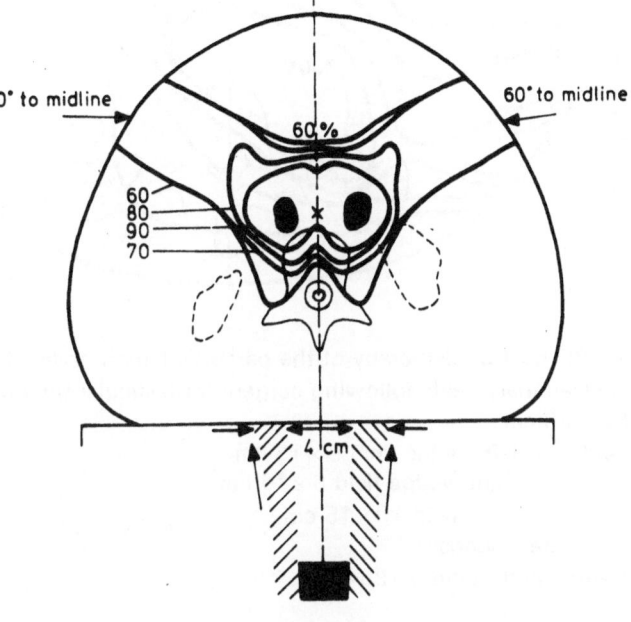

Fig. 297. 60-Co teletherapy of
the paraaortic lymph nodes
through three stationary fields
(section at the height of the
3rd lumbar vertebra)
    SSD 50 cm
    field size
        6 × 15 cm each ventral
           (at focus)
        8 × 15 cm dorsal
           (spinal cord
           shielded by a 4 cm
           wide satellite lead
           block)
    Calculated isodoses
    (Mau and Fürst 1973)

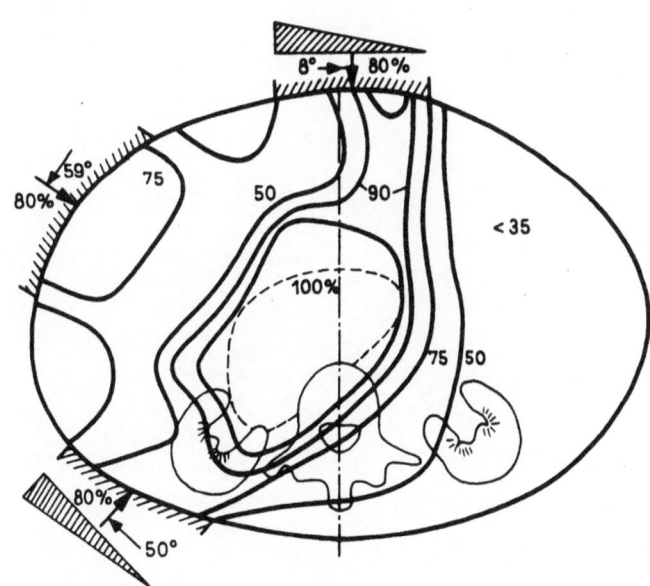

Fig. 298. 60-Co teletherapy of
the paraaortic lymph nodes
through three stationary fields
following surgery for testicular
tumour
    SSD 80 cm
    field size
        8 × 10 cm each
           wedge field
        10 × 15 cm
           open field
    Calculated isodoses
    (Notter and Ranudd 1964)

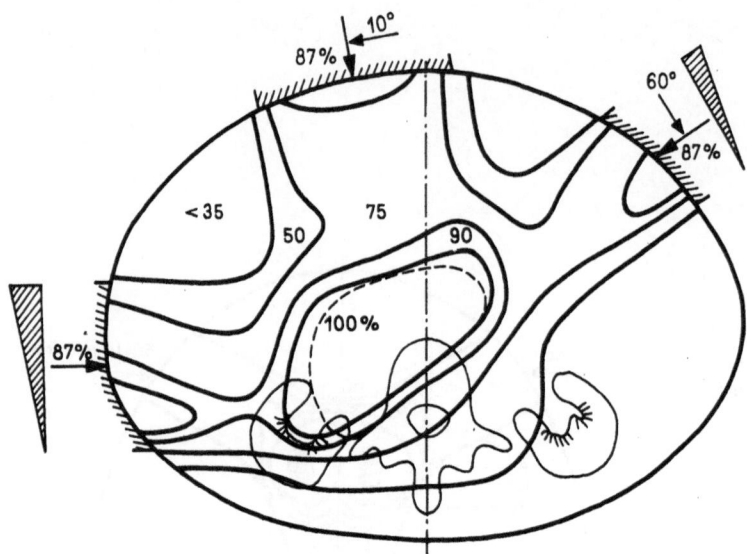

Fig. 299. 60-Co teletherapy of the paraortic lymph nodes through three stationary fields following surgery for testicular tumour
 SSD 80 cm
 field size: left wedge field 8 × 15 cm
         right wedge field 6 × 15 cm
         open field 10 × 15 cm
 Calculated isodoses
 (Notter and Ranudd 1964)

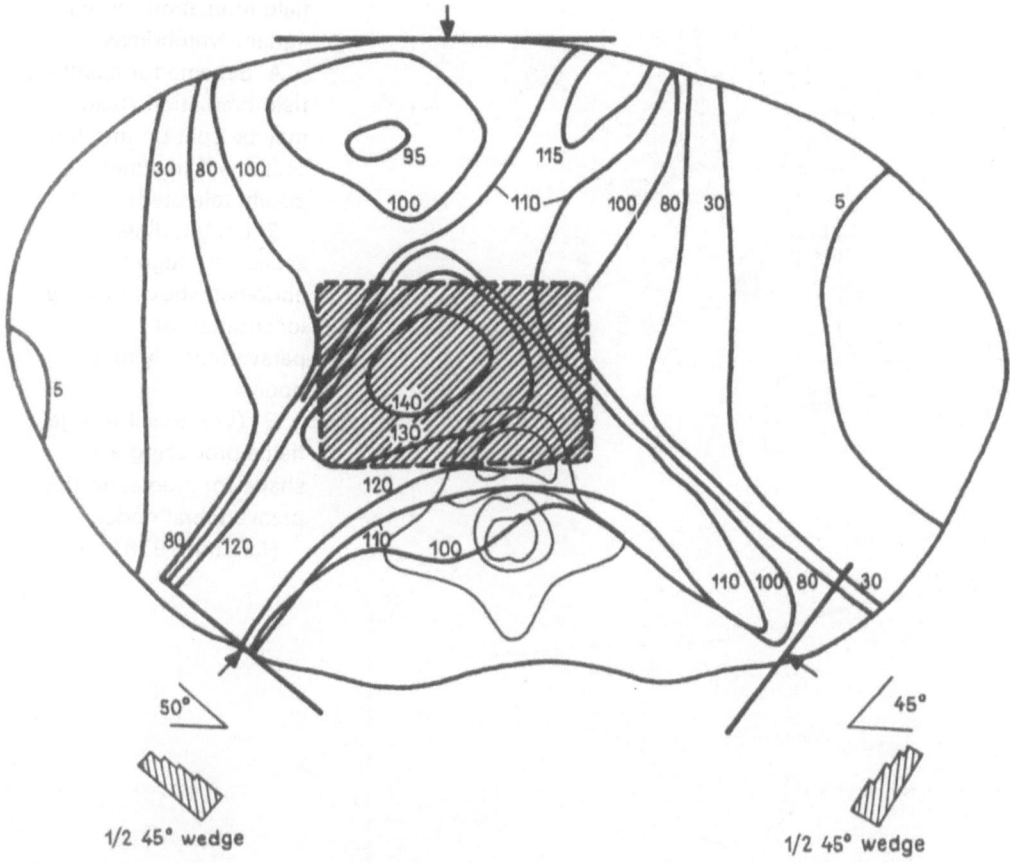

Fig. 300. 60-Co teletherapy of the paraaortic lymph nodes through a ventral field and two dorsal fields

Ventral field: SSD 70 cm
field size 10 × 15 cm
Dorsal fields: SSD 60 cm
field size 5 × 15 cm each
two 45° half-wedges
Water phantom
(Fletcher 1956a)

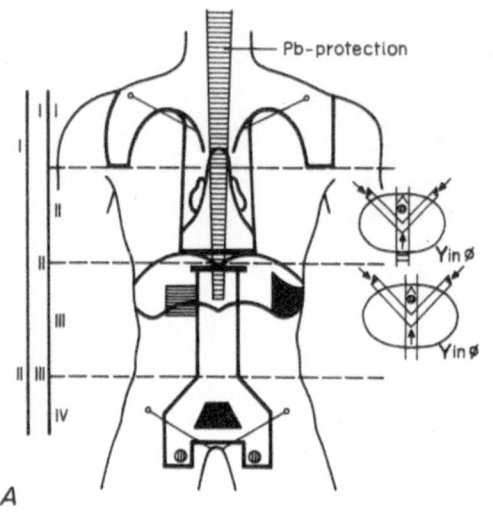

Pb-protection

I | I
I
II
II
III
II | III
IV

A

Yin ∅

Yin ∅

Fig. 301. 60-Co mantle field irradiation for malignant lymphomas

A. Scheme for mantle field irradiation (field may be split up into four sections if treatment is poorly tolerated)

B. Longitudinal section through the abdomen showing deep localization of paravertebral lymph nodes

C. Two dorsal wedge fields producing a V shape for irradiating the paravertebral nodes
    (Kärcher 1976)

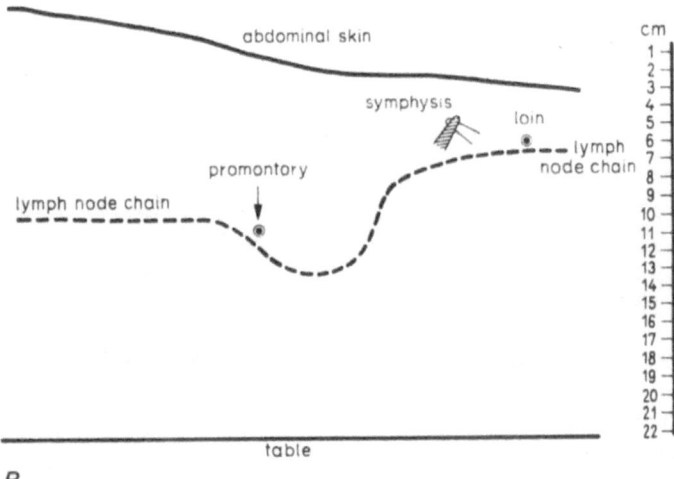

abdominal skin

symphysis

loin

promontory

lymph node chain

lymph node chain

cm
1
2
3
4
5
6
7
8
9
10
11
12
13
14
15
16
17
18
19
20
21
22

table

B

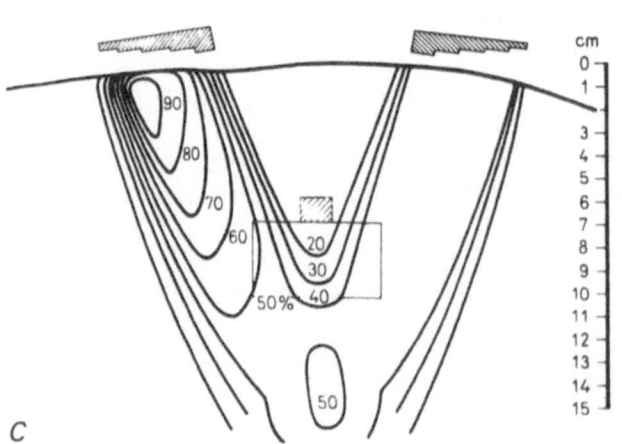

cm
0
1

3
4
5
6
7
8
9
10
11
12
13
14
15

90
80
70
60
50%
20
30
40
50

C

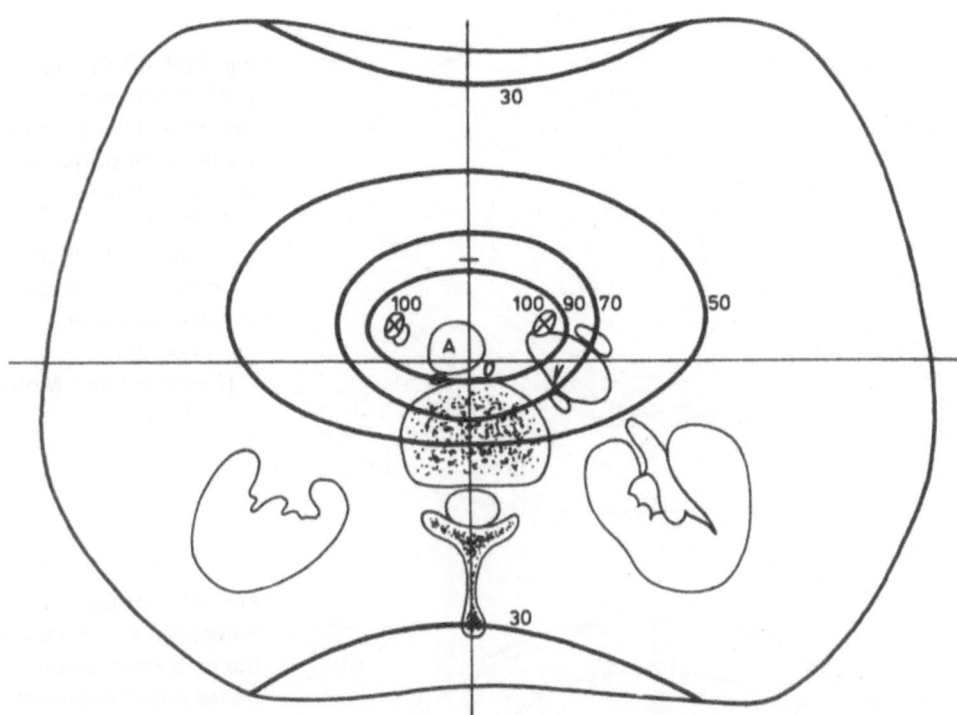

Fig. 302. 60-Co two-arc therapy of the paraaortic lymph nodes using wedge filter
SAD 65 cm
axis depth 6.5 cm from ventral
arcs 160° (±20°/±180°)
field size 6 × 14 cm at axis
wedge 17.5°, apex pointing posteriorly at 90° position of source
Plexiglas–water phantom
(Beduhn and Kuttig 1967)

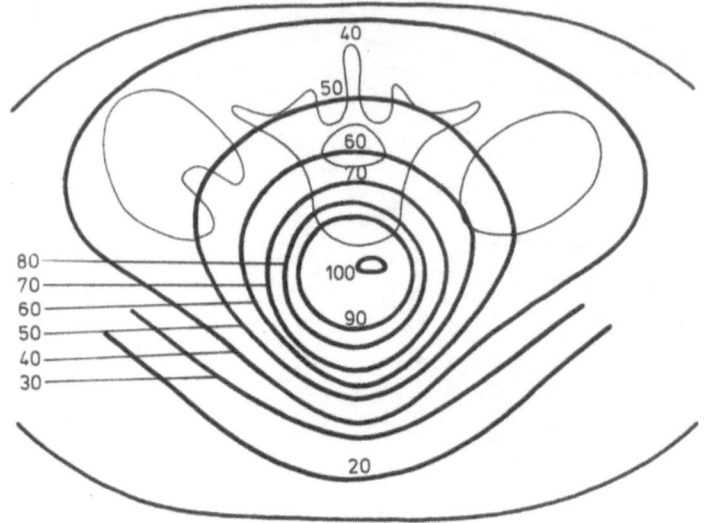

Fig. 303. 60-Co arc
(180°) therapy of the
paraaortic lymph nodes
(at the level of the 3rd
lumbar vertebra)
　　SAD 60 cm
　　axis depth 12.5 cm
　　field size 4 × 15 cm
　　Plexiglas–water
　　　phantom
　　(Frischbier and Möhle
　　　1967)

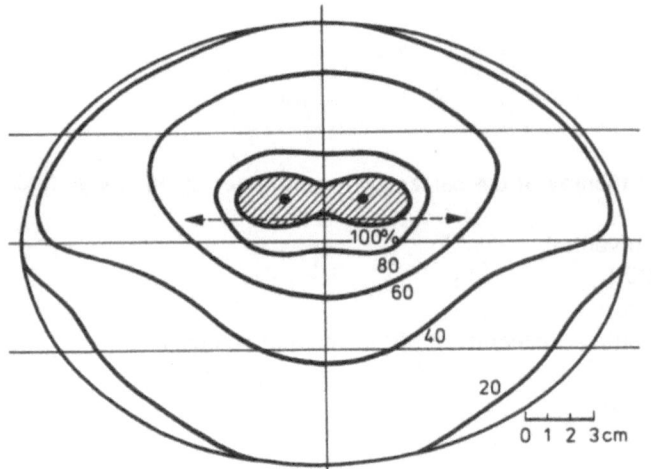

Fig. 304. 60-Co
translation arc therapy of
the paraaortic lymph
nodes with transversal
displacement of the axis
　　SAD 60 cm
　　axis depth 9 cm
　　arc 200°
　　translation distance of
　　　axis 12 cm
　　translation of table
　　　2.69 cm/min
　　field size 4 × 8 cm
　　Plexiglas phantom
　　(Kuttig and Becker
　　　1968)

Fig. 305. Two-centre two-arc
60-Co irradiation of the
paraaortic lymph nodes
   SAD 65 cm
   axis 2 cm before the anterior
      edge of vertebra
      3 cm left and right to the
      midline
   distance of axes 6 cm
   arcs 200° (±100°)
   field size 4 × 14 cm on the
      surface
   Alderson–Rando phantom
   (Rödel et al. 1969)

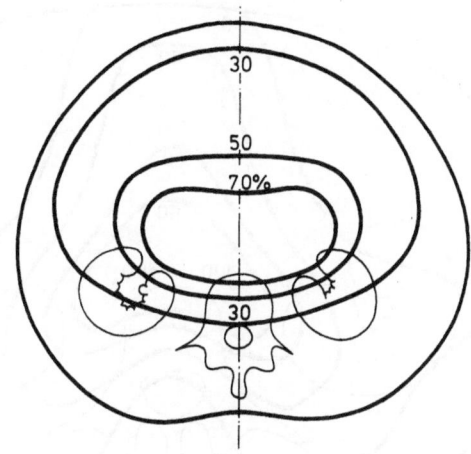

Fig. 306. Two-centre two-arc
60-Co treatment of the
paraaortic lymph nodes
   SAD 60 cm
   distance of axes 5 cm
   arcs 160°
   field size 5 × 15 cm at focus
   Calculated isodoses
   (Mau and Fürst 1973)

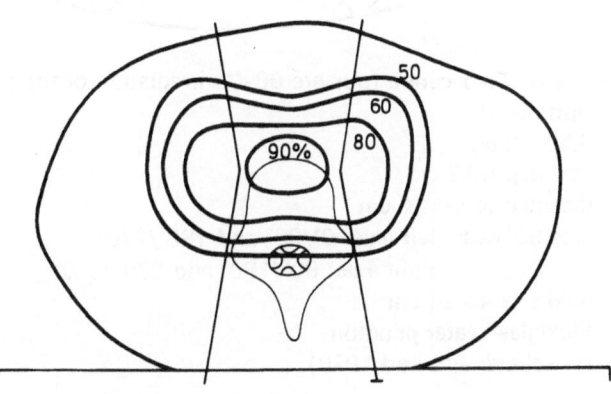

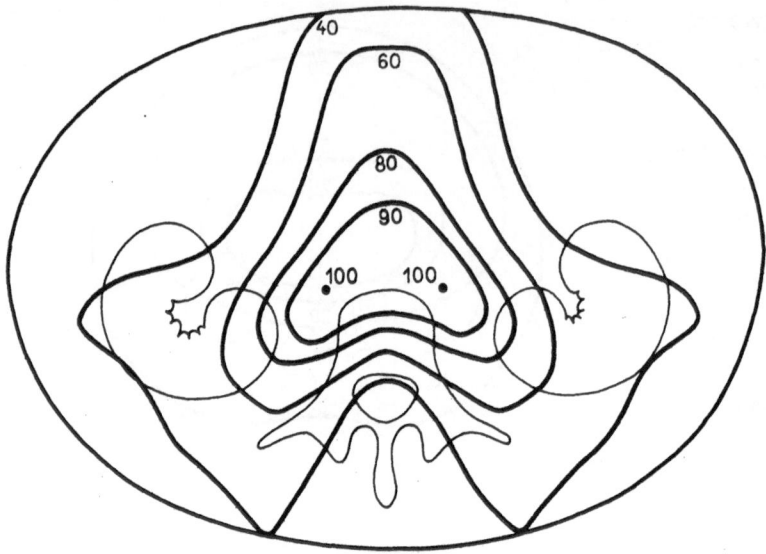

Fig. 307. Two-centre four-arc 60-Co irradiation of the paraaortic lymph nodes
   SAD 60 cm
   axis depth 12 cm
   distance of axes 6 cm
   arcs 90° each, left axis: 0°/90° and 180°/270°
                 right axis: 90°/180° and 270°/360°
   field size 4 × 14 cm
   Plexiglas–water phantom
   (Frischbier and Karl 1970)

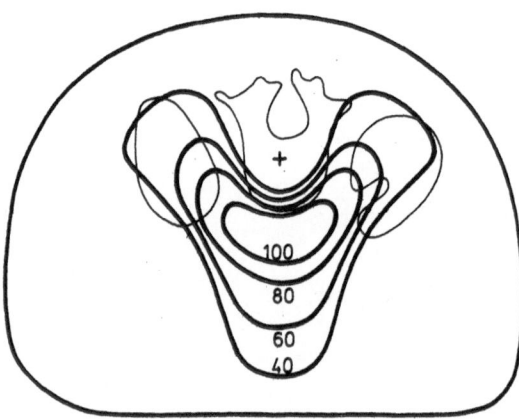

Fig. 308. One-centre two-arc eccentric irradiation of the paraaortic lymph nodes with high-energy X-rays (42 MV)
   FAD 120 cm
   axis depth 8 cm in the midline
   arcs 70° (±5°/±75°)
   field size 3 × 16 cm
   central beam tilted to produce a
     ±3 cm shift on the surface
   Alderson–Rando phantom
   (Heuss and Hoeffken 1972)

Fig. 309. Two-centre two-arc excentric irradiation of the paraaortic lymph nodes with 42 MV X-rays
  FAD 105 cm
  axis depth 11 cm, 7 cm on each side of the midline
  distance of axes 14 cm
  arcs 40° (±10°/±50°)
  central beam tilted to produce a ±5 cm shift on the surface
  field size 3 × 16 cm
  Alderson–Rando phantom
  (Heuss and Hoeffken 1972)

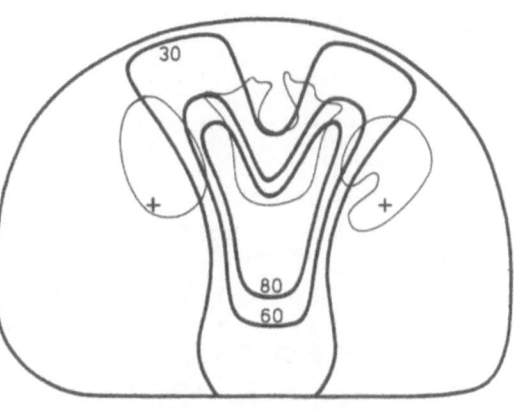

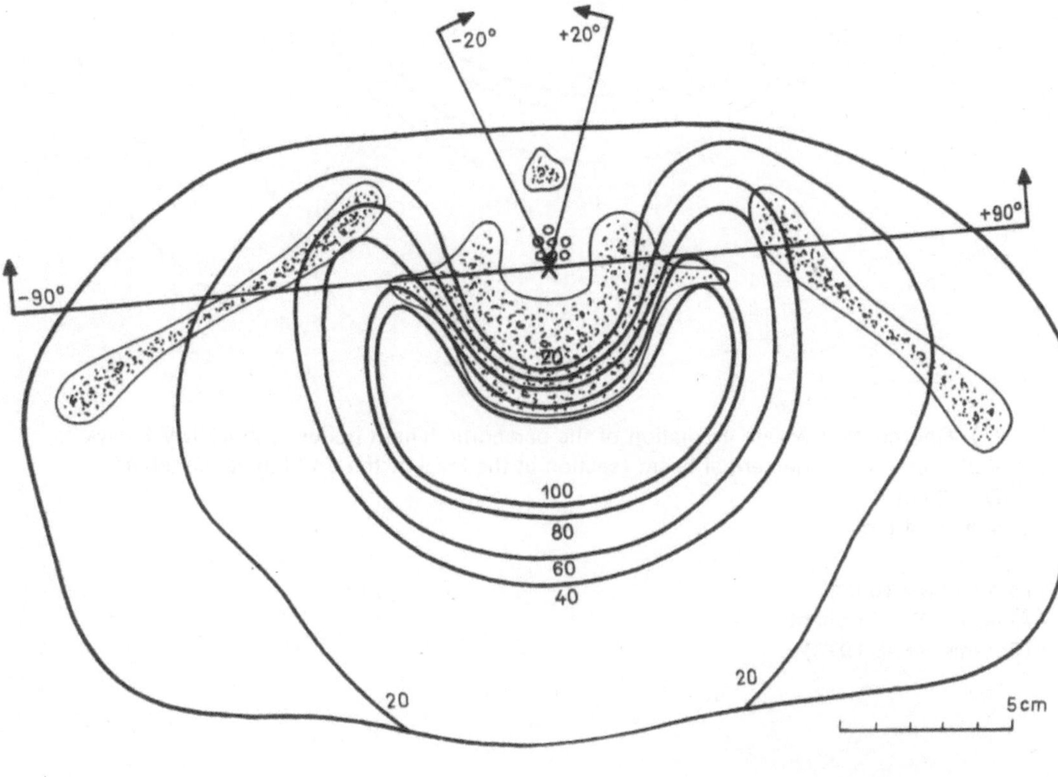

Fig. 310. One-centre two-arc irradiation of the paraaortic lymph nodes with 42 MV X-rays with a 2° lateral tilt of the central beam (section at the level of aortic bifurcation)
  FAD 120 cm
  axis depth 4 cm
  arcs 110°
  field size 3 × 10 cm
  Alderson–Rando phantom
  (Fournier et al. 1973)

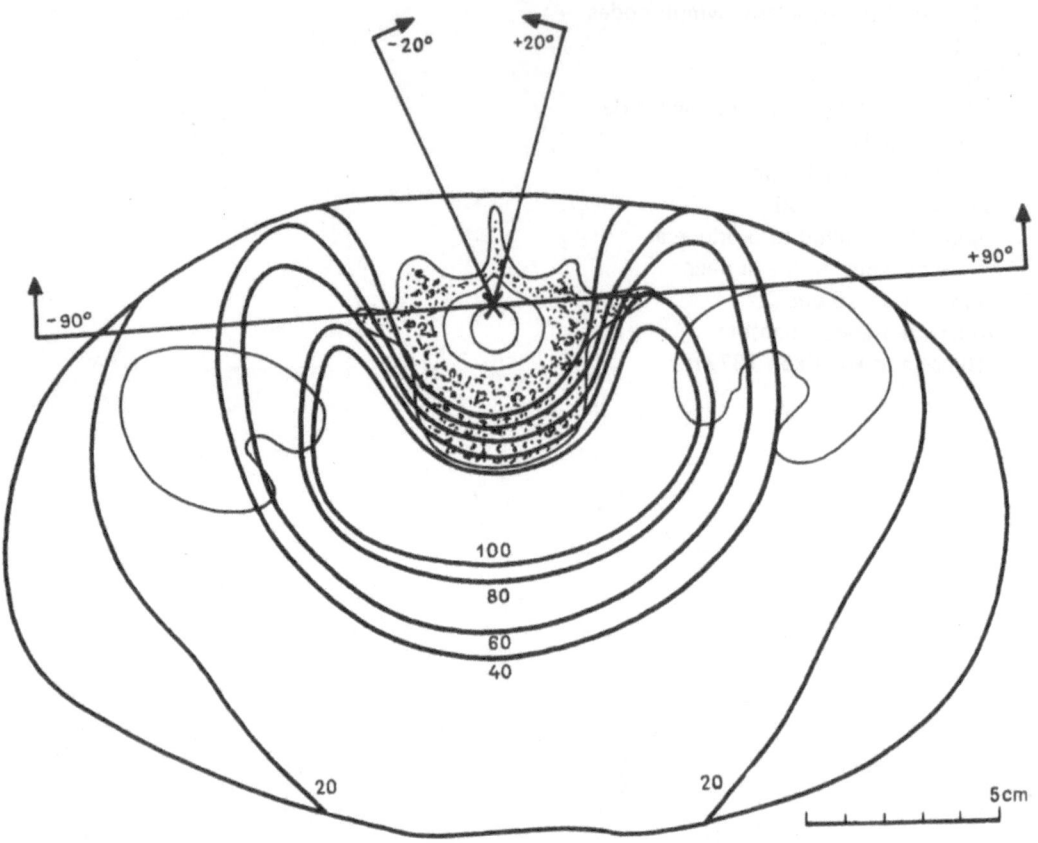

Fig. 311. One-centre two-arc irradiation of the paraaortic lymph nodes with 42 MV X-rays
with a 2° lateral tilt of the central beam (section at the level of the 2nd lumbar vertebra)
  FAD 120 cm
  axis depth 4 cm
  arcs 110°
  field size 3 × 10 cm
  Alderson–Rando phantom
  (Fournier et al. 1973)

Skeletal system

Mandible

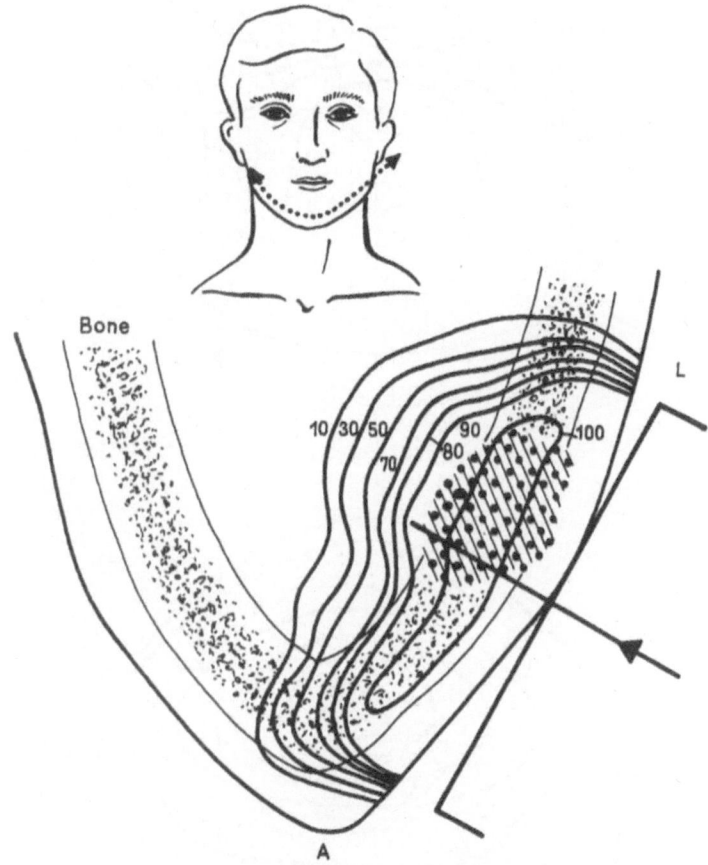

Fig. 312. Irradiation of a
mandibular tumour with
10 MeV electrons
  FSD 90 cm
  field size 8 × 5 cm
  Inhomogeneous
    phantom with bone
  (Laughlin et al. 1965)

Vertebral column

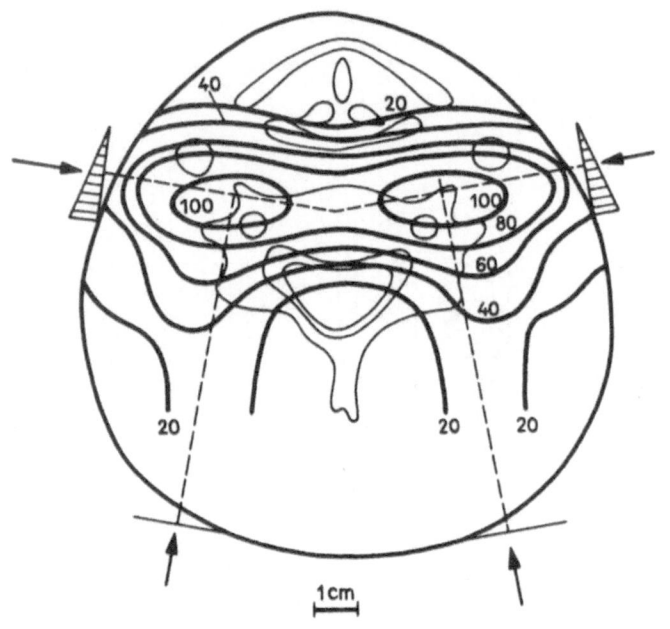

Fig. 313. 60-Co tele-
therapy of the cervical
spine through four
stationary fields (section
at the level of the 4th
cervical vertebra).
Ventral fields are wedge
filtered (15°)
  SSD 50 cm.
  field size 2 × 4 cm
  angles of incidence
    ventral fields 80° to
    the vertical
    oblique dorsal fields
    angulating at 170°
Paraffin and MgO
    phantom
  (Kuttig and Schäfer
    1968)

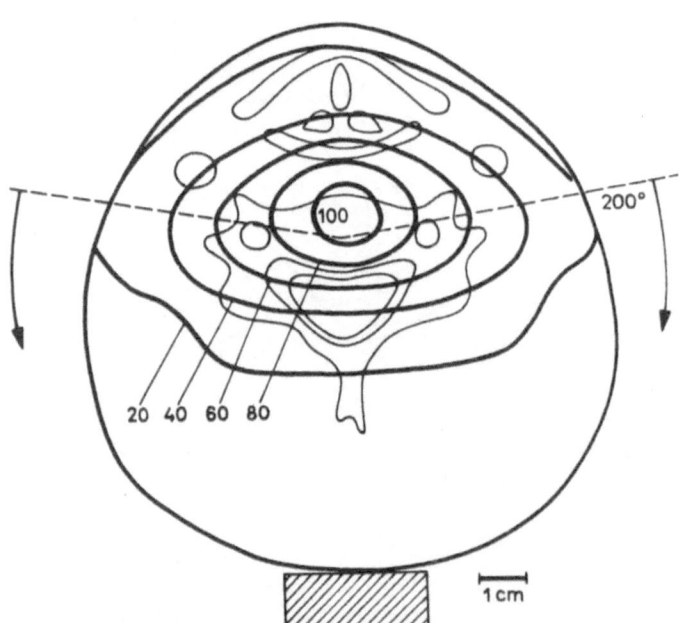

Fig. 314. 60-Co arc
(200°) therapy of the
cervical spine at the
level of the 4th cervical
vertebra (surface over
the spine protected with
a 3 cm wide 6 cm thick
lead block).
  SAD 60 cm
  axis depth 7 cm from
    dorsal in the
    midline
  field size 2 × 4 cm
Paraffin and MgO
    phantom
  (Kuttig and Schäfer
    1968)

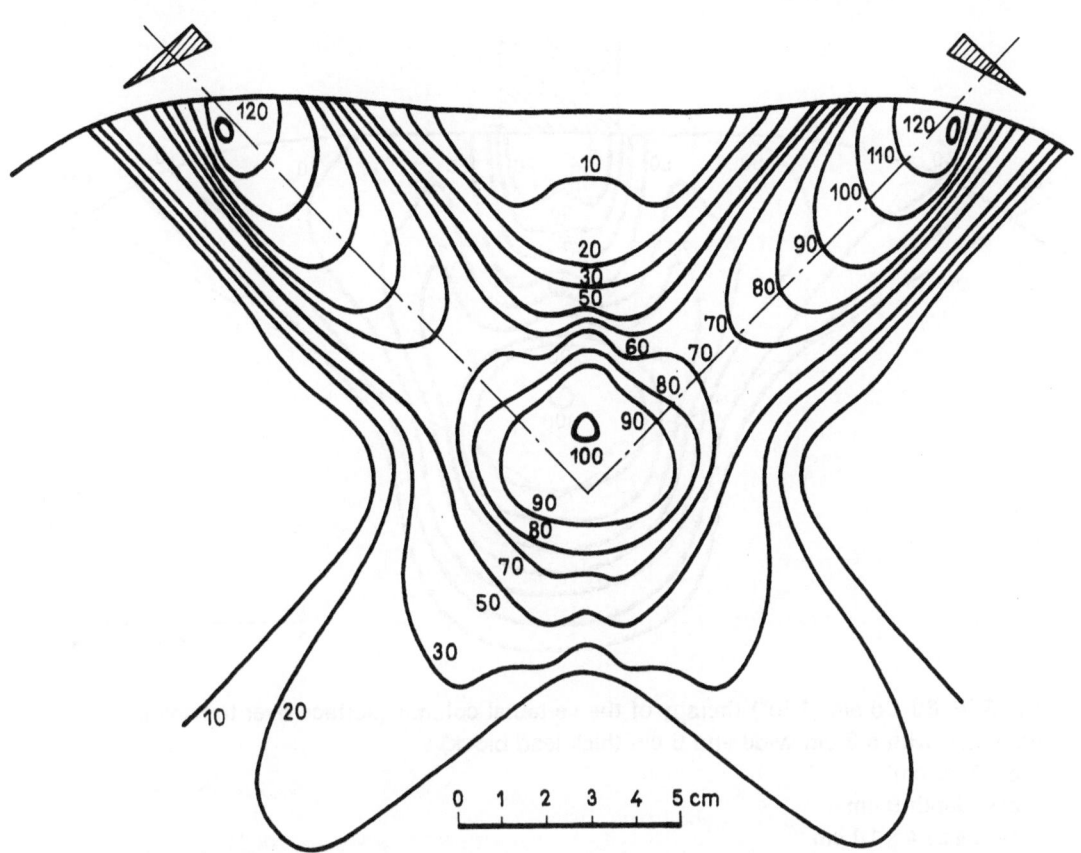

Fig. 315. 60-Co teletherapy of the spine through two 15° wedge fields
SSD 50 cm
field size 4 × 10 cm
focussing on 8 cm depth
Plexiglas–water phantom
(Kuttig et al. 1965)

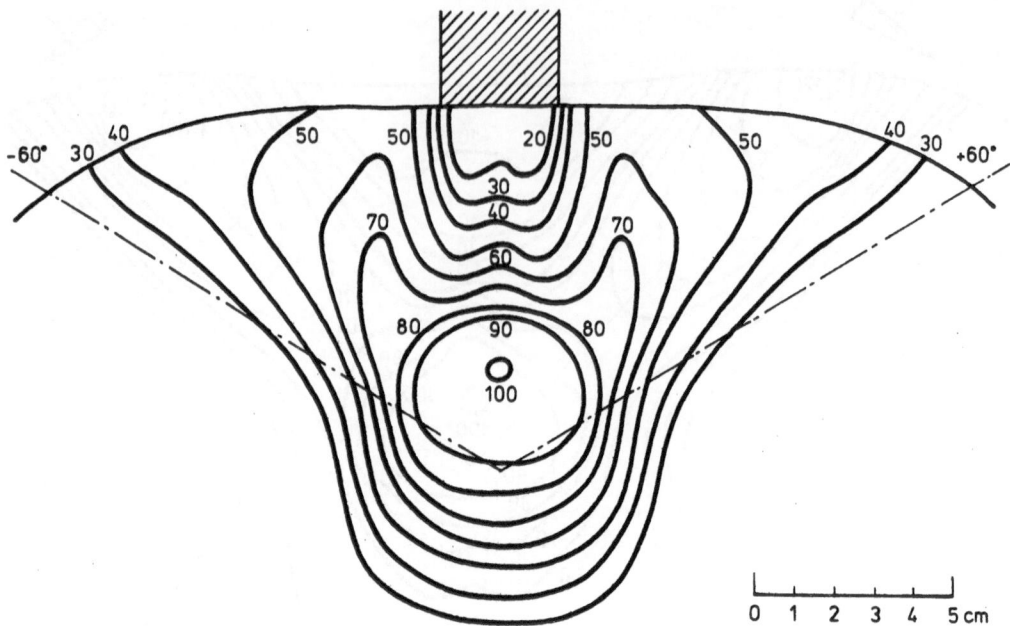

Fig. 316. 60-Co arc (120°) therapy of the vertebral column (surface over the spine protected with a 3 cm wide and 6 cm thick lead block)
    SAD 60 cm
    axis depth 9 cm
    field size 4 × 10 cm
    Plexiglas–water phantom
    (Kuttig et al. 1965)

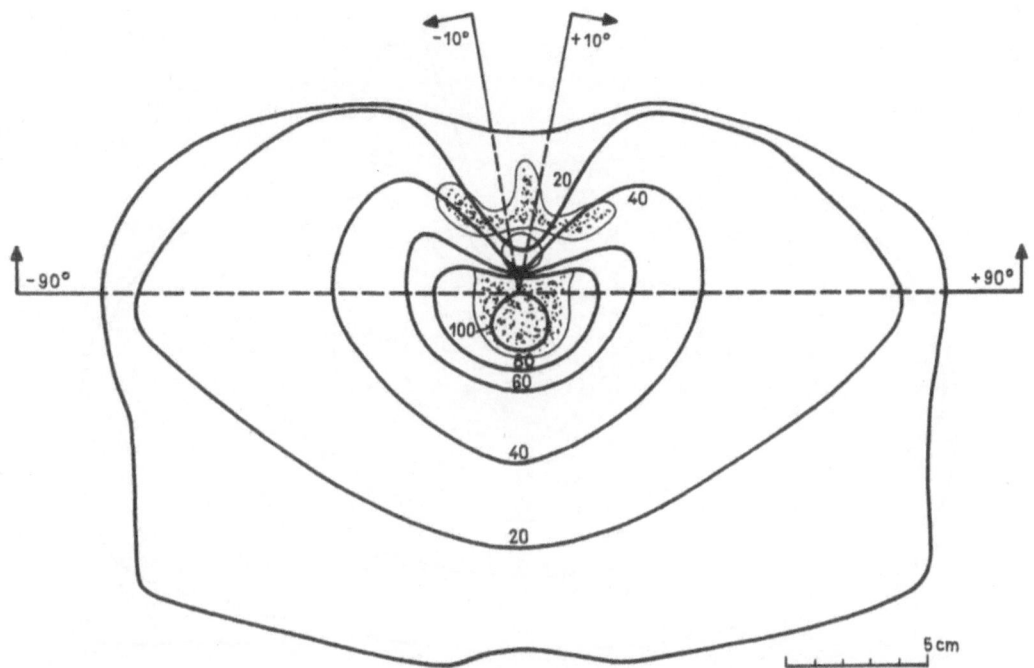

Fig. 317. One-centre two-arc irradiation of the spine with 42 MV X-rays at the level of the 8th thoracic vertebra
    FAD 120 cm
    axis depth 5.5 cm
    arcs 80°
    1° lateral tilt of the central beam
    field size 3 × 10 cm at axis
    Alderson–Rando phantom
    (Scheidel et al. 1973)

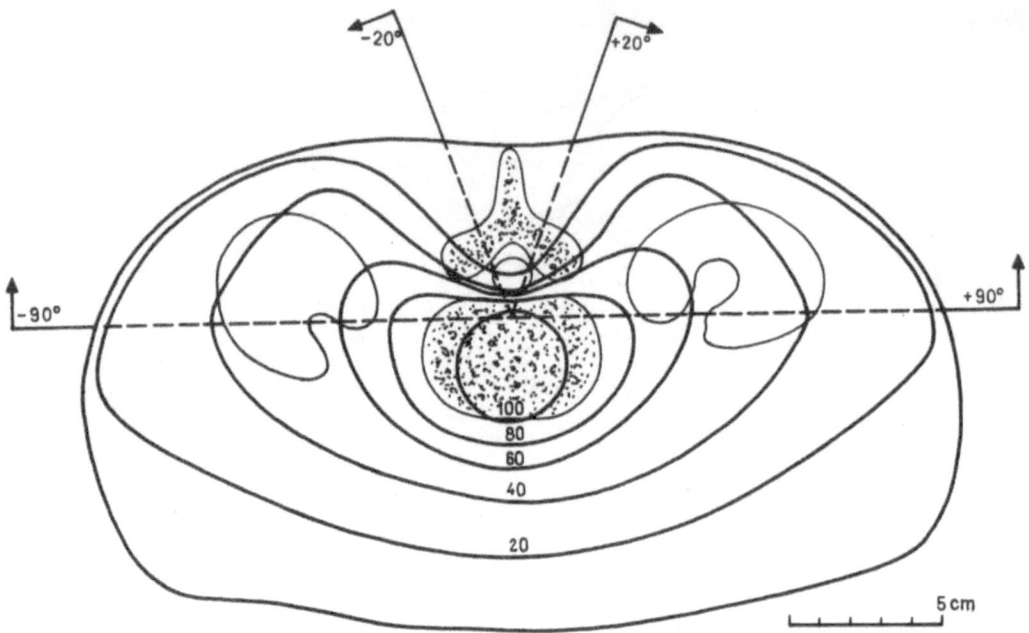

Fig. 318. One-centre two-arc (both 70°) irradiation of the spine with 42 MV X-rays at the level of the 2nd lumbar vertebra
    FAD 120 cm
    axis depth 5.5 cm
    1° lateral tilt of the central beam
    field size 4 × 10 cm at axis
    Alderson–Rando phantom
    (Scheidel et al. 1973)

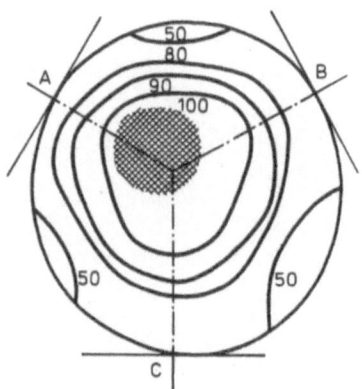

Fig. 319. 60-Co teletherapy of the femur through three stationary fields
    SSD 60 cm
    field size 7.2 × 12 cm
    central beams enclose angles of 120°
    (Becker and Schubert 1961)

Central nervous system

Anterior cranial cavity

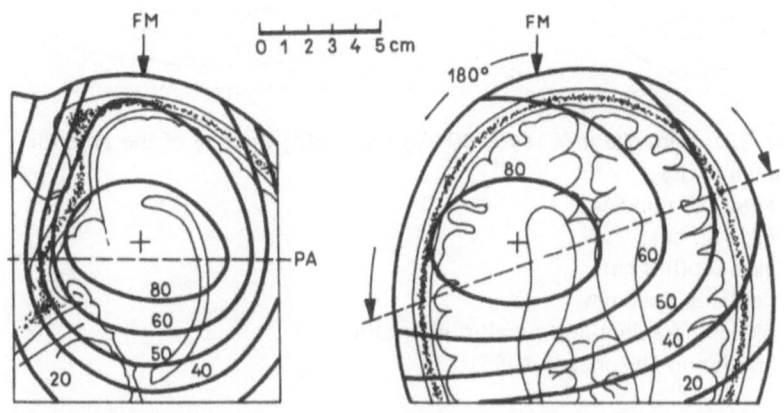

Fig. 320. Arc (180°) therapy of the anterior cranial cavity with 200 kV
X-rays
  Filter 0.5 mm Cu
  FAD 50 cm
  axis depth 8 cm
  field size 4 × 6 cm
  Skeletal cranium and paraffin phantom
  (Breit and Hirschauer 1955)

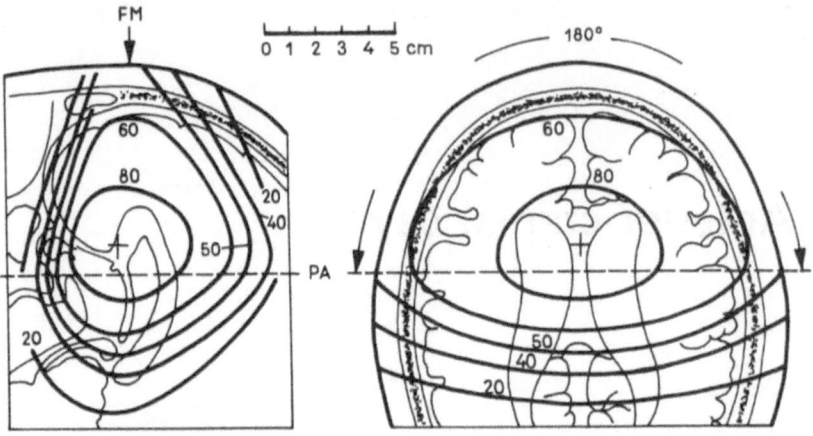

Fig. 321. Kilovoltage X-ray (200 kV) arc (180°) therapy of the anterior
cranial cavity
    Filter 0.5 mm Cu
    FAD 50 cm
    axis depth 8 cm
    field size 4 × 6 cm
    Skeletal cranium and paraffin phantom
    (Breit and Hirschauer 1955)

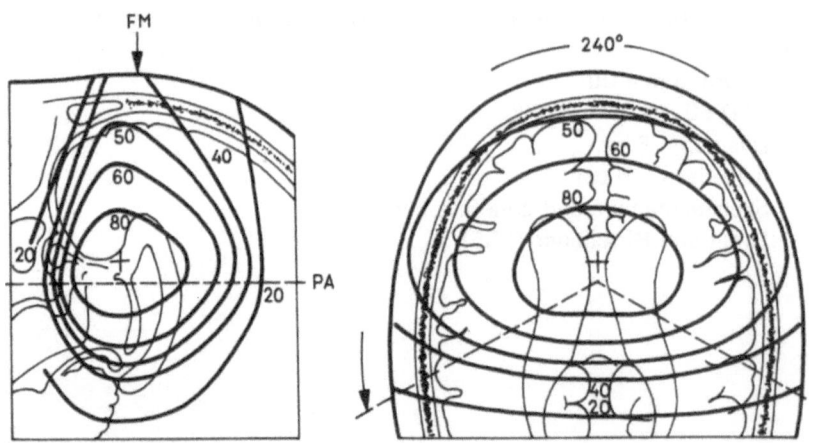

Fig. 322. Kilovoltage X-ray (200 kV) arc (240°) therapy of the anterior
cranial cavity
    Filter 0.5 mm Cu
    FAD 50 cm
    axis depth 8 cm
    field size 4 × 6 cm
    Skeletal cranium and paraffin phantom
    (Breit and Hirschauer 1955)

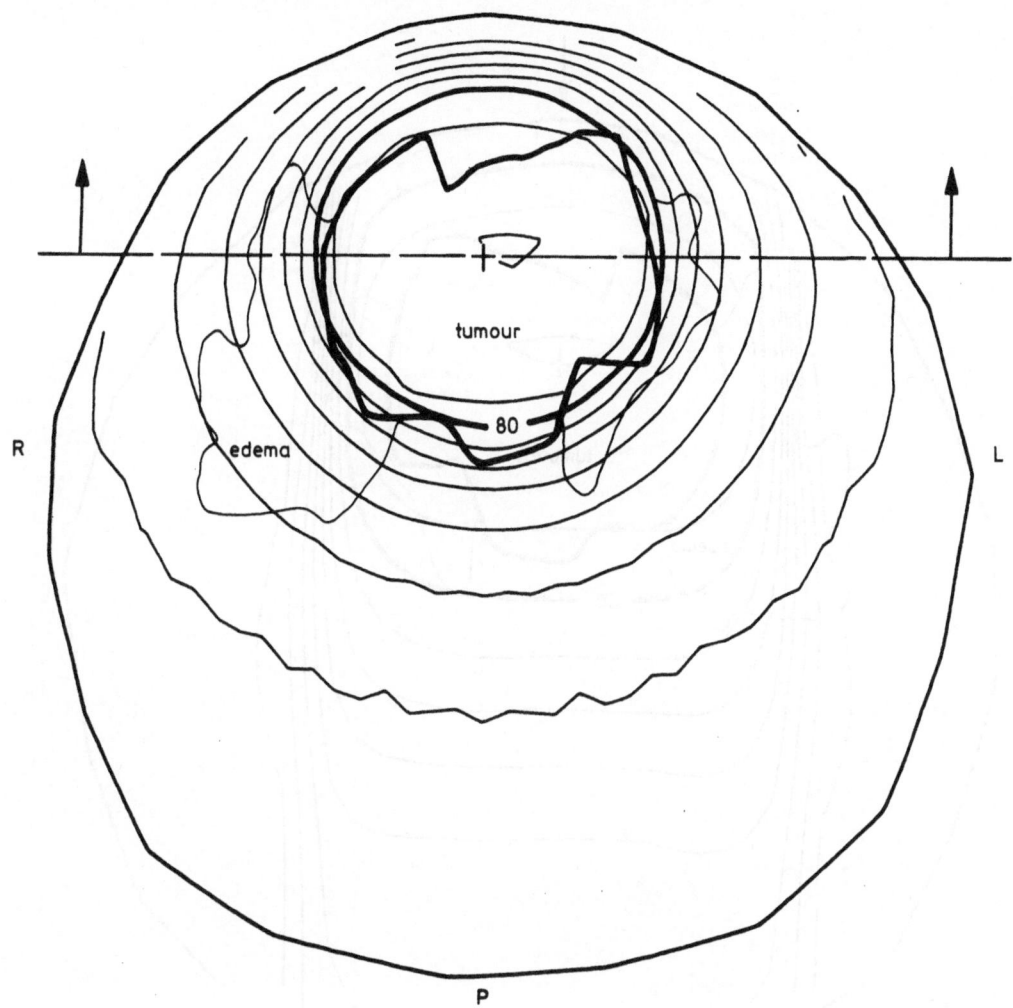

Fig. 323. Arc therapy of the anterior cranial cavity with 42 MV X-rays
FAD 120 cm
axis depth 5 cm
arc 180° (90°/90°)
field size 6 × 8 cm
Computer calculated isodoses

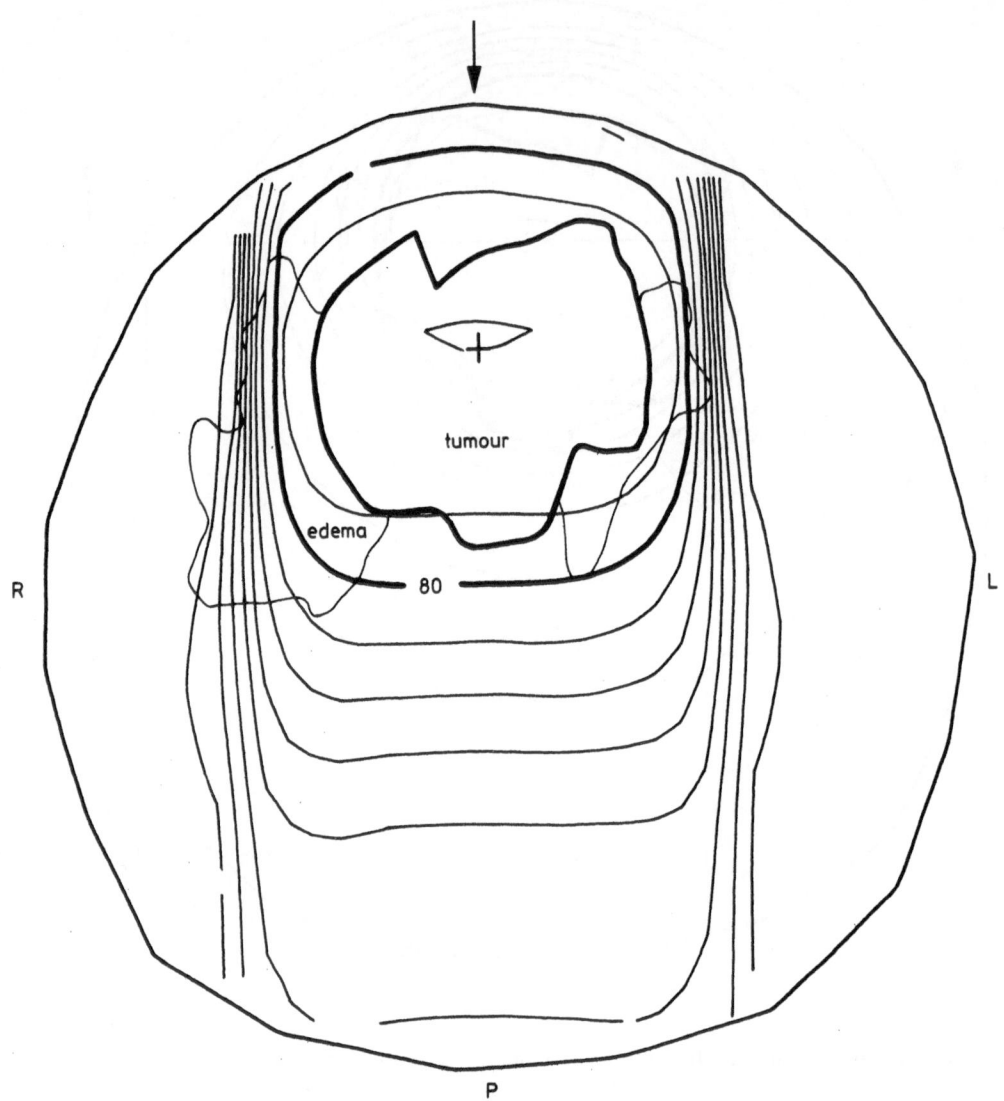

Fig. 324. Combined electron beam and high-energy X-ray irradiation of the anterior cranial cavity
  Electron beam: 25 MeV
                 FSD 100 cm
                 field size 8 cm diam
  X-rays: 42 MV
          FSD 100 cm
          field size 8 × 8 cm
  Loading 1 : 1
  Computer calculated isodoses

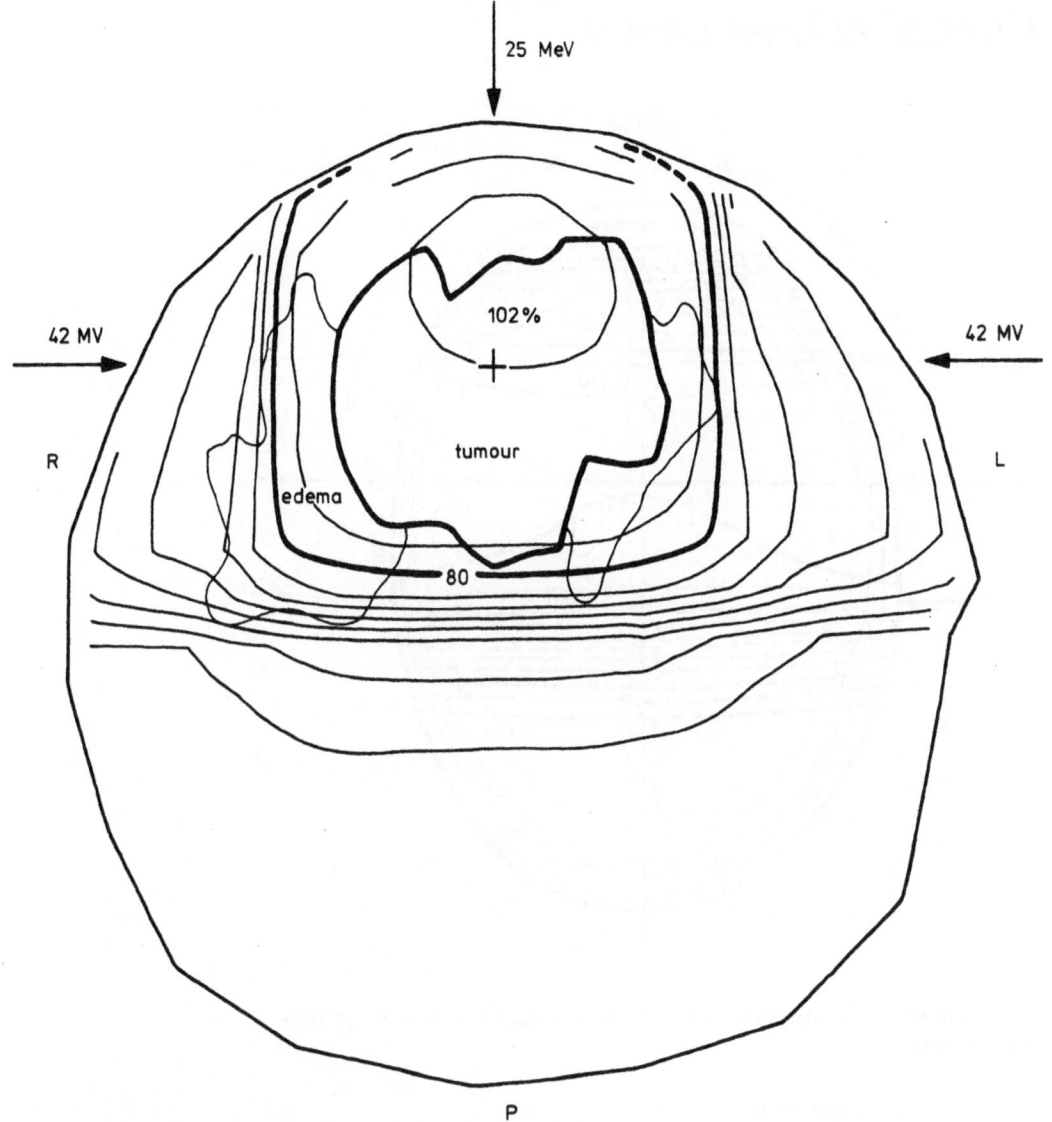

Fig. 325. Combined electron beam and high-energy X-ray irradiation of the anterior cranial cavity through two lateral photon fields and a sagittal electron field
Electron beam: 25 MeV
                FSD 100 cm
                field size 8 cm diam
X-rays: 42 MV
        field size 8 × 8 cm
Computer calculated isodoses

Central cranial cavity

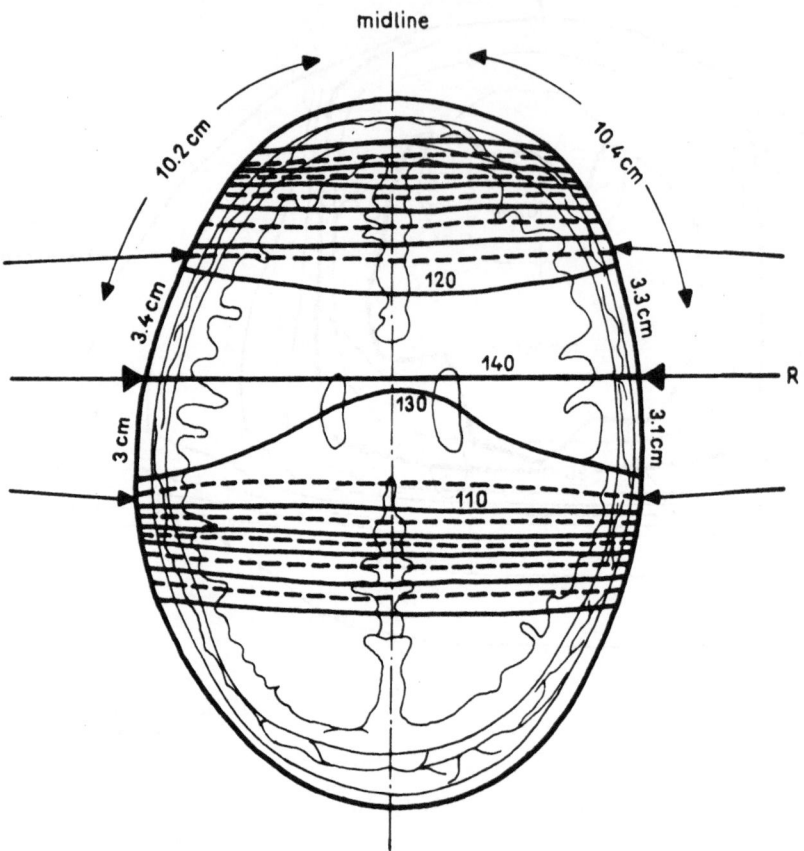

Fig. 326. 60-Co teletherapy of the central cranial cavity through two
lateral fields
  SSD 60 cm
  field size 6 × 8 cm each
  (Gyenes, personal communication)

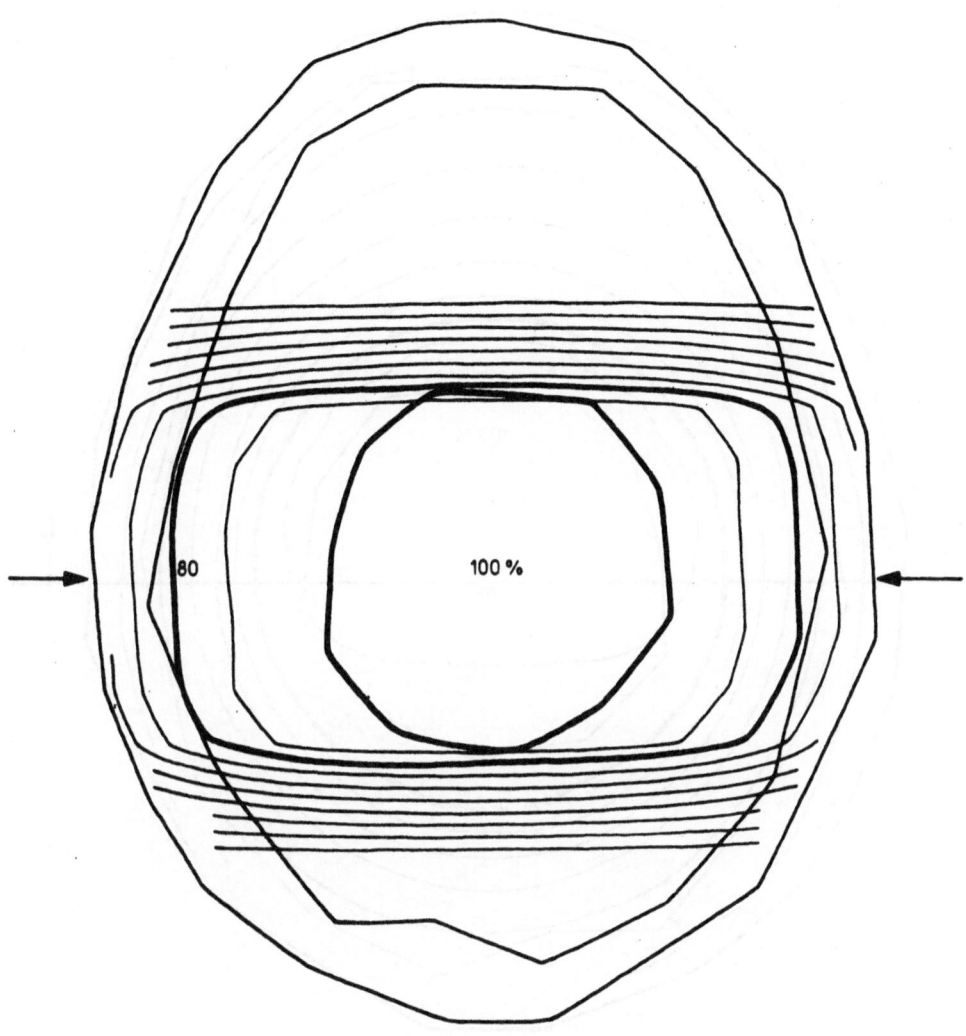

Fig. 327. High-energy X-ray (42 MV) irradiation of the central cranial cavity through two lateral isocentric photon fields
   FID 120 cm
   field size 8 × 8 cm
   Computer calculated isodoses

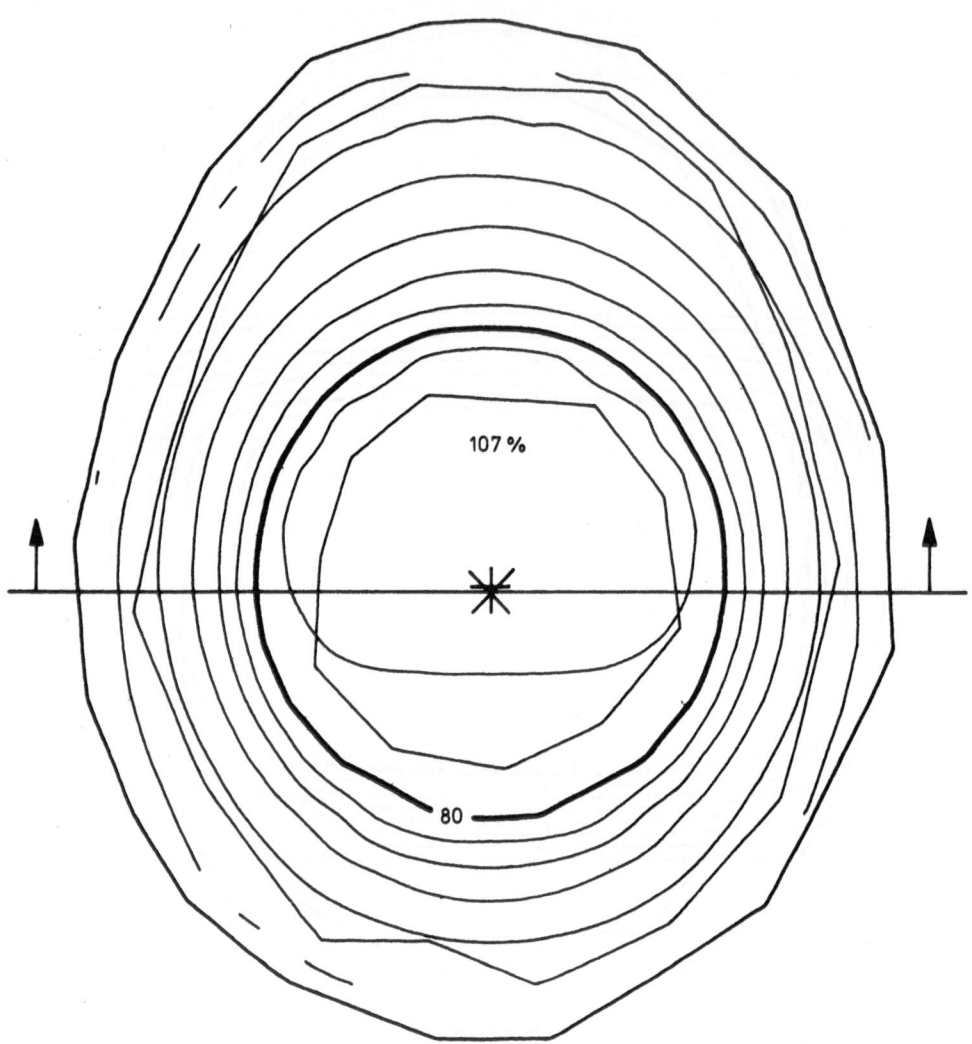

Fig. 328. Arc therapy of the central cranial cavity with 42 MV X-rays
FAD 120 cm
axis depth 9 cm
arc 180° (90°/90°)
field size 8 × 8 cm
Computer calculated isodoses

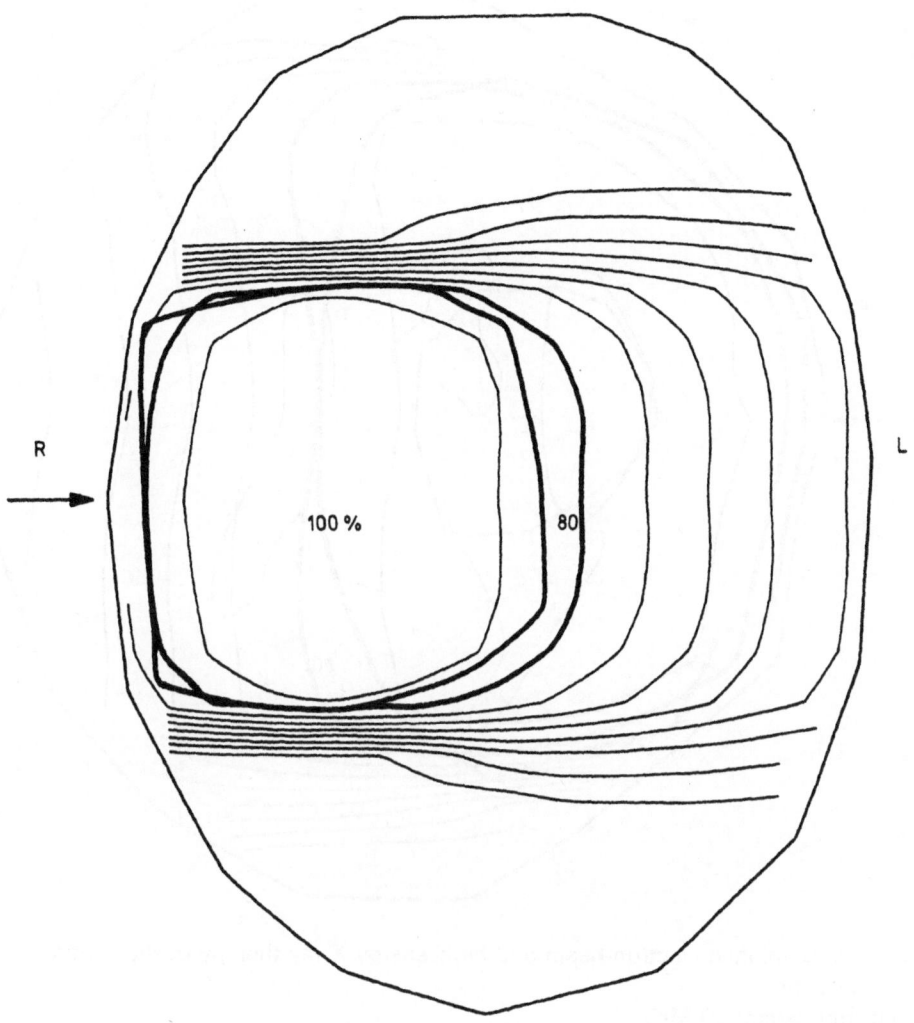

R

L

100 %

80

Fig. 329. Combined electron beam and high-energy X-ray therapy of the central cranial cavity

Electon beam: 30 MeV
        FSD 100 cm
           field size 8 cm diam

X-rays: 42 MV
     FSD 100 cm
     field size 8×8 cm

Loading 1 : 1

Computer calculated isodoses

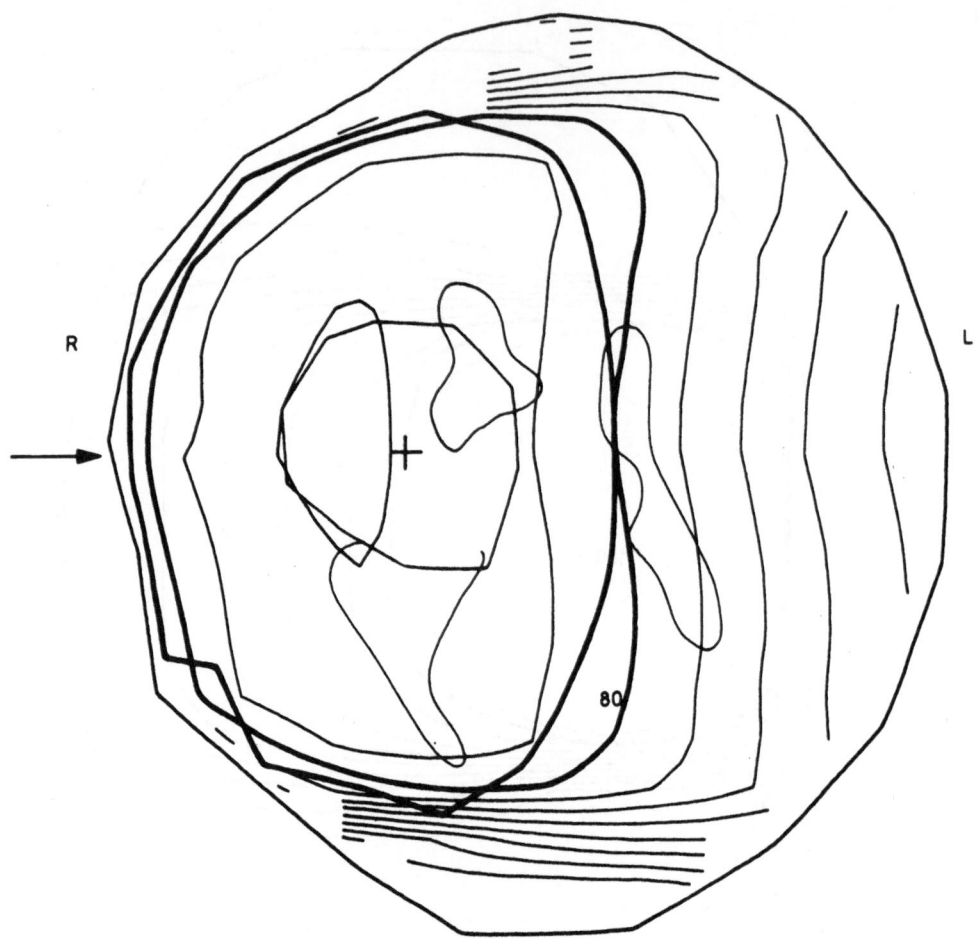

R   L

Fig. 330. Combined electron beam and high-energy X-ray therapy of the central cranial cavity
    Electron beam: 30 MeV
                        FSD 100 cm
                        field size 12 cm diam
    X-rays: 42 MV
                FSD 100 cm
                field size 12 × 12 cm
    Loading 1 : 1
    Computer calculated isodoses

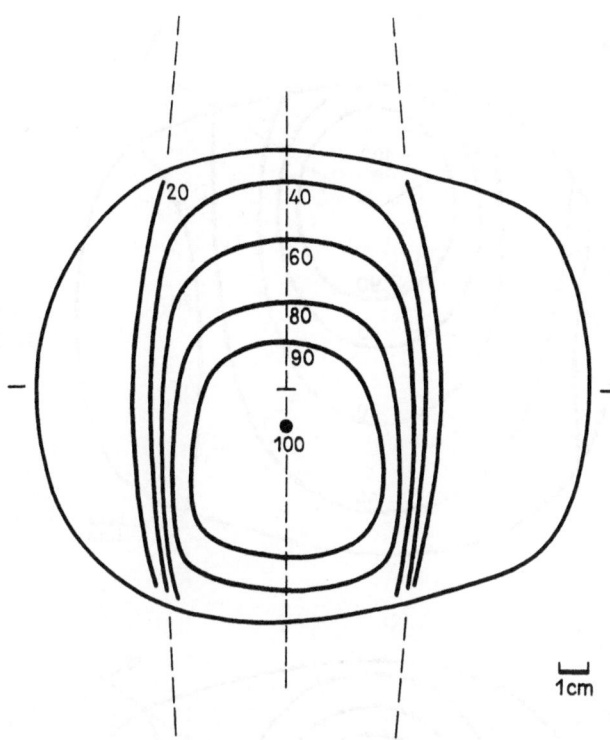

Fig. 331. Electron beam therapy of the central cranial cavity through two oblique lateral fields (the affected side receives two-thirds of the maximum dose)
    Affected side:
       25 MeV electrons
       FSD 100 cm
       field size 8 × 6 cm
    Intact side:
       42 MeV electrons
       FSD 100 cm
       field size 8 × 6 cm
    Alderson–Rando phantom
    (Herbig et al. 1971)

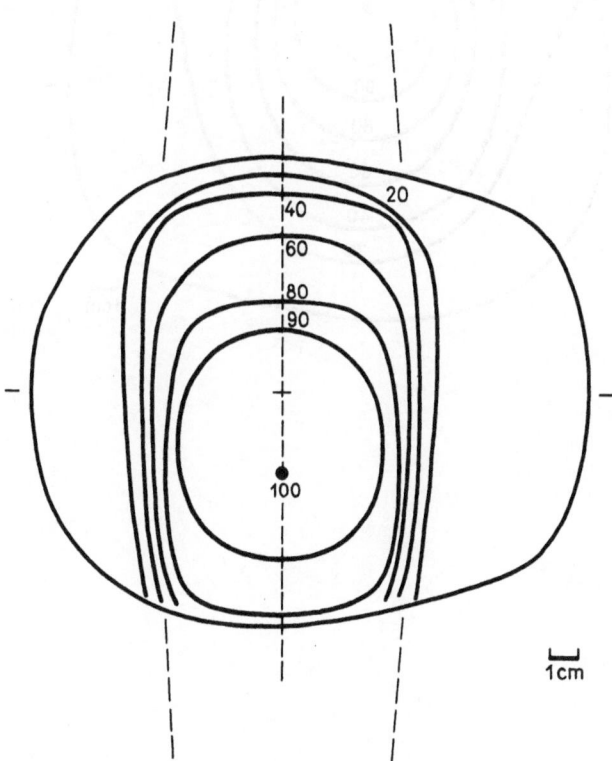

Fig. 332. Combined electron beam and high-energy X-ray irradiation of the central cranial cavity through two lateral cranial fields
    Electron beam:
       25 MeV (affected side)
       FSD 100 cm
       field size 8 × 6 cm
    X-rays:
       42 MV (intact side)
       FSD 100 cm
       field size 8 × 6 cm
    Alderson–Rando phantom
    (Herbig et al. 1971)

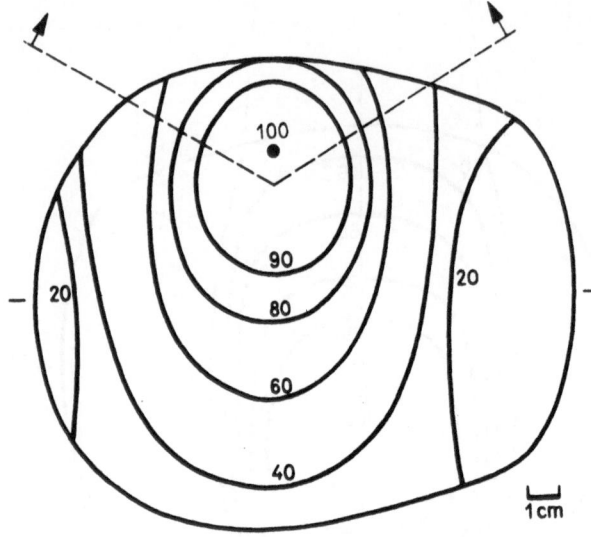

Fig. 333. Arc (120°) treatment of the central cranial cavity with 25 MeV electrons
FAD 120 cm
axis depth 4 cm
field size 6 × 8 cm
Alderson–Rando phantom
(Herbig et al. 1971)

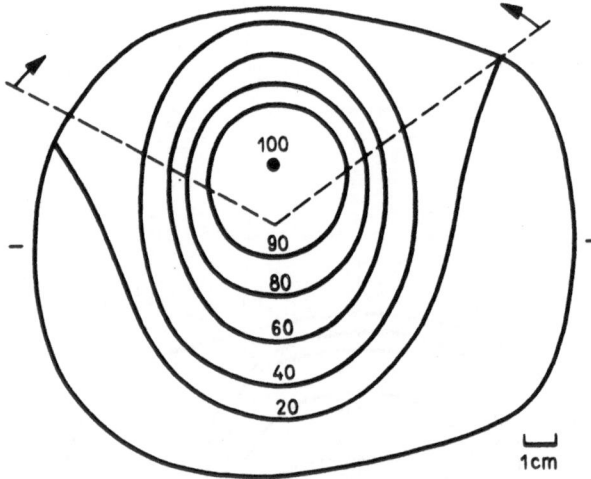

Fig. 334. Arc (120°) treatment of the central cranial cavity with 42 MeV electrons
FAD 120 cm
axis depth 7 cm
field size 6 × 8 cm
Alderson–Rando phantom
(Herbig et al. 1971)

Sellar region

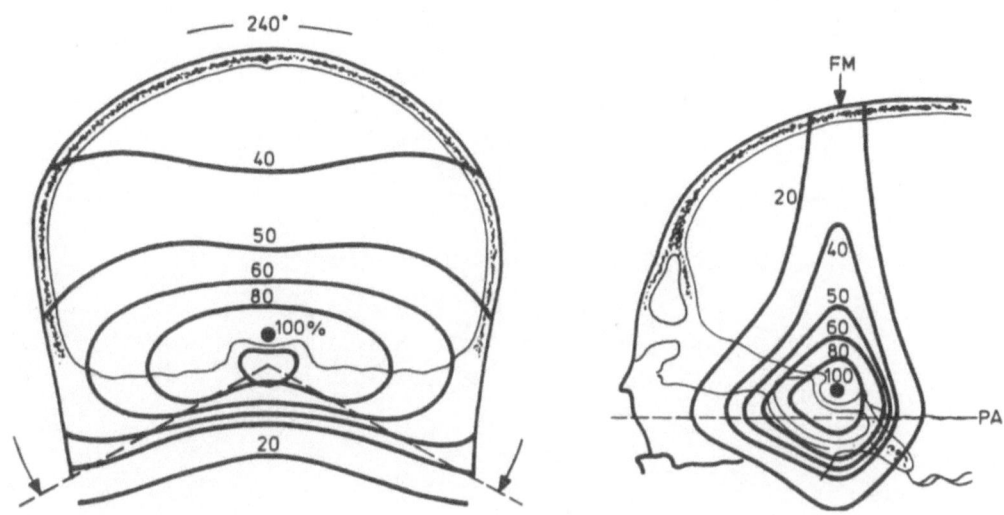

Fig. 335. Kilovoltage X-ray (200 kV) arc (240°) therapy of the sellar region
FAD 50 cm
axis depth 11 cm
field size 2 × 4 cm
Skeletal cranium and paraffin phantom
(Breit and Hirschauer 1955)

Fig. 336. 137-Cs
teletherapy of a
centrally localized
suprasellar tumour
through three
stationary fields
SSD 40 cm
field size 6 × 8 cm
Cranial phantom
(Scherer et al.
1965)

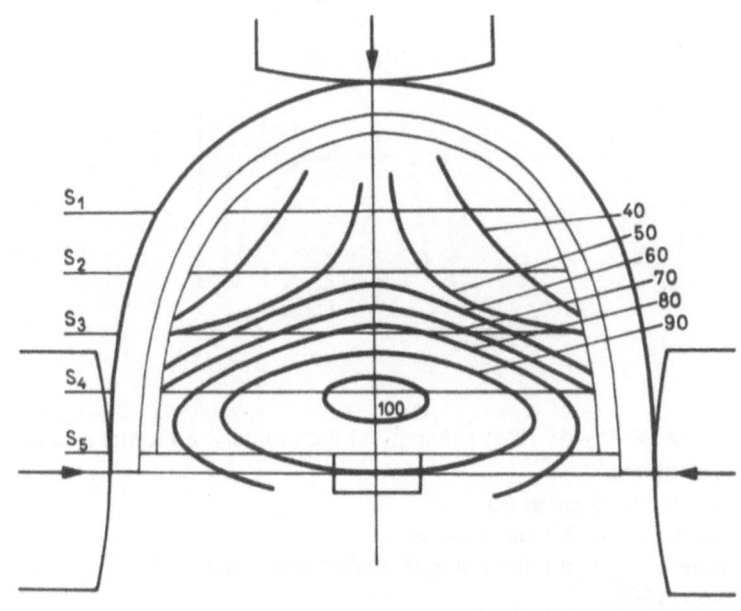

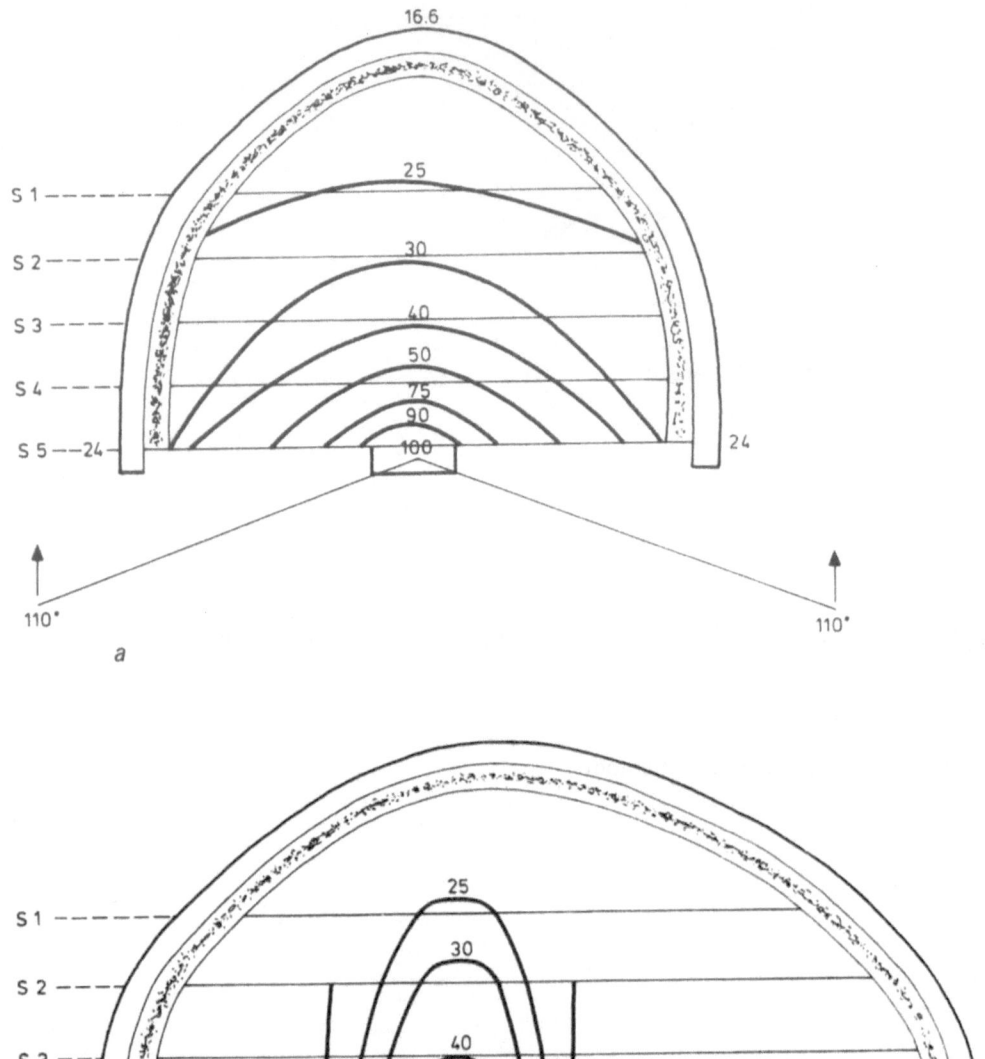

Fig. 337. 60-Co arc (220°) therapy of the pituitary. *a* Frontal section. *b* Sagittal section
SAD 65 cm
axis depth 10 cm at 90°
field size 2.6 × 3.2 cm at focus
Skeletal cranium phantom with Araldit and Leguval
(Löhr 1962)

254 | Sellar region

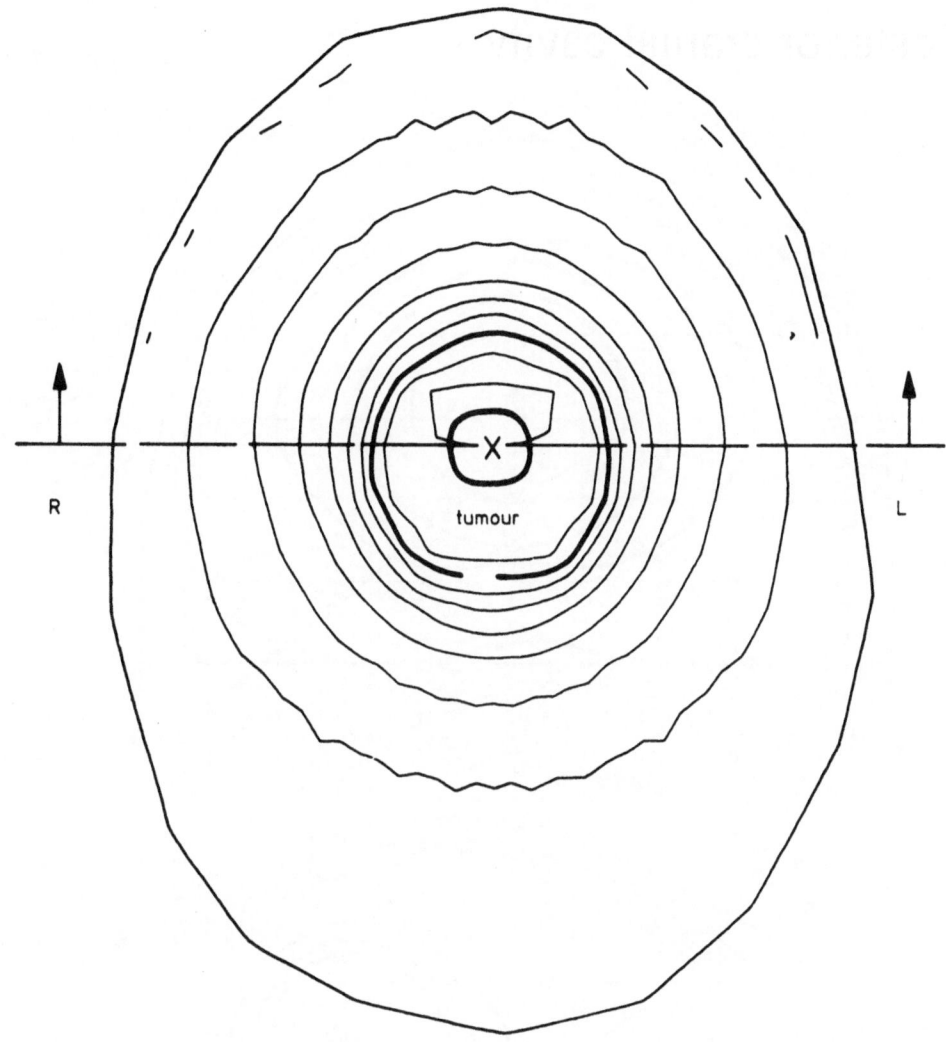

R

L

tumour

X

Fig. 338. Arc therapy of the sellar region with high-energy X-rays (42 MV)
FAD 120 cm
axis depth 8 cm
arc 180° (90°/90°)
field size 4 × 4 cm
Computer calculated isodoses

Posterior cranial cavity

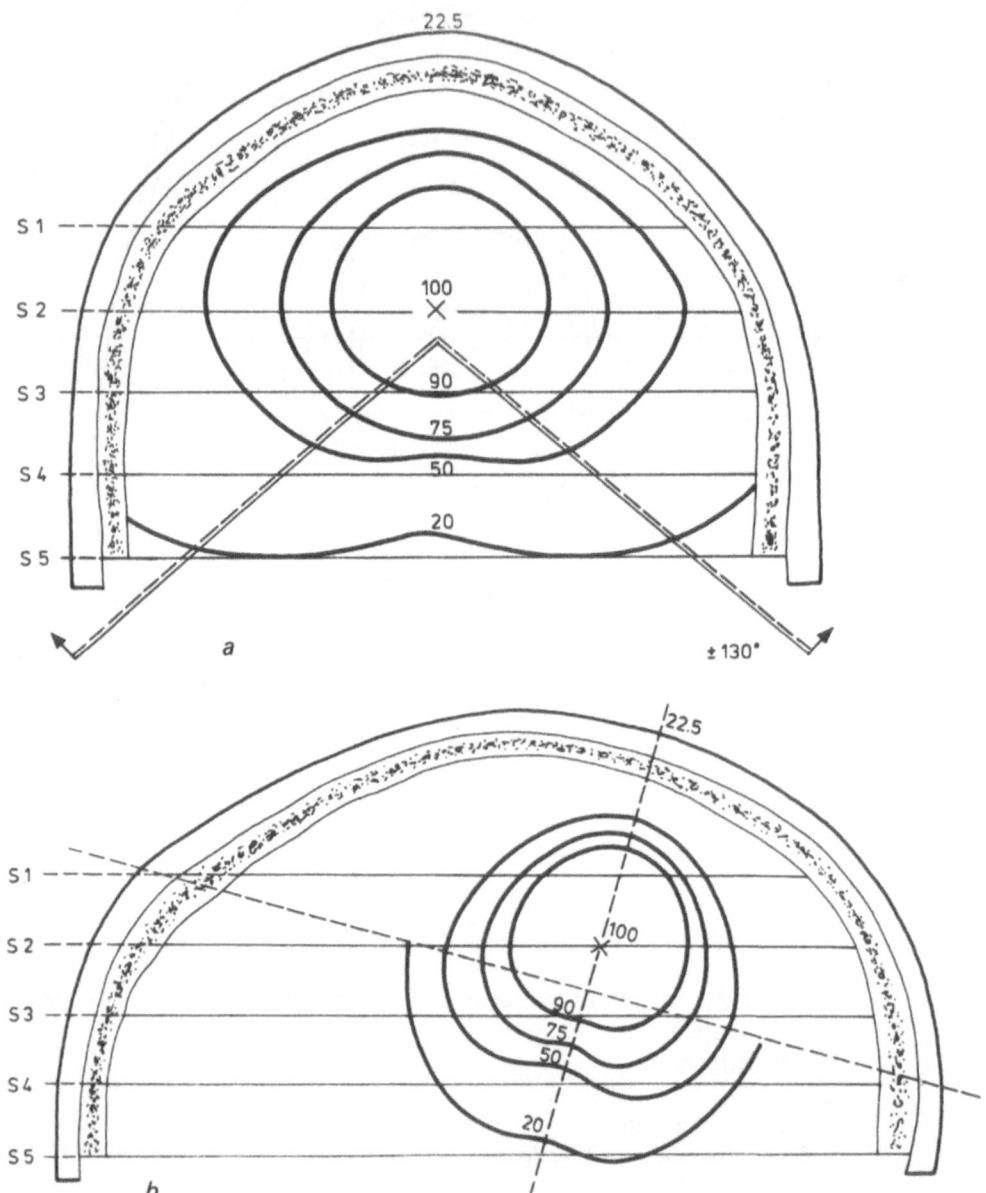

Fig. 339. 60-Co arc (260°) therapy of the posterior cranial cavity. *a* Frontal section
b Sagittal section
   SAD 65 cm
   axis depth 5.5 cm
   field size 3.5 × 4.8 cm on the surface
   Skeletal cranium phantom with Araldit and Leguval
   (Bottler and Löhr 1961)

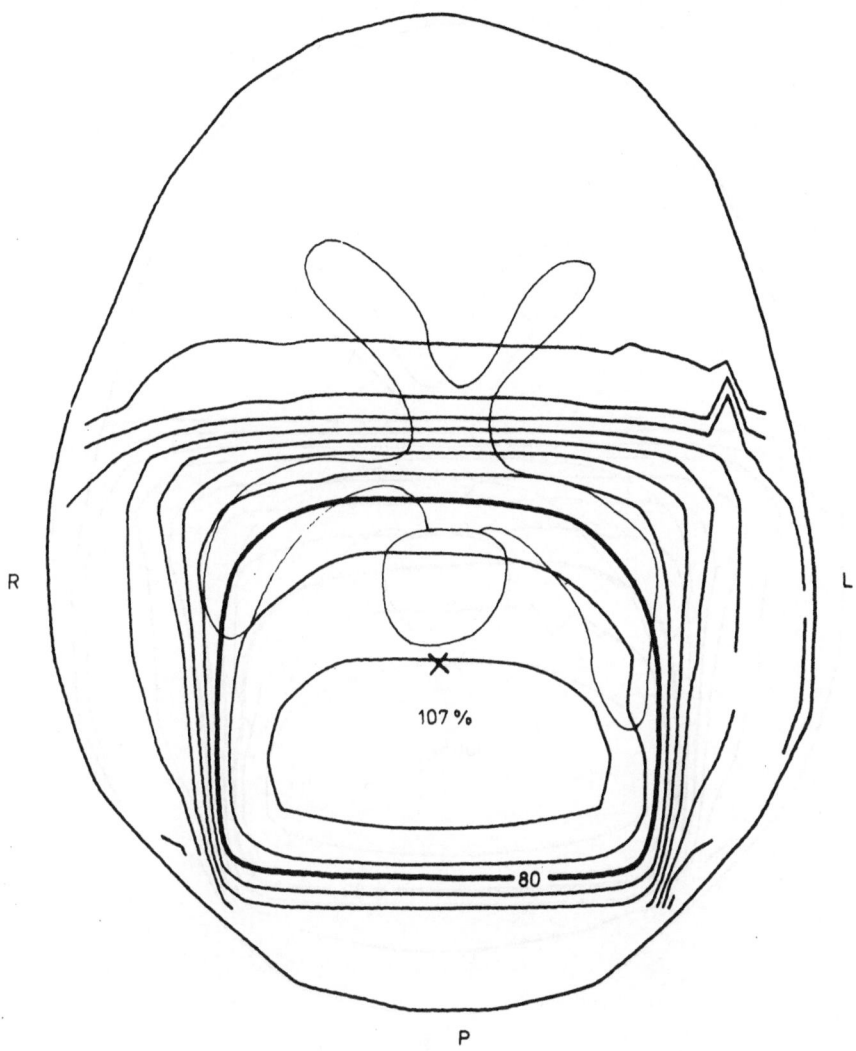

Fig. 340. Combined electron beam and high-energy X-ray irradiation of the posterior cranial cavity through an occipital field and two lateral isocentric photon fields

Electron beam: 20 MeV
FSD 100 cm
field size 8 cm diam
X-ray: 42 MV
FID 120 cm
field size 8 × 8 cm
Loading 1 : 1 : 1
Computer calculated isodoses

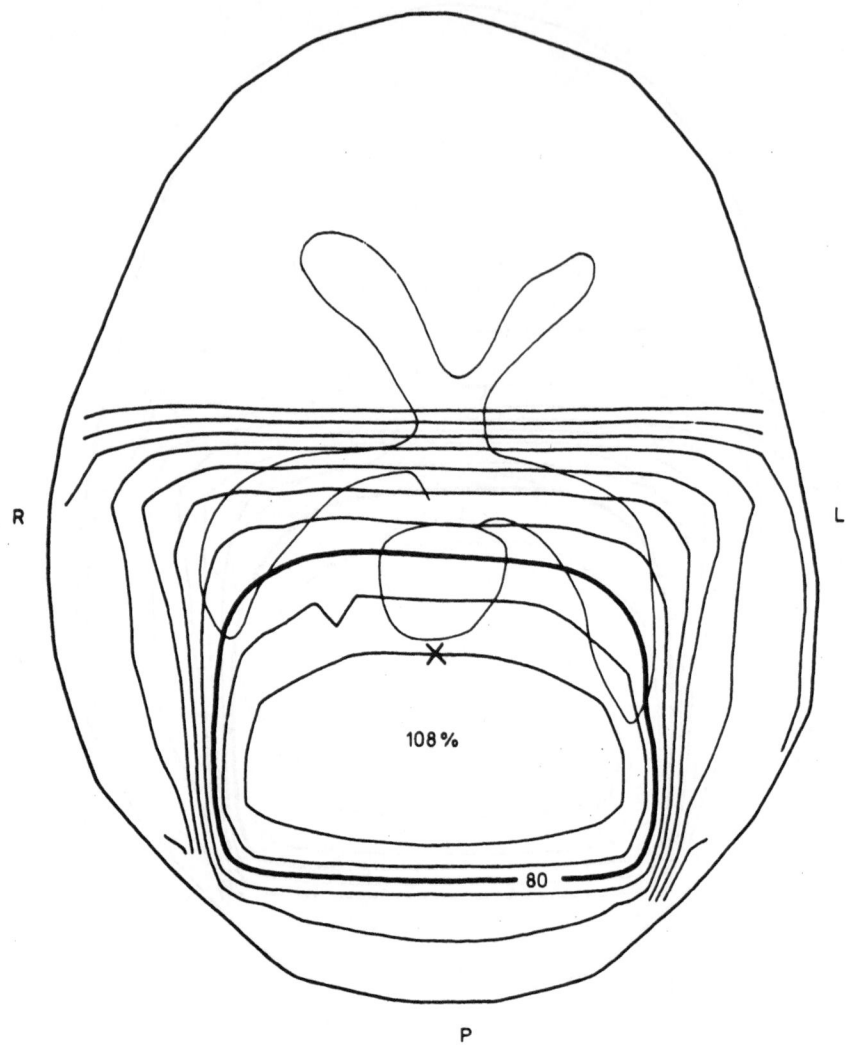

Fig. 341. Combined electron beam and high-energy X-ray irradiation of the posterior cranial cavity through an occipital electron field and two lateral isocentric photon fields

Electron beam: 25 MeV
      FSD 100 cm
      field size 8 cm diam
X-rays: 42 MV
    FID 120 cm
    field size 8 × 8 cm
Loading 1 : 1 : 1
Computer calculated isodoses

Medulloblastoma

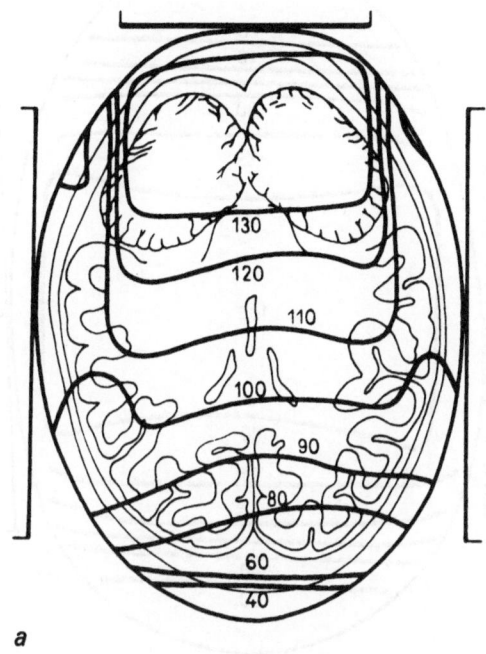

a

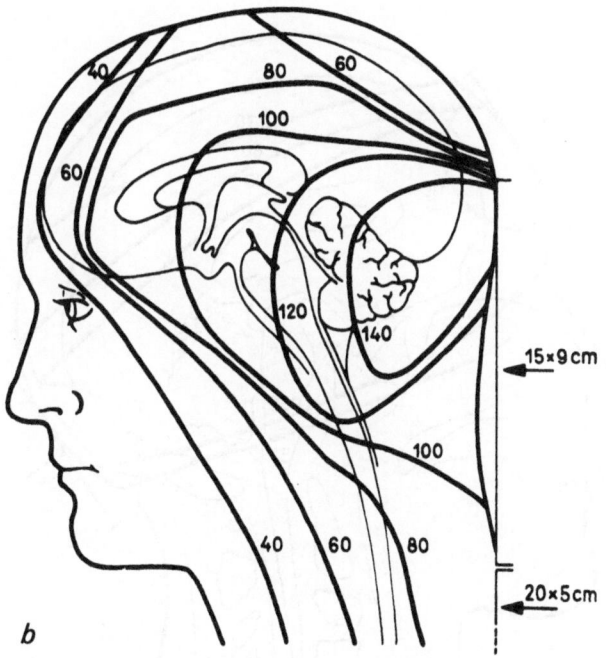

Fig. 342. X-ray (250 kV) therapy
of the brain and spinal cord for
medulloblastoma. Cerebral irradiation through three stationary
fields, spinal cord irradiation
through a dorsal stationary field.
a Frontal section. *b* Sagittal
section
   HVT 3.4 mm Cu
   FSD 40 cm
   field size
     cerebral: 15 × 9 cm
      dorsal 10 × 9 cm
      each lateral
    spinal cord: 5 × 20 cm
(Bloom et al. 1969)

b

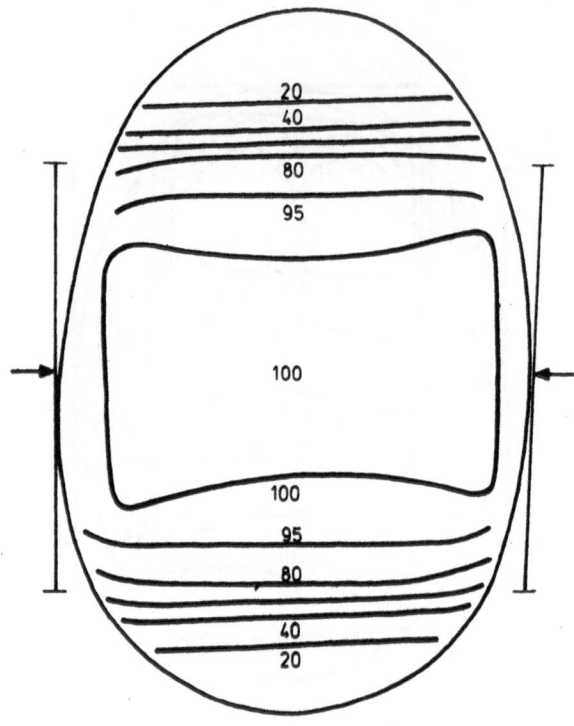

Fig. 343. 60-Co teletherapy of the brain for medullo-blastoma through two opposing stationary fields
SSD 50 cm
field size 8 × 10 cm each
Alderson–Rando phantom
(Kuttig and Beduhn 1967)

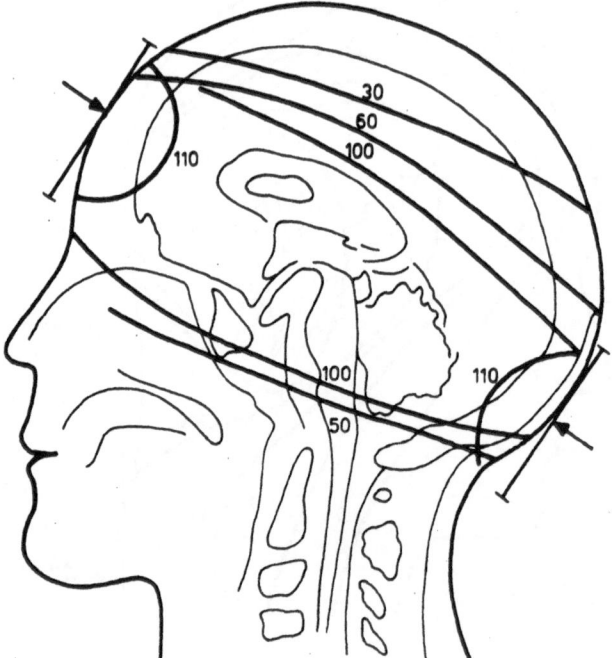

Fig. 344. 60-Co teletherapy of the brain for medullo-blastoma through a ventral and a stationary dorsal field
SSD 50 cm
field size 8 × 8 cm each
Alderson–Rando phantom
(Kuttig and Beduhn 1967)

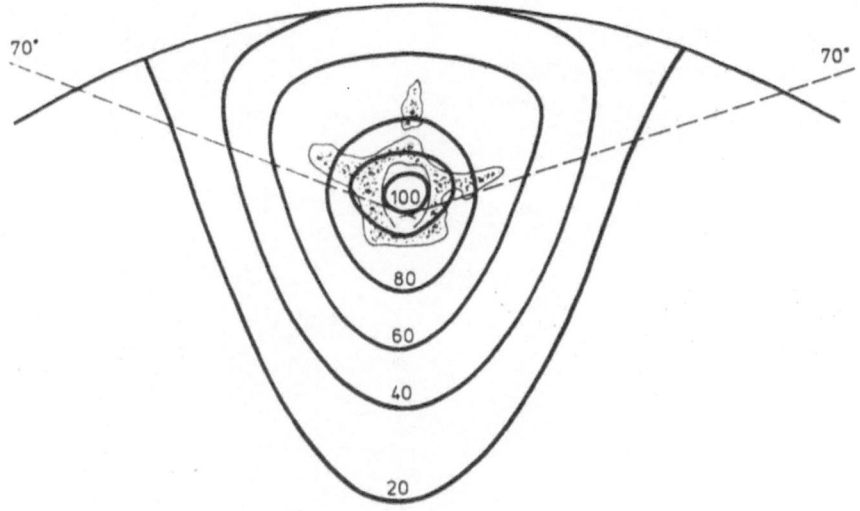

Fig. 345. 60-Co arc (150°) treatment of the spine in medulloblastoma (axis displaced along the longitudinal axis of the patient's body)
   SAD 60 cm
   axis depth 6 cm
   displacement of table 24 cm/9 min
   arcing of the source 180°/min
   field size 4 × 4 cm
   (Kuttig and Beduhn 1967)

References

Bagshaw, M. A., Kaplan, H. S., Sagerman, R. H., Linear accelerator supervoltage radiotherapy. *Radiology* **85**, 121–129 (1965).

Barth, G., Römmert, F., Schneider, W., Zur Methode der Rotationsbestrahlung des Magenkarzinoms. *Strahlentherapie* **95**, 66–70 (1954).

Baštecký, J., Chvojka, Z., Die Ergebnisse der Telekobaltbestrahlung des Bronchialkrebses. *Radiobiologia Radiotherapia* **5**, 35–44 (1964).

Becker, J., Baum, F.-K., Der Schutz der Augenlinse bei Bestrahlung intraorbitaler Tumoren mit schnellen Elektronen. *Strahlentherapie* **113**, 351–355 (1960).

Becker, J., Kärcher, K.-H., Weitzel, G., Elektronentherapie mit Supervoltgeräten, in *Strahlenbiologie, Strahlentherapie, Nuklearmedizin und Krebsforschung. Ergebnisse 1952–1958*. pp. 431–510. Georg Thieme Verlag, Stuttgart (1959).

Becker, J., Schubert, G., *Die Supervolttherapie*. Georg Thieme Verlag, Stuttgart (1961).

Beduhn, D., Kuttig, H., Die Bewegungsbestrahlung der paraaortalen Lymphknoten mit Co^{60}-Gammastrahlen. *Strahlentherapie* **132**, 481–486 (1967).

Birkner, R., Dietz, G., Hinz, G., Puppe, D., Die Mehrfeldbestrahlung von Blasentumoren in der Telekobalttherapie. *Strahlentherapie* **124**, 493–512 (1964).

Bloom, H. J. G., Wallace, E. N. K., Henk, J. M., The treatment and prognosis of medulloblastoma in children. *Amer. J. Roentgenol.* **105**, 43–62 (1969).

Boone, M. L. M., Harle, T. S., Higholt, H. W., Fletcher, G. H., Malignant disease of the paranasal sinuses and nasal cavity. *Amer. J. Roentgenol.* **102**, 627–636 (1968).

Bottler, E., Löhr, E., Messungen des Isodosenverlaufes bei Kobalt-60-Pendelbestrahlung an einem Schädelphantom. *Strahlentherapie* **115**, 326–332 (1961).

Breit, A., Hirschauer, A., Die Dosisverteilung bei der Pendelbestrahlung der Sellagegend. *Strahlentherapie* **98**, 398–403 (1955).

Breit, A., Hirschauer, A., Messergebnisse am Phantom bei der Pendelbestrahlung der vorderen Schädelgrube. *Strahlentherapie* **104**, 103–109 (1957).

Brizel, H. E., Lanzi, L. H., Duthorn, E. M., A comparison of techniques for parametrial irradiation using cobalt 60. *Amer. J. Roentgenol.* **89**, 101–107 (1963).

Burkell, C. C., Watson, T. A., Some observations on the clinical effects of cobalt–60 telecurie therapy. *Amer. J. Roentgenol.* **76**, 895–904 (1956).

Campos, J. L., Lampe, I., Fayos, J. V., Radiotherapy of carcinoma of the floor of the mouth. *Radiology* **99**, 677–682 (1971).

Castro, V., Whitcomb, W. P., Short axis rotation with cobalt 60 teletherapy unit, using copper wedge filters and square fields. *Amer. J. Roentgenol.* **89**, 117–119 (1963).

Chance, O., Five years' experience of arc therapy. *Brit. J. Radiol.* **31**, 293–298 (1958).

Chu, F. C. H., Scheer, A. C., Gaspar-Landero, J., Electron-beam therapy in the management of carcinoma of the breast. *Radiology* **75**, 559–567 (1960).

Dalley, V. M., Malignant disease of the antrum. *Brit. J. Radiol.* **32**, 378–385 (1959).

Edsmyr, F., Jacobsson, F., Dahl, O., Walstam, R., $Cobalt^{60}$ teletherapy in treatment of carcinoma of the bladder. *Radiobiologia Radiotherapia* **5**, 641–648 (1964).

Fehrentz, D., Kuttig, H., Hymmen, U., Fornusek, A., Bewegungsbestrahlung mit schnellen Elektronen zur Tiefentherapie. *Strahlentherapie* **137**, 509–517 (1969).

Fletcher, G. H., Clinical stationary field therapy with a cobalt-60 unit. *Amer. J. Roentgenol.* **75**, 91–116 (1956a).

Fletcher, G. H., A clinical program to evaluate the practical significance of higher energy levels than the 1–3 MeV. *Amer. J. Roentgenol.* **76**, 866–894 (1956b).

Fletcher, G. H., Supervoltage radiotherapy for cancers of the uterine cervix. *Brit. J. Radiol.* **35**, 5–17 (1962).

Fletcher, G. H., *Textbook of Radiotherapy*. Lea-Febiger, Philadelphia (1973).

Fletcher, G. H., MacComb, W. S., Chau, P. M., Farnsley, W. G., Comparison of medium voltage and supervoltage roentgen therapy in the treatment of oropharynx cancers. *Amer. J. Roentgenol.* **81**, 375–401 (1959).

Fornusek, A. H., Kuttig, H., Fehrentz, D., Vergleichende Untersuchungen über die Dosisverteilung bei Megavolttherapie im Bereich der Schädelbasis. *Strahlentherapie* **143**, 1–11 (1972).

Fournier, D., Kuttig, H., Curland, St., Zur Elektronen-Pendelbestrahlung der Thoraxwand. *Strahlentherapie* **144**, 393–397 (1972).

Fournier, D., Németh, G., Kuttig, H., Bisegmentale Pendelbestrahlung der aortalen Lymphknoten unter Auslenkung des Nutzstrahlenbündels mit ultraharten Röntgenstrahlen des 42-MeV Betatrons. *Strahlentherapie* **146**, 43–51 (1973).

Fowler, J. F., Farmer, F. T., Measured dose distributions in arc and rotation therapy: a critical comparison of moving and fixed field techniques. *Brit. J. Radiol.* **30**, 653–659 (1957).

Franke, H., Die räumliche Dosisverteilung im Kehlkopfbereich bei Bewegungsbestrahlung. *Strahlentherapie* **102**, 617–628 (1957).

Friedman, A. B., Benninghoff, D. L., Alexander, L. L., Aron, B. S., Total abdominal irradiation using cobalt 60 moving strip technique. *Amer. J. Roentgenol.* **108**, 172–177 (1970).

Friedman, M., Southard, M., Ellett, W., Supervoltage (2 MeV) rotation irradiation of carcinoma of the head and neck. *Amer. J. Roentgenol.* **81**, 402–419 (1959).

Frischbier, H.-J., Karl, B., Zur Telekobaltbestrahlung der aortalen Lymphknoten. *Strahlentherapie* **140**, 32–36 (1970).

Frischbier, H.-J., Kuttig, H., Die Telekobalttherapie des Mammakarzinoms. *Strahlentherapie* **120**, 512–524 (1963).

Frischbier, H.-J., Kuttig, H. Die Anwendung von Ausgleichsfiltern zur Verbesserung der Dosisverteilung bei der Telekobalttherapie des Kollumkarzinoms. *Strahlentherapie* **125**, 161–172 (1964).

Frischbier, H.-J., Möhle, G., Möglichkeiten zur Telekobalttherapie des lumbalen Lymphsystems. *Strahlentherapie* **132**, 487–496 (1967).

Frischbier, H.-J., Seifert, A., Zur Dosisverteilung bei der kombinierten Radium- und Telekobalttherapie des Kollumkarzinoms. *Strahlentherapie* **127**, 347–357 (1965).

Frischkorn, R., Erste Erfahrungen mit der routinemässigen Anwendung der Kobaltfernbestrahlung in der gynäkologischen Strahlentherapie. 42. Tagung der Deutschen Röntgengesellschaft. *Sonderbände zur Strahlentherapie* **49**, 149–156 (1962).

Frössler, H., Ahlmeyer, A., Dissmann, R., Schütz, J., Kobalt-60-Teletherapie im kleinen Becken. Dosismessungen am Phantom. *Strahlentherapie* **144**, 156–163 (1972).

Gale, N. H., Innes, G. S., The advantages of employing mixed high energy X-ray and electron beams in radiation therapy. *Brit. J. Radiol.* **33**, 261–264 (1960).

Gauwerky, F., Adam, K., Die Rolle der Radiotherapie bei der Behandlung der malignen Nierentumoren Erwachsener. *Strahlentherapie* **142**, 629–643 (1971).

Gauwerky, F., Frommhold, H., Zur Strahlentherapie der Epipharynxtumoren. *Strahlentherapie* **146**, 125–139 (1973).

Gietzelt, F., Degner, W., Fürst, G., zur Horst-Meyer, H., Schmidt, H., Roth, A., Die biaxiale Pendelbestrahlung des Kollumkarzinoms mit Kobaltgammastrahlung. *Radiobiologia Radiotherapia* **3**, 521–529, (1962).

Gough, J. J., The use and extensions of one-centre, one-arc techniques. *Brit. J. Radiol.* **35**, 94–100 (1962).

Gyenes, Gy., Strahlenbehandlung von Blasentumoren mit Telekobalttherapie und Röntgensiebbestrahlung. *Radiobiologia Radiotherapia* **3**, 579–584 (1962).

Gyenes, Gy., Über die Telekobaltbestrahlung des Blasenkarzinoms mit Hinsicht auf die Dosisverteilung. *Radiobiologia Radiotherapia* **10**, 715–718 (1969).

Gyenes, Gy., Dose distribution with high voltage irradiation of mediastinal Hodgkin's disease. *Strahlentherapie* **144**, 591–594 (1972).

Halama, J., Rassow, J., Methodischer Beitrag zur Hochvolttherapie des Vulvakarzinoms. *Strahlentherapie* **138**, 129–136 (1969).

Hanks, G. E., Bagshaw, M. A., Kaplan, H. S., The management of cervical lymph-node metastasis by megavoltage radiotherapy. *Amer. J. Roentgenol.* **105**, 74–82 (1969).

Hellriegel, W., Strahlentherapie des Rektumkarzinoms. *Strahlentherapie* **145**, 243–255 (1973).

Herbig, W., Kuttig, H., Schnabel, K., Möglichkeiten und Dosisverteilung bei Elektronentherapie und kombinierter Elektronen- und Röntgentherapie von Gehirntumoren. *Strahlentherapie* **142**, 412–416 (1971).

Heuss, K., Beitrag zur Bestrahlungsplanung bei der Elektronentherapie des Bronchialkarzinoms. *Strahlentherapie* **141**, 25–31 (1971)

Heuss, K., Hoeffken, W., Zur Anwendung der Pendelbestrahlung mit schnellen Elektronen in der Tiefentherapie. *Strahlentherapie* **138**, 40–49 (1969).

Heuss, K., Hoeffken, W., Zur Anwendung exzentrischer Pendelbestrahlungen mit einem 42-MeV-Betatron in der Tiefentherapie. *Strahlentherapie* **143**, 485–493 (1972).

Howarth, J., Wilson, C. W., Moving-beam therapy with cobalt 60: its adaptability to the lesion shape to be treated. *Amer. J. Roentgenol.* **85**, 53–58 (1961).

Johns, H. E., Darby, E. K., Watson, T. A., Burkell, C. C., Comparison of dosage distributions obtainable with 400 kVp X rays and 22 MeV X rays. *Brit. J. Radiol.* **23**, 290–299 (1950).

Kärcher, K. H., *Krebsbehandlung als interdisziplinäre Aufgabe.* Springer Verlag, Berlin, Heidelberg, New York (1975).

Kärcher, K. H., in Scherer, E. (ed.), *Strahlentherapie, Radiologische Onkologie.* Springer Verlag, Berlin, Heidelberg, New York (1976)

Kärcher, K. H., Heckenthaler, W., Binder, W., Dimopoulos, J., Seitz, W., Indikationen zur Strahlentherapie in der Ophthalmologie. *Strahlentherapie* **142**, 381–389 (1971).

Kitagawa, T., 10 MeV Betatron electron beam therapy adapted to a case of mycosis fungoides. *Amer. J. Roentgenol.* **88**, 229–234 (1962).

Kiviniitty, K., Unnérus, C.-E., Die Strahlenbehandlung der Parametrien bei gynäkologischen Tumoren. *Strahlentherapie* **136**, 416–419 (1968).

Klein, H. D., Heuss, K., Hoeffken, W., Pendelbestrahlung des Rektumkarzinoms mit schnellen Elektronen eines 42-MeV-Betatrons. *Strahlentherapie* **142**, 644–652 (1971).

Kling, G., Ringleb, D., Rödel, K., Radiologische Klinik und Telekobaltbestrahlung des Prostatakarzinoms. *Strahlentherapie* **141**, 531–539 (1971).

Koeck, G. P., Jacobson, L. E., Hillsinger, W. R., Description of a method and results of treatment of breast carcinoma with cobalt 60 teletherapy. *Amer. J. Roentgenol.* **91**, 67–79 (1964).

Kozlova, A. V., Strahlentherapie inoperabler Krebsmetastasen in Halslymphknoten. *Radiobiologia Radiotherapia* **6**, 717–721 (1965).

Kriester, A., Arndt, J., Albert, L., Standardisierte Bestrahlungsplanung für Telekobalt- und ultraharte Bremsstrahlung bei Harnblasentumoren. *Radiobiologia Radiotherapia* **10**, 729–736 (1969).

Krüger, H., Gietzelt, F., Degner, W., Erste Erfahrungen in der Anwendung hochenergetischer Elektronen beim Larynxkarzinom. *Radiobiologia Radiotherapia* **5**, 385–397 (1964).

Kuhn, E., Gyüdi, S., Eine neue Methode zur Bestrahlung des bilateralen Halslymphsystems mit Kobalt-60-Gammastrahlen. *Strahlentherapie* **144**, 398–406 (1972).

Kuttig, H., Die Strahlentherapie beim Wilms-Tumor. *Radiobiologia Radiotherapia* **9**, 247–252 (1968).

Kuttig, H., Beduhn, D., Neue Bestrahlungsmethoden beim Medulloblastom. Deutscher Röntgenkongress 1967, Teil B *Sdbd. 66 zur Strahlentherapie* 236–240 (1967).

Kuttig, H., Becker, H., Die Pendeltranslation mit Transversalverschiebung der Achse in der Kobalt-60-Teletherapie. *Strahlentherapie* **135**, 528–533 (1968).

Kuttig, H., Brands, K., Schnabel, K., Elektronen-Tiefentherapie im Thoraxbereich. *Strahlentherapie* **142**, 621–628 (1971).

Kuttig, H., Brenner, G., Zunter, F., Verbesserung der Dosisverteilung bei kombinierter Radium-Kobalt-60-Teletherapie des Kollumkarzinoms durch biaxiale, bisegmentale Pendelbestrahlung der Parametrien. *Strahlentherapie* **136**, 131–137 (1968).

Kuttig, H., Harbst, H., Lachmann, U., Misri, H., Zunter, F., Die postoperative Strahlentherapie des Mammakarzinoms unter Verzicht auf die Bestrahlung der Thoraxwand. *Strahlentherapie* **140**, 27–31 (1970)

Kuttig, H., Herbig, W., Die Anwendung von Keilfiltern in der Telekobalttherapie. *Strahlentherapie* **127**, 336–346 (1965).

Kuttig, H., Liebe, A., Meybier, G., Problematik und Möglichkeiten der Elektronentherapie der parasternalen Lymphbahnen. *Strahlentherapie* **144**, 649–655 (1972).

Kuttig, H., Németh, Poser, H., Die Elektronen-Pendelbestrahlung der beidseitigen Halslymphabflussgebiete mit Jalousietubus. *Strahlentherapie* **145**, 396–400 (1973).

Kuttig, H., Pini, M., Sunaric, D., Möglichkeiten zur Telekobalttherapie der Wirbelsäule mit kurativen Dosen. *Strahlentherapie* **128**, 241–246 (1965).

Kuttig, H., Schäfer, G., Methoden zur Kobalt-60-Teletherapie von Metastasen in der Halswirbelsäule. *Strahlentherapie* **135**, 666–669 (1968).

Landberg, T., Nordberg, U.-B., Olivecrona, H., Lindgren, M., Henrickson, H., Treatment of inoperable pulmonary tumours with high-energy electrons. *Acta Radiol. Ther. Phys. Biol.* **11**, 172–191 (1972).

Laughlin, J. S., Physical aspects of high energy electron therapy. *Amer. J. Roentgenol.* **99**, 915–923 (1967).

Laughlin, J. S., Lundy, A., Phillips, R., Chu, F., Sattar, A., Electron-beam treatment planning in inhomogenous tissue. *Radiology* **85**, 524–531 (1965).

Lederman, M., Technique of radiation treatment of orbital tumours. *Brit. J. Radiol.* **30**, 469–476 (1957).

Lederman, M., Jones, C. H., Mould, R. F., Cancer of the middle ear: technique of radiation treatment. *Brit. J. Radiol.* **38**, 895–905 (1965).

Lederman, M., Jones, C. H., Mould, R. F., Carcinoma of the oesophagus with special reference to the upper third. Part II. Physical considerations. *Brit. J. Radiol.* **39**, 197–204 (1966).

Lindgren, M., Nordberg, U.-B., Record from external beam therapy designed specially for 60-Co treatment with stationary fields. *Acta Radiol. Ther. Phys. Biol.* **3**, 457–462 (1965).

Lintner, L., Chládek, V., Abrahamovič, M., Unsere Ergebnisse bei der Behandlung des Kehlkopfkrebses durch Bestrahlung und Operation (1949 bis 1958). *Radiobiologia Radiotherapia* **5**, 273–283 (1964).

Löhr, E., Die 60-Co-Kleinfeld-Pendelbestrahlung der Hypophyse. *Strahlentherapie* **118**, 386–392 (1962).

Malinowski, Z., Wasilewski, M., Results of Co-60-therapy of carcinoma of the larynx. *Radiobiologia Radiotherapia* **9**, 599–602 (1968).

Maruyama, Y., Radiotherapy of tympanojugular chemodectomas. *Radiology* **105**, 659–663 (1972).

Matschke, S., Richter, J., Vergleichende Untersuchung der Dosisverteilung bei verschiedenen Methoden der Ösophagusbestrahlung. *Radiobiologia Radiotherapia* **4**, 385–399 (1963).

Matschke, S., Welker, K., Die individuelle Isodosenanpassung bei der biaxialen Pendelbestrahlung gynäkologischer Tumoren. *Radiobiologia Radiotherapia* **4**, 401–409, (1963).

Mau, S., Fürst, G., Strahlentherapiepläne für klassifizierte Blasenkarzinome. *Radiobiologia Radiotherapia* **14**, 111–116 (1973).

Miller, J. D. R., Results of treatment in glomus jugulare tumors with emphasis on radiotherapy. *Radiology* **79**, 430–434 (1962).

Morrison, R., Deeley, T. J., The treatment of carcinoma of the bladder by supervoltage X rays. *Brit. J. Radiol.* **38**, 449–458 (1965).

Morrison, R., Deeley, T. J., Bewley, D. K., The relative biological efficiency of 8 MV X rays and radium gamma rays, with reference to buccal mucosa. *Brit. J. Radiol.* **34**, 308–312 (1961).

Morrison, R., Newbery, G. R., Deeley, T. J., Preliminary report on the clinical use of the medical research council 8 MeV linear accelerator. *Brit. J. Radiol.* **29**, 177–186 (1956).

Németh, G., Fournier, D., Kuttig, H., Die Bewegungsbestrahlung der Parametrien und des Lymphabflussgebietes des Beckens mit ultraharten Röntgenstrahlen. *Strahlentherapie* **146**, 166–173 (1973a).

Németh, G., Kuttig, H., Methoden und Dosisverteilung der Elektronentherapie maligner Schilddrüsentumoren. *Strahlentherapie* **146**, 289–295, (1973).

Németh, G., Kuttig, H., Poser, H., Die Anwendung der Elektronen-Pendelbestrahlung mit Jalousietubus im Beckenbereich. *Strahlentherapie* **145**, 533–537 (1973b).

Németh, G., Wulff, W., A hypopharynx területén kialakuló dózisviszonyok különböző minőségű sugárzások alkalmazása során. *Magyar Onkologia* **14**, 161–166 (1970).

Nobler, M. P., Efficacy of a perineal teletherapy portal in the management of vulvar and vaginal cancer. *Radiology* **103**, 393–397 (1972).

Nordberg, U.-B., Olivecrona, H., Roentgen irradiation at 200 kV of neoplasms of the nasopharynx. *Acta Radiol. Ther. Phys. Biol.* **4**, 305–310 (1966).

Notter, G., Ranudd, N. E., Treatment of malignant testicular tumours. *Acta Radiol. Ther. Phys. Biol.* **2**, 273–301 (1964).

Nowakowski, W.: Recurrences of cervical carcinoma treated with Co-60. *Radiobiologia Radiotherapia* **9**, 609–614 (1968).

Okumura, Y., Mori, T., Kitagawa, T., Modification of dose distribution in high-energy electron beam treatment. *Radiology* **99**, 683–686 (1971).

Perry, H., Tsien, K. C., Nickson, J. J., Laughlin, J. S., Treatment planning in therapeutic application of high energy electrons to head and neck cases. *Amer. J. Roentgenol.* **88**, 251–261 (1962).

Phillips, R., Karnofsky, D. A., Hamilton, L. D., Nickson, J. J., Roentgen therapy of hepatic metastases. *Amer. J. Roentgenol.* **71**, 826–834 (1954).

Poser, H., Németh, G., Kuttig, H., Die Anwendung der Elektronen-Pendelbestrahlung im Bereiche der Halslymphknoten. *Strahlentherapie* **145**, 277–281 (1973a).

Poser, H., Németh, G., Kuttig, H., Telezentrische Kleinwinkel-Pendelbestrahlung der Harnblase mit schnellen Elektronen. *Strahlentherapie*. **145**, 390–395 (1973b).

Rassow, J., Sack, H., Beitrag zur Elektronentiefentherapie mittels Pendelbestrahlung *Strahlentherapie* **141**, 5–12 (1971).

Ratner, T. G., Bibergal, A. V., Palicyna. N. A., Besonderheiten der Dosisverteilung bei Mehrzonenkonvergenzbestrahlung in der Gammatherapie. *Radiobiologia Radiotherapia* **8**, 598–605 (1967).

Richter, J., Schirrmeister, D., Neue Ergebnisse bei der Ermittlung von Dosisverteilung mit Rechenautomaten. *Radiobiologia Radiotherapia* **6**, 371–375 (1965).

Robbins, R., Tsien, K. C., Rotation therapy at 250 kV. *Amer. J. Roentgenol.* **79**, 394–399 (1958).

Rödel, K., Ringleb, D., Barth, G., Biaxiale Telekobalt-Pendelbestrahlung der paraaortalen Lymphknoten. *Strahlentherapie* **138**, 641–644 (1969).

Rödel, K., Ringleb, D., Einstelltechnik bei Nierenmalignomen unter Telekobaltbedingungen. *Strahlentherapie* **140**, 366–373 (1970).

Rodriguez-Antunez, A., Cooks, S. A., Jelden, G. L., Hunter, I. W., Straffon, R. A., Stewart, B. H., Management of primary and metastatic carcinoma of the prostate by the radiotherapist. *Amer. J. Roentgenol.* **118**, 876–880 (1973).

Sack, H., Rassow, J., Beitrag zur Elektronentiefentherapie mittels Pendelbestrahlung. *Strahlentherapie* **144**, 641–648 (1972).

Sack, H., Scherer, E., Klinisch-methodische Überlegungen zur postoperativen Strahlenbehandlung des Brustkrebses mit konventionellen und Hochvoltmethoden. *Strahlentherapie* **143**, 473–484 (1972).

Scheidel, A., Németh, G., Kuttig, H., Möglichkeiten zur kurativen Behandlung der Wirbelsäule mit ultraharten Röntgenstrahlen. *Strahlentherapie* **146**, 36–42 (1973).

Scherer, E., Rassow, J., Methodische Grundlagen der perkutanen Strahlenbehandlung von Lymphknotenmetastasen des Halses. *Strahlentherapie* **141**, 523–530 (1971).

Scherer, E., Halama, J., Kaufmann, H., Klinische Erfahrungen bei der Telegammabehandlung mit Caesium 137. *Strahlentherapie* **127**, 161–169 (1965).

Scherer, E., Kaufmann, H., Rassow, J., Sack, H., Erfahrungen mit dem 43-MeV-Betatron bei Bestrahlung von Abdominaltumoren unter besonderer Berücksichtigung von Ovarial- und Blasenkarzinomen. *Radiobiologia Radiotherapia* **13**, 151–160 (1972).

Schnabel, K., Oeftering, T., Pereyra, J., Kuttig, H., Elektronen-Tiefentherapie im Thoraxbereich. *Strahlentherapie* **144**, 566–572 (1972).

Schuhknecht, H.-J., Tietze, D., Zur Telekobalttherapie der Tumoren des Larynx und Hypopharynx. *Radiobiologia Radiotherapia* **11**, 375–379 (1970).

Smith, I. H., Lott, J. S., Some observations on the effect of cobalt 60 beam therapy on epidermoid carcinoma during the first five-year study period. *Amer. J. Roentgenol.* **79**, 406–414 (1958).

Spechter, H. J., Experimentelle Studien über die Bewegungsbestrahlung im kleinen Becken bei gynäkologischen Tumoren. Part II. *Strahlentherapie* **102**, 629–661 (1957).

Spechter, H. J., Bewegungsbestrahlung beim Carcinoma colli uteri. *Radiobiologia Radiotherapia* **3**, 331–337 (1962).

Starzynska, T., Appreciation of the value of telegammatherapy in the treatment of lung cancer. *Radiobiologia Radiotherapia* **9**, 603–608 (1968).

Stauch, G. W., Glaeser, L., Dosimetrische Studie und methodische Überlegungen zur Strahlenbehandlung des Kollumkarzinoms. *Strahlentherapie* **143**, 164–171 (1972).

Stratev, I., Rödel, K., Exzentrische Supervolt-Pendeltherapie wirbelsäulennaher Tumoren. *Strahlentherapie* **132**, 362–369 (1967).

Trump, J. G., Granke, R. C., Wright, K. A., Evans, W. W., Hare, H. F., Ewert, E. E., Conlon, W. L., Treatment of tumors of the pelvic cavity with supervoltage radiation. *Amer. J. Roentgenol.* **72**, 284–292 (1954).

Trump, J. G., Wright, K. A., Evans, W. W., Hare, H. F., Lippincott, S. W., Two million volt roentgen therapy using rotation. *Amer. J. Roentgenol.* **66**, 613–623 (1951).

Van Vaerenbergh, P. M., Schelstraete, K., Simons, M., Die Kombinationstherapie von Tumoren der Lippe, der Zunge und der Larynx mit schnellen Elektronen (6 bis 17,5 MeV). *Strahlentherapie* **137**, 264–266 (1969).

Ward, H. W. C., Electron therapy at 15 MeV. *Brit. J., Radiol.* **37**, 225–230 (1964).

Wasilewski, M., Jablonska, M., Gajl, D., 3 year results of Co-60 treatment of advanced carcinoma of the bladder. *Radiobiologia Radiotherapia* **9**, 615–620 (1968).

Welker, K., Die individuelle Bestrahlungsplanung. *Radiobiologia Radiotherapia* **6**, 49–54 (1965).

Welker, K., Eichhorn, H.-J., Untersuchungen zur Standardisierung der bi- und vieraxialen Co^{60}-Pendelbestrahlung des kleinen Beckens. *Strahlentherapie* **141**, 655–661 (1971).

Welker, K., Eichhorn, H.-J., Untersuchungen über Raumdosis und relative Herdraumdosis in der Tumortherapie. *Strahlentherapie* **143**, 377–385 (1972a).

Welker, K., Eichhorn, H.-J., Untersuchungen zur Frage der bestrahlungstechnischen Optimierung bei der Co^{60}-Strahlentherapie des Kollumkarzinoms. *Radiobiologia Radiotherapia* **13**, 523–532 (1972b).

Williams, I. G., Horwitz, H., The primary treatment of adenocarcinoma of the rectum by high voltage roentgen rays (1,000 kV). *Amer. J. Roentgenol.* **76,** 919–928 (1956).

Wood, C. A. P., Techniques and early results of treatment of carcinoma of the larynx and pharynx by supervoltage radiation. *Brit. J. Radiol.* **32,** 661–668 (1959).

Wright, K. A., Granke, R. C., Trump, J. G., Physical aspects of megavolt electron therapy. *Radiology,* **67,** 553–561 (1956).

Zatz, L. M., Von Essen, C. F., Kaplan, H. S., Radiation therapy with high-energy electrons. *Radiology* **77,** 928–939 (1961).

Zwicker, H., Felix, R., Dosimetrie am Alderson-Phantom bei der Kobalt-60-Teletherapie von Nasen- und Nasennebenhöhlentumoren. *Strahlentherapie* **143;** 494–502 (1972).

Index of authors

Italic page numbers indicate that the author referred to is included in et al.